"The Third Edition of the *Comprehensive Textbook of Geriatric Psychiatry* is an instant classic. It is a must buy for fellows in geriatric psychiatry and medicine. This third edition will also be an indispensable reference for any health care professional hoping to stay current with the mental health needs of senior patients. The reviews are up-to-date and the section on the history of geriatrics and geriatric psychiatry is indeed comprehensive. The editors have achieved a near perfect balance in covering biomedical and psychosocial research, clinical practice, and public policy. This is truly an encyclopedia of geriatric mental health care divided into sections on the aging process, psychiatric evaluation, mental disorders of late life, and treatment, with the medical-legal, ethical, and financial issues combined in the financial sector."

— Gary J. Kennedy, M.D., Professor of Psychiatry,
Montefiore Medical Center

Comprehensive Textbook of Geriatric Psychiatry

Third Edition

STUDY GUIDE

Comprehensive Textbook of Geriatric Psychiatry

Third Edition

STUDY GUIDE

Edited by

Joel Sadavoy, MD, FRCP(C)
Lissy F. Jarvik, MD, PhD
George T. Grossberg, MD
Barnett S. Meyers, MD

Associate Editors

William Burke, MD
Nathan Herrmann, MD, FRCP(C)

AAGP
American
Association
for Geriatric
Psychiatry

W. W. Norton and Company
New York • London

Sponsored by the
American Association for
Geriatric Psychiatry

For information about permission to reproduce selections from this book, write to Permissions, W. W. Norton & Company, Inc., 500 Fifth Avenue, New York, NY 10110

Production Manager: Jean Blackburn, Bytheway Publishing Services, Norwich, NY
Manufacturing by Quebecor World Fairfield Graphics, Fairfield, PA

ISBN 0-393-70428-9 (pbk.)

W. W. Norton & Company, Inc., 500 Fifth Avenue, New York, N.Y. 10110
www.wwnorton.com

W. W. Norton & Company Ltd., Castle House, 75/76 Wells St., London W1T 3QT

1 3 5 7 9 0 8 6 4 2

Contents

QUESTIONS

I: THE AGING PROCESS

II: PRINCIPLES OF EVALUATION

III: PSYCHIATRIC DISORDERS OF THE ELDERLY

IV: TREATMENT

V: MEDICAL-LEGAL, ETHICAL, AND FINANCIAL ISSUES

ANSWERS

IV: TREATMENT

V: MEDICAL-LEGAL, ETHICAL, AND FINANCIAL ISSUES

Editors and Associate Editors

Joel Sadavoy, MD, FRCP(C)
Professor, Sam and Judy Pencer and Family Chair in Applied General Psychiatry, and faculty, Graduate Institute of Medical Sciences, University of Toronto; Psychiatrist-in-Chief and Head of Geriatric Psychiatry Services, Mount Sinai Hospital

Lissy F. Jarvik, MD, PhD
Professor Emerita of Psychiatry and Biobehavioral Sciences, University of California Los Angeles School of Medicine; Distinguished Physician Emeritus, US Department of Veterans Affairs of the Greater Los Angeles Area

George T. Grossberg, MD
Samuel W. Fordyce Professor and Director of Geriatric Psychiatry, St. Louis University School of Medicine

Barnett S. Meyers, MD
Professor of Psychiatry, Weill Medical College of Cornell University; Professor of Clinical Epidemiology, Graduate School of Health Sciences, Weill Medical College of Cornell University, New York Presbyterian Hospital–Westchester Division

William Burke, MD
Professor and Vice Chair, Department of Psychiatry, University of Nebraska

Nathan Herrmann, MD, FRCP(C)
Head of the Division of Geriatric Psychiatry and Professor of Psychiatry, University of Toronto; Head of the Division of Geriatric Psychiatry, Sunnybrook, and Women's Health Sciences Centre, Toronto

Preface

Thing book was prepared to allow students and practitioners dealing with
mental health in the elderly to assess their knowledge of the subject.
The questions highlight key areas for each aspect of the field. Each set of
questions was prepared by the authors of the corresponding chapter of the
Comprehensive Textbook of Geriatric Psychiatry, Third Edition, and have
been carefully reviewed to ensure that they are both clear and correspond to
current standards of examination questions. The answers are all derived from
material in the *Comprehensive Textbook of Geriatric Psychiatry*, Third Edition. Readers are directed to the relevant chapter in that textbook for more
detailed discussion of the subject areas raised by the questions. Each of the
questions in annotated with a brief explanation of why the correct answer is
appropriate and why the incorrect answers are not. Selected references are
attached to each question.

Every effort was made to ensure that the information is up-to-date and
state-of-the-art; however, geriatric psychiatry is a rapidly moving field so any
information may be overtaken by new data. This book will be appropriate
for use by specialists taking examinations for special competence in geriatric
psychiatry, residents and other trainees in psychiatry who are preparing for
exams, and other practitioners of geriatric mental health who want to assess
their knowledge of the field.

The senior editors are indebted to the associate editors Drs. William Burke
and Nathan Herrmann in the preparation of this book, as well as to our collab-
orators at W. W. Norton, Deborah Malmud, Michael McGandy, and Kevin
Olsen, who have worked so effectively with us on the preparation of both the
Comprehensive Textbook of Geriatric Psychiatry, Third Edition, and this self-
assessment manual.

Comprehensive Textbook of Geriatric Psychiatry

Third Edition

STUDY GUIDE

QUESTIONS

I The Aging Process

Chapter 1
Epidemiology of Psychiatric Disorders

Choose the best response to the following questions:

1. The risk of a depressive syndrome is *increased* by
   a. Poor quality of social supports
   b. Increase in number of medications
   c. Recent bereavement
   d. Caregiver burden
   e. All of the above
   f. None of the above

2. Which of the following disorders may begin in late life?
   a. Anxiety symptoms
   b. Agoraphobia
   c. Major depression
   d. Schizophrenia
   e. Only a and c
   f. All of the above

3. Risk for dementia of the Alzheimer or vascular types is *increased* by
   a. The presence of the APOE ε4 allele ✓
   b. Down syndrome ✓
   c. Stroke ✓
   d. Cigarette smoking ✓
   e. a, b, and c only
   f. All of the above

4. Dementia of the Alzheimer type often leads to
   a. Death
   b. Dependency
   c. Hip fractures
   d. Weight loss
   e. Only b and d
   f. All of the above

5. Later-onset schizophrenia is characterized by

    a. Increased thought disorder
    b. A negative history of lifelong isolation
    c. Increased levels of negative symptoms
    d. Relatively impaired premorbid levels of independent functioning
    e. All of the above
    f. None of the above

6. Patients with schizophrenia who have grown old in long-term mental hospitals have high rates of

    a. Auditory hallucinations
    b. Visual hallucinations
    c. Negative symptoms
    d. Severe aggressivity
    e. All of the above
    f. None of the above

7. In patients over 60 years of age admitted to psychiatry units, rates of alcohol abuse and related problems can be as high as

    a. 5%
    b. 40%
    c. 60%
    d. 85%

Chapter 2
Genetics of Dementia

Choose the best response to the following questions:

1. Males and females are equally likely to inherit a disease through all of the following transmission patterns *except*

    a. Autosomal recessive
    b. X-linked recessive
    c. Autosomal dominant
    d. None of the above

2. Which of the following is *not* an established risk factor for Alzheimer's disease (AD)?

    a. Positive family history
    b. Advancing age

   c. History of head trauma

   d. *Apolipoprotein E ε4 (APOE ε4)* allele

   e. Genetic mutations in the tau gene

3. A mature messenger ribonucleic acid (mRNA)

   a. Consists of exons

   b. Consists of introns

   c. Is derived from transfer RNA

   d. Is a large part of the human genome

4. Characteristics of polygenic traits include all of the following *except*

   a. Usually quantitative

   b. Indicate an interplay occurs between multiple genes

   c. Traits typically follow the normal distribution curve

   d. Traits typically follow a mitochondrial inheritance pattern

5. Direct DNA testing is currently available for all of the following *except*

   a. Early-onset familial AD

   b. Huntington's disease (HD)

   c. Cerebral autosomal dominant arteriopathy with subcortical infarcts and leukoencephalopathy (CADASIL)

   d. Vascular dementia

   e. Familial Creutzfeldt-Jakob (CJD) disease

6. All of the following should take place *prior* to genetic testing for asymptomatic persons at risk for HD *except*

   a. Obtain informed consent from the individual undergoing testing

   b. Establish the diagnosis of HD in a family member

   c. Determine that the individual has adequate health and disability insurance

   d. Offer psychiatric assessment for at-risk individuals

   e. Discuss the implications of genetic testing to other family members

   f. Avoid formal genetic counseling by a genetics professional

7. Tau mutations have been identified in which disease?

   a. Alzheimer's disease

   b. Frontotemporal dementia

   c. Huntington's disease

   d. Cerebral autosomal dominant arteriopathy with subcortical infarcts and leukoencephalopathy

   e. Familial Creutzfeldt-Jacob's disease

8. All of the following chromosomes harbor susceptibility genes for AD *except*

   a. 20
   b. 14
   c. 1
   d. 21

9. The prion gene (*PRNP*) that harbors mutations associated with CJD is on chromosome

   a. 19
   b. 20
   c. 21
   d. 1
   e. 10

For questions 10–14, match the following genetic findings with their specific disease(s):

   a. Valine-to-isoleucine amino acid substitution, codon 717
   b. CAG trinucleotide repeats
   c. Glutamic acid-to-lysine amino acid substitution, codon 200
   d. *APOE ε4* allele
   e. Trisomy 21

   10. Creutzfeldt-Jakob prion disease
   11. Early-onset AD (*APP* gene)
   12. HD
   13. Late-onset AD
   14. Down syndrome

Chapter 3
Genetics of Mood Disorders and Associated Psychopathology

Choose the best response to the following questions:

1. The single best study design for demonstrating the genetic basis of a human disease is

   a. Twin study
   b. Family study
   c. Linkage study

    d. Adoption study

    e. None of the above

2. Which statement best describes the current understanding of the etiology of mood disorders in the elderly?

    a. Mood disorders primarily result from adverse life events

    b. The same genetic factors are equally important in younger and older people

    c. Genetic diseases seen mostly in the elderly are sometimes important factors

    d. Mood disorders are primarily complications of degenerative brain diseases

    e. None of the above

3. Single-nucleotide polymorphisms (SNPs)

    a. Are rare genetic mutations that may lead to disease

    b. May have no impact on gene function

    c. Are widely used as genetic markers in linkage studies

    d. Can be used for case–control but not family-based association studies

    e. All of the above

4. Family studies show that, in relatives of probands with unipolar disorder, the risk is

    a. Not increased for unipolar or bipolar disorder

    b. Increased 2-fold for unipolar or bipolar disorder

    c. Increased 10-fold for unipolar or bipolar disorder

    d. Increased 15-fold for unipolar or bipolar disorder

    e. Increased for schizophrenia

5. Family studies show that the proportion of relatives with mood disorder

    a. Increases with increasing age of onset of affective disorder in the proband

    b. Increases with decreasing age of onset of affective disorder in the proband

    c. Decreases with decreasing age of onset of affective disorder in the proband

    d. Is unchanged by the age of onset of affective disorder in the proband

6. Compared to mood disorders at younger ages, late-onset mood disorders are characterized by

   a. Increased genetic loading
   b. Decreased genetic loading
   c. Decreased medical/neurological comorbidities
   d. Mutations on chromosome 11

For questions 7–10, the diseases listed below may present with symptoms of mood disorder. Match the abnormality with the disease.

7. *Notch3* mutations
8. *Amyloid precursor protein* (APP)
9. Chromosome 20 prion protein (PrP)
10. Presenilins

a. Frontotemporal dementia
b. Alzheimer's disease
c. Hereditary multiinfarct dementia (cerebral autosomal dominant arteriopathy with subcortical infarcts and leukoencephalopathy, CADASIL)
d. Creutzfeldt-Jakob disease (CJD)

Chapter 4
The Biology of Aging

Choose the best response to the following questions:

1. A 72-year-old woman has an average blood pressure of 164/91 measured on three different occasions without orthostatic changes. She eats an unrestricted diet and has a weight appropriate for her height. Fundoscopic examination reveals arteriovenous nicking without hemorrhages. Vibration sensation is decreased at the ankles, but pulses are normal. Random serum urea nitrogen, glucose, and electrolytes are normal, and serum creatinine is 1.2 mg/dL. What are the next steps in her evaluation?

   a. None, these are normal findings for her age
   b. Do a 24-hour urine collection for creatinine clearance
   c. Check fasting serum lipids and glucose level
   d. Exercise stress testing

2. Which of the following statements concerning changes in the aging skeleton is *not true*?

   a. Men do not lose significant bone mineral density with increasing age

    b. Women experience an accelerated rate of bone mineral density loss following menopause

    c. Gonadal hormones have an important role in maintaining trabecular bone mineral density

    d. Calcium and vitamin D are critical in maintaining bone integrity of cortical bone

    e. The increased rate of long-bone fractures with age occurs 10 years earlier in women compared to men

3. Dosing of psychotropic medications in the elderly must often be adjusted. Which of the following statements is *not* a correct explanation of why?

    a. Total body water declines with age, leaving a smaller volume of distribution for many medications

    b. Hepatic metabolism of phase I pathway drugs declines with age and may result in higher levels of some agents for a longer period of time

    c. Increase in central adipose tissue enhances the distribution of these highly lipid-soluble molecules and leads to prolonged elimination of many agents

    d. Older adults are less sensitive to some of these medicines and so often require higher doses

4. Choose which of the following statements about age-related changes in skin is false:

    a. Skin atrophies with loss of the subcutaneous fat cushion

    b. Cool temperatures and low humidity ameliorate the effects of reduced sebaceous and eccrine glands

    c. Elastin fragments with age

    d. Sun exposure encourages increased collagen deposition

    e. Age-related changes in elastin and collagen lead to skin wrinkling

5. Choose the incorrect statement regarding thyroid function in old age:

    a. Thyroxine (T_4) gradually declines

    b. 3,5,3′-Triiodothyronine (T_3) gradually declines

    c. Thyroid-stimulating hormone (TSH) is inconsistently elevated in some studies

    d. All of the above

    e. None of the above

Chapter 5
Normal Aging: Changes in Cognitive Abilities

Choose the best response to the following questions:

1. Functional abilities in the normal older adult are

   a. Impaired for their instrumental activities of daily living by age 70 years, but their ability to perform their activities of daily living is not impaired
   b. Unrelated to risk of nursing home placement
   c. Typically not impaired, although the speed of performance declines
   d. Impaired because of age-related changes in cognitive abilities

2. A 75-year-old Spanish-speaking woman who is a recent refugee from a South American country seeks consultation because of difficulty with her memory. Which of the following is true regarding assessment of her cognitive function?

   a. Results of intelligence tests will not be influenced by cultural background
   b. Administering the usual tests in Spanish ensures adequate assessment of verbal fluency
   c. As a Hispanic, she is likely to perform as well as English speakers on test of digit span
   d. The norms developed for Spanish versions of cognitive tests will likely be applicable to her
   e. None of the above

3. Although there can be several ways to define "successful aging," data indicate that the preservation of mental functioning is important because

   a. It is necessary to health and overall ability to function
   b. It is associated with greater wisdom
   c. It ensures adequate performance of instrumental activities of daily living
   d. All of the above

4. Exercise has been shown to

   a. Preserve cognitive function
   b. Improve cardiovascular fitness even in the very old
   c. Improve attentional capacity

d. Improve memory in depressed elders

e. All of the above

Chapter 6
Sociodemographic Aspects of Aging

Choose the best response to the following questions:

1. Which statement most accurately describes the current demographic landscape of aging in the United States?

    a. The population in the United States older than age 65 will both grow and age during the next 40 years because of the aging of the baby boomers

    b. Men and women are about equally represented in the older population

    c. Increases in life expectancy during the past 100 years have been caused primarily by life extension after 40 years of age

    d. The United States has the highest life expectancy in the world today

    e. All of the above

2. Which of the following statements about work and retirement is *false?*

    a. Labor force and retirement patterns were different for men and women during the 20th century

    b. Corporation workers who seek early retirement are more frequently motivated by health problems

    c. There is a correlation between a person's age at retirement and their propensity to work after their retirement

    d. Workers employed by businesses and corporations have greater variation in their age at retirement than workers who are self-employed

3. Which of the following statements concerning the economic and educational resources of persons over 65 is *true?*

    a. A higher proportion of older persons (than working-aged persons) feels that their income is inadequate—Ν

    b. Older adults are slightly less likely than younger adults to live in households with an income below the poverty level—Ν

    c. Older persons in the United States tend to have higher incomes than those younger than 65 years—Ν

d. Fewer than half of recent retirees have as much as a high school education

4. Concerning family and housing issues, which of the following statements is *not true*?

    a. Most older people own their own homes
    b. Over a third of persons over age 85 years are living alone
    c. Men and women over 65 years are living in family settings in about equal proportions
    d. Only about 5% of persons over age 60 years have moved across state lines in any 5-year period in recent decades according to US census data

5. Which of the statements about religion and older adults is *false*: Religion is important to the health of older adults . . .

    a. Despite the fact that a minority of older adults are affiliated with a church
    b. Because churches can promote social integration
    c. Particularly in rural communities
    d. Because of the tangible support churches provide older adults

6. The high rates of diabetes complications among minority elders reflect

    a. Greater rates of screening for complications among minority groups
    b. Refusal of minority elders to seek medical treatment for diabetes
    c. Less utilization of preventive services among minority elders
    d. The tendency for minority elders to be fatalistic about their health

7. The rates of health risk behaviors such as smoking and physical inactivity in the elderly population

    a. Are relatively unchanged over the past several decades
    b. Are equally characteristic of men and women
    c. Are lower in the old-old than the young-old
    d. Should improve over the next several decades

8. The cumulative health effects of lack of resources over the life course are shown by

    a. Higher rates of disability among blacks than whites
    b. Higher prevalence of diabetes complications among minority elders
    c. Tendency for elders of low socioeconomic status to rate their health as poorer than elders of high socioeconomic status
    d. All of the above

Chapter 7
Self, Morale, and the Social World of Older Adults

Choose the best response to the following questions:

1. A 70-year-old man, a successful lawyer with a love of ancient history, decides to return to graduate school for an advanced degree in classics. He reports this decision to his primary care physician, who determines that the patient appears to be well adjusted and aging successfully. However, despite the patient's enthusiasm and vigor, the physician questions the wisdom of the patient's decision to begin a new course of study so late in life and consults a colleague who is a geriatric psychiatrist. The psychiatrist is most likely to conclude

   a. The patient is trying to put off recognition of his own mortality
   b. The patient's goal reflects enhanced self-efficacy
   c. The patient is denying his own aging
   d. The patient is trying to find younger persons in order to feel younger

2. A scientist in his late 60s loves his work but wonders if he should retire because he is not sure he will ever match his earlier achievements. He is reassured to learn that

   a. Creative productivity continues into advanced old age for some scientists
   b. Creative productivity plateaus, but it does not decline with age on average
   c. Creative productivity shows no clear relationship to age on average
   d. Creative productivity does not diminish with age for career scientists

3. Well-being in later life has been associated in longitudinal studies with voluntary pursuit of creative activities such as painting or writing

   a. For men, but not for women
   b. For women, but not for men
   c. For neither men nor women
   d. For both men and women

4. Regarding relations with family and friends, older adults

   a. Become less concerned with the quality of social ties
   b. Prefer friends and confidants rather than offspring for social support

   c. Seem to tolerate restrictions on their own time posed by contact
      with adult children
   d. All of the above
   e. None of the above

Chapter 8
The Role of Religion/Spirituality in the Mental Health
of Older Adults

Choose the best response to the following questions:

1. Choose the correct answer that describes how *most* older persons view
   themselves in terms of religion and spirituality.

   a. As spiritual but not religious
   b. As religious but not spiritual
   c. As neither religious nor spiritual
   d. As both religious and spiritual

2. What proportion of older adults in America indicate that religion is
   "very important" to them?

   a. 10%–20%
   b. 30%–40%
   c. 50%–60%
   d. 70%–80%
   e. 90%–100%

3. Regarding trends between 1980 and 2000 in the importance of religion
   to older adults and in religious attendance, choose the answer that best
   describes this trend.

   a. Religious attendance and religious importance have been steadily
      decreasing during this time
   b. Religious attendance and religious importance have remained about
      the same
   c. Religious attendance has been increasing and religious importance
      decreasing
   d. Religious attendance has been significantly decreasing and religious
      importance increasing
   e. Religious attendance and religious importance have been steadily
      increasing

4. Choose the correct answer about the role religion played in psychiatry in 19th century America.

   a. Religion played little or no part in psychiatric care in America during the mid-1800s
   b. Religion was seen as having a neurotic influence on patients and was discouraged
   c. Attending religious services was used to reward good behavior
   d. Chaplains played little role in the psychiatric care of institutionalized patients
   e. Chaplains were not allowed to see patients without an order from the psychiatrist

5. Among older medical patients in the southeastern United States, what percentage use religious beliefs or practices to help them cope with the stress of their illness?

   a. 5% or less
   b. 30%
   c. 50%
   d. 70%
   e. Up to 90%

6. Choose the correct statement about the relationship between religious beliefs and practices and depression in later life.

   a. Religious practices are associated with a greater prevalence of depression in older adults
   b. Intrinsic religiosity is unassociated with speed of recovery from depression
   c. Intrinsic religiosity is associated with more rapid remission of depression
   d. Religious activities are not associated with lower rates of depressive symptoms
   e. Religious attendance is not as strongly related to depression as private religious activities

7. Choose the *incorrect* statement about how religion influences depressive symptoms in later life.

   a. Religious beliefs and practices increase guilty preoccupations among older adults
   b. Religious involvement is associated with increased social support
   c. Religious involvement is associated with greater hope and optimism
   d. Religious activities are associated with lower rates of substance abuse
   e. Religious beliefs are associated with greater meaning and purpose

8. Choose the correct statement about the relationship between religion and schizophrenia.

   a. Religious involvement predisposes to the development of schizophrenia in older patients
   b. Traditional religious beliefs and practices have a stabilizing influence in chronic psychosis
   c. Exorcism has been successful in the treatment of schizophrenia
   d. Religious interventions worsen psychotic symptoms in schizophrenic patients
   e. Religious delusions are rare among schizophrenic older patients

9. Choose the correct statement about psychiatric interventions that involve religion.

   a. Psychiatrists should take a spiritual history when evaluating older patients
   b. Psychiatrists should routinely offer spiritual advice to their older patients
   c. Psychiatrists should pray with all older patients when experiencing severe crisis
   d. Psychiatrists should regularly share their own religious beliefs with older patients
   e. All older patients should be encouraged to attend religious services if not already doing so

Chapter 9
Ethnocultural Aspects of Aging in Mental Health

Choose the best response to the following questions:

1. Which Asian ethnic group has over 60% American-born minority elderly?

   a. Chinese
   b. Japanese
   c. Korean
   d. Vietnamese
   e. Filipino

2. Which illness creates the highest risk of excess mortality for Native American elderly?

   a. Hypertension
   b. Alcoholism
   c. Tuberculosis
   d. Diabetes
   e. Stroke

3. Compared to Caucasians, immigrant Mexican American elderly in the epidemiologic catchment area (ECA) study had

   a. One half the lifetime prevalence for a psychiatric disorder
   b. Double the lifetime prevalence for a psychiatric disorder
   c. The same lifetime prevalence for a psychiatric disorder
   d. Slightly higher lifetime prevalence for a psychiatric disorder
   e. Slightly lower lifetime prevalence for a psychiatric disorder

4. Of the groups below, the highest rate of suicide in the elderly is seen in

   a. African Americans
   b. Japanese Americans
   c. Chinese Americans
   d. Caucasians
   e. Native Americans

5. Slow metabolizers of medications using cytochrome 2D6 are most likely to be

   a. Asian
   b. African American
   c. Native American
   d. Caucasians
   e. Native Hawaiian and other Pacific Islanders

6. The American Society on Aging has suggested that when programs are developed for minority elderly, these programs require

   a. A mission statement
   b. Proportional representation of minority groups on governing bodies
   c. Special programs (meaningful)
   d. All of the above

7. A key element in differentiating a culture-bound syndrome from a similar *Diagnostic and Statistical Manual of Mental Disorders, Fourth Edition (DSM-IV)* disorder in the elderly is

   a. Unusual symptoms
   b. Short duration of symptoms
   c. High frequency of occurrence (in the culture)
   d. Patient's explanatory model for symptoms
   e. Response to medication

8. A culture-fair dementia screening tool for non-English-speaking minority elderly is the

   a. MMSE (Mini-Mental State Examination)
   b. MSQ (Mental Status Questionnaire)
   c. MMPI (Minnesota Multiphasic Personality Inventory)
   d. CDT (Clock Drawing Test)
   e. CASI (Cognitive Abilities Screening Instrument)

9. Early findings showed significantly lower prevalence rates of Alzheimer's dementia in their native countries than in the United States for which groups?

   a. Cree Indians
   b. Nigerians
   c. Japanese
   d. Chinese
   e. All of the above

II Principles of Evaluation

Chapter 10
Comprehensive Psychiatric Evaluation

Choose the best response to the following questions:

1. Which of the following is true about an assessment for competence?

    a. Competence is best viewed as a task-specific assessment
    b. Geriatric psychiatrists are seldom required to assess a patient's capacity to make decisions
    c. Competence to consent to treatment is generally judged by the same criteria as competence to appoint a power of attorney
    d. Presence of delusions is never a sufficient reason to declare a patient incompetent

2. All of the following are true about an interview with a collateral source *except*

    a. The quality of the informant's relationship with the patient sometimes interferes with obtaining an accurate history ✔
    b. Informants are usually best interviewed when seeing the patient for the first time
    c. When the informant is the caregiver of a geriatric patient, the informant is at high risk of depression. ✔
    d. An interview with the informant is necessary when the patient has dementia ✔

3. On a mental status examination, an elderly person looking vacantly into space who is appropriately dressed but apparently uncaring about stained clothes and smelling of urine is least likely to be diagnosed with

    a. Affective disorder ✔
    b. Anxiety disorder
    c. Cognitive disorder ✔
    d. Paranoid disorder ✔

4. An interview of an elderly paranoid patient might effectively employ which following interview technique?

   a. Redirect the patient to the correct reality when delusions are expressed
   b. Sit close to the patient and touch the patient reassuringly to establish contact and a therapeutic alliance
   c. Always inquire about Schneider's criteria
   d. Acknowledge the patient's fears of others while inquiring about their feelings regarding those around them

5. All of the following statements regarding the cognitive assessment are false *except*

   a. The cognitive assessment is best conducted at the end of the examination as a discrete part of the assessment
   b. The cognitive assessment is always an active process characterized by systematic questioning
   c. The examiner tries to introduce the cognitive assessment in a noninvolved, objective manner to avoid influencing the patient
   d. Much of the basic cognitive assessment can be conducted informally throughout the initial interview.

6. All of the following are examples of frontal systems tests *except*

   a. Go/no go
   b. Similarities task
   c. Multiple loop copying
   d. Word list generation
   e. Ideomotor apraxia

7. The Mini-Mental State Examination (MMSE)

   a. Is a diagnostic test for Alzheimer's disease
   b. Subtests are fairly universal and unaffected by culture, age, and education
   c. Will decline, on average, by 3 points per year in patients with Alzheimer's disease
   d. Often produces false-negative results in frontotemporal dementias

Chapter 11
Medical Evaluation and Common Medical Problems
of the Geriatric Psychiatry Patient

Choose the best response to the following questions:

1. A 77-year-old man reports difficulty hearing. He has the most difficulty hearing conversation in crowded places, such as at restaurants and large gatherings. He has no known exposure to loud noises, and he has not had any recent illnesses or medication changes. Current daily medications include 81 mg aspirin, 25 mg hydrochlorothiazide, and 100 mg sertraline. On examination, he seems to hear you only when you speak slowly and clearly. When you whisper softly in each ear, he has difficulty hearing in both ears. Examination of the ear canal is within normal limits. At this time, you should recommend

   a. No further testing
   b. Discontinuation of the aspirin
   c. Meclizine 25 mg po q 6 hours as needed
   d. Referral for audiological testing
   e. Magnetic resonance imaging (MRI) of the brain

2. A month ago, you began treating a 76-year-old man with depression. He has a history of hypertension for many years, for which he takes 25 mg hydrochlorothiazide each day. On review of symptoms at that time, he did mention that for 1 year he has had some difficulty initiating urination, and he reported needing to get up two to three times each night to urinate. He also reported two to three episodes of urinary incontinence each week. You begin treatment with 50 mg sertraline each day for his depression and order a urinalysis, which is normal. After discussion with his primary care doctor, you also begin 5 mg oxybutinin po bid for the urinary incontinence.

   Now, 1 month later, the patient reports that his mood is improving. However, he has decreased many of his social activities, remaining home most days. After much questioning, he admits that his urinary incontinence has worsened, to the point that he is afraid to leave the house because he may have an accident in public. He reports often feeling a sensation of bladder fullness. What should you do next?

   a. Increase the oxybutinin to 5 mg po tid
   b. Discontinue oxybutinin and begin treatment with 2 mg tolterodine bid
   c. Discontinue the oxybutinin and refer for further urological evaluation

    d. Discontinue the sertraline and refer for further urological evaluation

    e. Order a prostate-specific antigen test and intravenous pyelogram

3. An 85-year-old woman with Alzheimer's disease comes to your office with her daughter for a routine follow-up visit. The patient appears well groomed and is pleasant and cooperative during the interview. She was started on donepezil 1 month ago, with 0.5 mg clonazepam each night for sleep. On further questioning, the daughter reports her mother has had four falls over the last month. The falls occur at various times during the day and do not seem to be associated with changes in body position or with environmental hazards in the home. The last fall resulted in a visit to the emergency room, but there were no serious injuries.

    On physical examination, the patient has a blood pressure of 136/72 and pulse of 72 while lying. On standing, her blood pressure is 132/70 and pulse is 80. She has an ecchymosis over her left flank, which the patient and daughter both report occurred with the last fall. There are no other ecchymoses. Her gait is normal. During mental status testing, you note that the patient seems to have difficulty with her vision. What should you do next?

    a. Report the patient and daughter to Adult Protective Services

    b. Discontinue the clonazepam, request vision testing, and refer the patient back to her primary care provider for further evaluation of her falls

    c. Discontinue the clonazepam and encourage the patient to decrease her physical activity

    d. Begin 0.1 mg fludrocortisone po three times per week

    e. Refer the patient to physical therapy for gait training

4. A 65-year-old woman who is a long-term resident at a psychiatric residential facility is noted to have an elevated thyroid-stimulating hormone (TSH) level of 8.2 µU/mL (normal 0.5–4.0) on routine laboratory testing. Her vital signs are within normal limits, and she is without physical complaints. Physical examination is within normal limits. Additional testing is ordered, with the following results:

Serum thyroxine (total)	6.4 µg/dL (normal 5–12)
Free thyroxine index (FTI)	10 (normal 5–12)
Antimicrosomal antibody	Negative

What is the best approach to these laboratory findings?

    a. Begin 0.5 mg levothyroxine po each day and increase dose weekly by 0.25 mg until the TSH level is within normal limits

b. Begin intravenous levothyroxine therapy immediately

c. Order thyroid nuclear medicine scan

d. Order thyroid ultrasound

e. No therapy indicated; recheck thyroid function studies in 6 months

5. A 70-year-old woman is being treated in your clinic for depression. During a routine visit, she reports that she has had gradually worsening discomfort of her hips, hands, and knees over the past 2 years. She has had no treatment for this condition in the past. Recent screening laboratory testing was all within normal limits, including a complete blood count, erythrocyte sedimentation rate, and kidney and liver panel testing. She recently began use of an over-the-counter pain reliever containing ibuprofen, with some relief of her symptoms. What medication change(s) would you recommend to this patient?

a. Discontinue the ibuprofen and begin a trial of 1000 mg acetaminophen po tid

b. Discontinue the ibuprofen and begin trial of 5 mg prednisone po qd

c. Discontinue the ibuprofen and begin the cyclooxygenase-2 (COX-2) inhibitor celecoxib at 100 mg po bid

d. Continue the ibuprofen and prescribe 100 mg misoprostol μg po bid

e. Continue the ibuprofen and prescribe 20 mg omeprazole po qd

6. You are asked to evaluate a 65-year-old woman with dementia. As part of your evaluation for potentially reversible causes of her illness, you find the patient has positive Venereal Disease Research Laboratory (VDRL) test and antitreponemal antibody testing. There is no record of prior syphilis treatment. She has no other health problems and is not on medications. On mental status testing, the patient has abnormalities in language, memory, and executive functioning. Physical examination is notable for generalized weakness and brisk reflexes. What would you do next?

a. Lumbar puncture with cerebrospinal fluid evaluation for evidence of neurosyphilis

b. Therapeutic trial of 2.4 million units benzathine penicillin im as a single dose, with repeat mental status testing in 6 months

c. Hospitalization and 10-day course of intravenous penicillin followed by three weekly doses of benzathine penicillin

d. Repeat antitreponemal antibody testing every 3 months for 1 year

e. Repeat VDRL testing every 3 months for 1 year

7. A 75-year-old man is referred to you for treatment of depression. Several trials of different antidepressant medications have been unsuccessful. The patient remains depressed and has lost 20 pounds over the

past 6 months. He has a long history of hypertension and diabetes mellitus. He had a myocardial infarction 2 years ago, permanent pacemaker placement 1 year ago for symptomatic bradycardia, and an ischemic stroke 6 months ago with a residual mild hemiparesis. During evaluation by his primary care doctor for medical causes of weight loss, he was noted to have mild anemia, but other testing (chemistry panel, liver panel, and thyroid function tests) was within normal limits. Which of the following would be a contraindication to electroconvulsive therapy (ECT) in this patient?

a. Permanent pacemaker
b. Symptomatic ischemic stroke within the past year
c. Myocardial infarction within the past 3 years
d. Anemia
e. None of the above

8. You are called to evaluate an 80-year-old widowed woman who was brought in to the emergency room by her son. He reports she has been increasingly reclusive, and although previously very active, over the past 6 months she has not attended her usual church groups and functions at the local senior center.

On examination, her blood pressure is 160/72 with a pulse of 82 (lying). On standing, her blood pressure is 134/62 with a pulse of 104. The remainder of her physical examination is unremarkable. She scores 28/30 on Mini-Mental Status Examination, missing points on the day of the week and missing the calendar date by 4 days. She does acknowledge feelings of sadness, depression, and anhedonia. Screening laboratory work is within normal limits. An electrocardiogram shows first-degree atrioventricular block.

She is being discharged from the emergency room. Arrangements are made for her to live with her son for the time being, and she is referred to a new family physician in her area. You make arrangements to see her at your office in 1 week. At this time, you wish to prescribe an antidepressant medication. Which of the following factors in this patient is the most important predictor of the development of clinically significant postural hypotension with antidepressant therapy?

a. A history of hypertension
b. Preexisting orthostatic hypotension
c. A history of vertebral compression fractures
d. An abnormal electrocardiogram
e. None of the above

Chapter 12
The Neurological Evaluation in Geriatric Psychiatry

Choose the best response to the following questions:

1. Parkinson's disease (PD) is associated with

   a. Bradykinesia, myoclonus, and ataxia
   b. Characteristic loss of dopaminergic neurons in the locus ceruleus
   c. Age-associated increase in prevalence, rising rapidly with each decade after 40 years of age
   d. Greater concordance between monozygotic twins than between dizygotic twins, suggesting a significant component of heritability

2. Dementia with Lewy bodies (DLB) can be reliably distinguished from Alzheimer's disease by which of the following:

   a. Fluctuating mental status
   b. Parkinsonian features
   c. Hallucinations
   d. All of the above
   e. None of the above

3. The following interventions have been shown to help in the primary prevention of stroke:

   a. Carotid endarterectomy in patients with greater than 40% stenosis
   b. Warfarin therapy in postmyocardial infarction patients who also have atrial fibrillation, decreased left ventricular ejection fraction, or left ventricular thrombus
   c. Lowering homocysteine with B vitamin therapy
   d. Answers b and c only

4. Head trauma is

   a. Unlikely to produce persistent behavioral changes even when the duration of posttraumatic amnesia exceeds 1 week
   b. Less likely to produce persistent symptoms in younger victims compared to older
   c. An established risk factor for Alzheimer's disease
   d. Often followed by depression in cases of right-side injuries

5. Which of the following statements is true?

    a. Creutzfeldt-Jakob disease and "mad cow" disease are both apparently caused by excessive transmembrane version of the prion protein called CtmPrP
    b. Amyotrophic lateral sclerosis (ALS) is a trinucleotide expansion disease
    c. Subacute combined degeneration can be detected by a very low serum B_{12} level
    d. Human immunodeficiency virus type 1 (HIV-1)–associated dementia can be expected to occur in about 50% of patients with acquired immunodeficiency syndrome (AIDS)

6. Neurological changes commonly associated with apparently normal aging include all of the following *except*

    a. Loss of ankle jerks
    b. Spontaneous buccolingual dyskinesias
    c. Dysmetria on finger-to-nose testing
    d. Impaired lateral gaze

7. The following clinical feature helps distinguish motor system dysfunction of different etiologies:

    a. Neuroleptic-induced parkinsonism is associated with more resting tremor than is idiopathic PD
    b. The psychomotor retardation of depression is usually associated with less rigidity than is the bradykinesia of idiopathic PD
    c. Neuroleptic-induced akathisia usually produces less shifting from foot to foot than psychogenic hyperactivity
    d. Progressive supranuclear palsy (PSP) frequently exhibits both rigidity and ophthalmoplegia
    e. Answers b and d only

8. Which of the following statements is correct?

    a. Unilateral resting tremor is seen in idiopathic PD
    b. Brain tumors usually produce papilledema in the elderly
    c. Gait disorders affect less than 5% of the elderly
    d. Alcoholic cerebellar degeneration produces more appendicular than truncal ataxia

9. Frontal release signs

    a. Reveal frontal lobe pathology
    b. Are common in the healthy aged

c. Include patellar hyperreflexia

d. Do not occur with frontal lobe pathology

e. Can distinguish basal ganglia from frontal lobe pathology

Chapter 13
Neuropsychological Testing of the Older Adult

Choose the best response to the following questions:

1. Following open heart surgery, a 72-year-old woman presents in her hospital room with irritability, delusions, disorientation, and memory dysfunction. During the consultation with the family, family members noted that there has been no history of memory or psychiatric dysfunction prior to the current presentation. In evaluating the cognitive functioning of the patient, it was noted that her attention was severely impaired (she could only recall two digits forward, and she was unable to perform digits backward). Given the pattern of her symptoms, the most likely diagnosis is

   a. Vascular dementia

   b. Delirium

   c. Alzheimer's disease

   d. Psychotic disorder not otherwise specified

2. A 56-year-old man, currently hospitalized on the inpatient psychiatric ward for evaluation, presents with memory disturbances. On evaluation, it is noted that he also presents with several parkinsonian features, including a shuffling gait and a bilateral hand tremor. A neuropsychological evaluation was administered to determine the nature and severity of his memory dysfunction. What is a common heuristic for differentiating cortical from subcortical memory disturbances?

   a. Rapid loss of learned information versus total loss of learned information

   b. Rapid loss of learned information versus no loss of learned information

   c. Rapid loss of learned information versus impaired retrieval of learned information

   d. Intact recognition of learned information versus total loss of learned information

3. A 71-year-old African American woman is brought into the emergency room by her son, who reported that over the past 2 weeks his mother has been leaving the stove unattended, "losing" objects around the house, and just yesterday, he was called to the local police department after his mother became lost at the mall. She is ambulatory and demonstrated no language disturbance. What is the most likely etiology of this woman's cognitive difficulties?

   a. Alzheimer's disease
   b. Parkinson's disease
   c. Huntington's disease
   d. Vascular dementia

4. A recent neuropsychological evaluation on a 66-year-old Caucasian man reported that mild-to-moderate deficits were noted on measures of verbal fluency, drawing, and visual memory. A task of fine motor skill was noted to be slow, particularly with the left hand. The neuropsychologist concluded that there was no gross deficit in any cognitive domain, but the cognitive performance was "spotty." Which is the likely diagnosis?

   a. Alzheimer's disease
   b. Vascular dementia
   c. Huntington's disease
   d. Parkinson's disease

5. Intellectual functioning is often thought to decline with increasing age. However, research has demonstrated that certain aspects of intellectual functioning are affected differentially. The cognitive profile associated with aging, often termed the *classic aging pattern*, is thought to present with the following:

   a. Greater decline in performance IQ in comparison to verbal IQ
   b. An equal decline in both verbal and performance IQ
   c. No decline in performance and verbal IQ
   d. A greater decline in verbal IQ in comparison to performance IQ

6. During a yearly physical, a 65-year-old retiree expressed some concern over what she perceives is a decline in her cognitive abilities. The patient reported that several of her friends were recently diagnosed with Alzheimer's disease, and she is concerned that, since her retirement, her cognitive abilities have declined. A neuropsychological evaluation concluded that there were no gross deficits in her cognitive abilities. Cognitive changes associated with normal aging are best described as

a. Moderate memory decline with a noticeable decline in language functions
b. Psychomotor slowing and subtle memory changes
c. No discernible cognitive changes
d. A general decline in all cognitive domains

Chapter 14
Neuroimaging in Late-Life Mental Disorders

Choose the best response to the following questions:

1. Positron emission tomography (PET) can be used to assess

   a. Regional glucose metabolism
   b. Cerebral blood flow
   c. Receptor density
   d. Neurotransmitter metabolism
   e. All of the above

2. The classical pattern of glucose hypometabolism seen early in the course of Alzheimer's disease (AD) is

   a. Cerebellar hypometabolism
   b. Frontotemporal hypometabolism
   c. Temporal-parietal hypometabolism
   d. None of the above

3. Parietal hypometabolism in the absence of formal diagnosis or family history of AD may be seen in patients with subjective memory complaints and

   a. High spinal fluid amyloid levels
   b. Mutations in the amyloid precursor gene (*APP*)
   c. The apolipoprotein E 4 (APOE 4) allele
   d. Hyperphosphorylated tau

4. Magnetic resonance spectroscopy (MRS)

   a. Is helpful as a marker of neuronal structure and function
   b. Can be used to monitor the impact of pharmacological intervention
   c. Provides information that is complementary to brain structural data
   d. Uses the same principles of physics as magnetic resonance imaging (MRI)
   e. All of the above

5. Neuroimaging findings that characterize late-life depression include

   a. Small brain volumes in the prefrontal lobes, hippocampus, and cau-
      date nucleus
   b. Larger high-intensity lesion volumes
   c. Smaller whole brain volume
   d. Increased amyloid binding in the hippocampus
   e. Both a and b

6. Cerebral blood flow in depression

   a. Is lower than blood flow in controls in the resting, pretreatment
      state
   b. Changes with treatment
   c. Cannot be estimated in humans
   d. Does not change with treatment
   e. Both a and b

7. Functional magnetic resonance imaging (fMRI) is

   a. Useful clinically
   b. Used in the study of genes
   c. A research tool in cognitive neuroscience
   d. Inexpensive and easy to perform

8. In vivo amyloid imaging

   a. Is readily available as a diagnostic tool
   b. Is specific for the diagnosis of vascular dementia.
   c. Is still in the development stages
   d. Can be used to effectively monitor pharmacological treatment in AD
   e. Both a and c

Chapter 15
Electroencephalography

Choose the best response to the following questions:

1. The electroencephalogram (EEG) in the elderly

   a. Does not differ at all from that of young adults
   b. Defines the diagnostic gold standard in cases of dementia
   c. May be used to rule out seizures

d. May normally show temporal slow waves

e. Should be routinely performed in depressed patients

2. Common normal findings in the EEG of subjects over the age of 80 years include

a. A posterior dominant rhythm of 8–9 Hz

b. Isolated temporal slow waves

c. Rare spike-and-wave foci

d. All of the above

e. Answers a and b only

3. In the evaluation of cognitive impairment, an EEG should be performed

a. Only when delirium is suspected

b. Whenever there are focal neurological signs

c. To document the presence of an underlying, secondary mental disorder

d. Only to rule out possible seizures

e. Even when the diagnosis of dementia appears to be clear

4. In an elderly patient, the presence of a normal EEG

a. Is inconsistent with the presence of dementia

b. Rules out the presence of an encephalopathy

c. Is seen rarely after the age of 70 years

d. Suggests the possibility of an underlying depression if there are co-existing severe cognitive deficits

e. Usually lacks an alpha rhythm

5. The EEG in delirious patients

a. Typically shows triphasic waves following overdoses with anticholinergic agents

b. Often shows slowing that is proportional to the level of confusion

c. Shows many features similar to those of a demented patient

d. All of the above

e. Answers b and c only

6. Normal EEGs may be seen in

a. Dementia

b. Delirium

c. Aging

d. Seizure disorders

e. All of the above

Matching set questions

   a. Repeated loss of consciousness with generalized tonic–clonic move-
      ments
   b. Spike-and-wave complexes in the EEG
   c. Frontally predominant intermittent rhythmic delta activity
   d. Occipital spikes
   e. Focal slowing
   f. Posterior dominant rhythm of less than 10 Hz
   g. Paroxysmal lateralizing epileptiform discharges
   h. Bancaud's phenomenon

   7. Which EEG abnormality is highly suggestive of Creutzfeldt-Jakob
      disease in a patient with myoclonus and a rapidly progressive de-
      mentia?
   8. What is the single most reliable indicator of a seizure disorder?
   9. What finding most reliably distinguishes between the EEGs of
      normal older and young adults?
  10. Which is the most common EEG abnormality in vascular de-
      mentia?

III Psychiatric Disorders of the Elderly

Chapter 16
Alzheimer's Disease

Choose the best response to the following questions:

1. A 76-year-old woman presents to her physician with the following complaint: "My memory is not as good as it used to be." She also complains that, "I cannot remember names as well as I could 5 years ago" and "I forget where I put things." The patient reports that she retired from her job as a teacher 17 years ago and now volunteers for a special education program in a primary school. She reports no difficulty with her volunteer work. Her husband says he has not noticed any problem in his wife's mental condition, and that she still drives to her volunteer job and has continued to pay her household bills. She scores in the normal range on screening cognitive testing. The medical workup is unremarkable, and magnetic resonance imaging (MRI) shows cortical atrophy, ventricular dilatation, and white matter changes. Which of the following is the most probable diagnosis?

   a. Normal pressure hydrocephalus
   b. Mild cognitive impairment
   c. Alzheimer's disease (AD)
   d. Age-associated memory impairment

2. An 89-year-old man with AD is referred by his physician to a geriatric psychiatrist for treatment. His wife reports that he can no longer pay his bills and needs considerable help in dressing and bathing himself. Cognitive assessment indicates that he knows his name and his wife's name, but he has difficulty counting backward from 10, says the president is Kennedy, and cannot recall his prior occupation. He is not receiving any medication for his dementia or other psychotropic medications. His wife says that he is manageable and asks if there is any medication that would be helpful. Which of the following medications is approved for use in persons with this degree of dementia?

   a. Risperidone
   b. Donepezil
   c. Memantine
   d. Rivastigmine

3. Which of the following symptoms is most commonly observed in patients with AD?

   a. The belief that someone has been stealing their belongings
   b. Olfactory hallucinations, such as smelling something burning
   c. Auditory hallucinations, such as hearing the voices of dead relatives
   d. The belief that the spouse or other relatives are unfaithful
   e. The belief that people, such as the spouse, are not really who they say they are

4. Hyperphosphorylated tau is most commonly found in the hippocampus in which of the following conditions?

   a. Lewy body dementia
   b. Cerebrovascular dementia
   c. Mild cognitive impairment
   d. Age-associated memory impairment
   e. AD

5. You are asked to provide a one-time consultation on a 91-year-old woman who was diagnosed with AD 3 years ago and who has had high blood pressure for many years, which is under control with medication. She has been taking donepezil, sertraline, amlodipine, hydrochlorothiazide, aspirin, gingko biloba, coenzyme Q, multivitamins, and homocysteine modulators. Recently, her local physician added memantine. Her live-in caregiver states that the patient is able to bathe and dress by herself, although she needs help in selecting clothes. When she goes shopping with the caregiver, she is only able to pick items off the supermarket shelves when they are pointed to and cannot pay for them. She cannot cook but helps set the table and can feed herself. She toilets independently and is "clean" and meticulous in toileting. However, for several months she has been incontinent at night and sometimes during the day. Which of the following recommendations should be made to her referring physician?

   a. Discontinue the gingko biloba
   b. Discontinue the coenzyme Q
   c. Suggest an alternative be found for the amlodipine
   d. Suggest an alternative be found for the aspirin
   e. Suggest an alternative be found for the hydrochlorothiazide

6. Severe, end-stage AD is commonly associated with all of the following findings *except*

   a. Marked slowing of electrical activity on electroencephalographic evaluation with marked delta and theta activity

b. Presence of marked rigidity in response to range-of-motion assessment of both elbows
c. Presence of an abnormal plantar reflex on neurological examination
d. Presence of marked anemia
e. Loss of ambulatory capacity

Chapter 17
Vascular Dementias

Choose the best response to the following questions:

1. A 67-year-old man is brought for evaluation by his family because they think he is "getting Alzheimer's" and should make plans to wind down his business. He makes clear his feeling that their concerns are overblown but agrees to be examined to placate them. He reports he has "always been in good health," although he admits his memory "is not as good as it used to be." Which of the following historical features would provide the strongest presumption of "evidence of cerebrovascular disease . . . judged to be etiologically related to the disturbance" of cognition to support a diagnosis of vascular dementia?

   a. Elevated score (8) on the Hachinski Ischemia Scale
   b. Sudden onset of symptoms following an episode of severe arrhythmia accompanied by transient "confusion"
   c. A magnetic resonance imaging (MRI) study demonstrating "deep white matter opacities, probably ischemic"
   d. Concomitant diagnosis of diabetes mellitus with microvascular complications
   e. Identification of depressed mood and articulation of fears of "losing it"

2. A 59-year-old man is seen in consultation in a stroke rehabilitation unit because of concern about depression and vascular dementia— without a prior history of major psychiatric disorder or cognitive impairment. He is 6 weeks post–left frontal stroke with nonfluent aphasia and right hemiparesis. He is able to comprehend and communicate and has begun to regain movement and activity in his right arm and leg. He is observed to be indifferent to the tasks of rehabilitation. He has a very poor appetite, has lost nearly 20 pounds, and sleeps up to 18 hours a day. The rehabilitation staff is frustrated by his lack of

motivation and energy; he consistently "agrees" to make an effort but then begs off therapy sessions after only a few minutes and only very rarely initiates "homework."

After you waken him for the interview, you find him to be physically lethargic, but gracious; he comprehends questions and can make himself well understood despite significant and effortful difficulty expressing his thoughts. He is able, however, to convey a realistic assessment of his situation, including understanding of the importance of rehabilitation efforts. Although he appears sad, he denies overt feelings of sadness, depression, or despair but is unable to convey hope. He convincingly denies suicidal ideation. He has little emotional response, however, to this discussion and is unable to commit to modifying his behavior. Which of the following is the best diagnostic premise for initiating treatment in this case?

a. Major depressive episode
b. Apathy as a result of frontal lobe stroke injury
c. Other intercurrent medical complications
d. Vascular dementia, possibly with depression

3. Which of the following would be the best choice for treatment of major depression following a stroke?

a. Tricyclic antidepressant
b. Selective serotonin reuptake inhibitor
c. Stimulant medication
d. Problem-solving therapy

4. A home health care agency cares for an 82-year-old widowed woman with multiple physical problems who has "developed Alzheimer's and hallucinations" since she suffered a right hemisphere stroke several months before. Her hemiparesis persists, but her function has improved overall. Her primary care doctor added 2 mg olanzapine bid along with 2 mg benztropine mesylate bid to a regimen of 13 medications, but this has made her "worse," leading to consultation with you.

You find a woman who is inattentive, focuses on multiple physical symptoms (diarrhea/constipation, headache, backache, loss of energy), but who clearly can recall episodes of vivid, usually pleasant visual images that she recognizes to be hallucinations. She is inattentive, but with cues can recall all three words you give her to remember. Your most likely initial recommendation will be

a. Initiate 1 mg risperidone bid
b. Obtain MRI

   c. Discontinue olanzapine and benztropine
   d. Arrange admission to a nearby experienced geriatric hospital
   e. Contact Adult Protective Services to arrange for a conservator

5. A 73-year-old psychotherapist is referred for evaluation of "memory
   loss." She and her family are discussing whether she should retire from
   her sharply reduced but still professionally rewarding practice she
   maintains at an office in her home. She reports having suffered two
   strokes that she emphasizes were "small," and an MRI report describes three lacunar lesions plus a mild degree of white matter opacity. She and her family agree, however, that she has regained energy
   since she had a pacemaker placed 6 months previously, and that there
   has been no further decline. You have records from her referring physician documenting normal results on metabolic studies, and she takes
   no medications that would be likely to affect cognition adversely. On
   examination, she has mild deficits in memory testing and has difficulty
   copying complicated figures, scoring 26 on the Mini-Mental State Examination. However, her language functions and reasoning are fully
   intact, except that she complains about her ability to write since the
   second stroke episode. You diagnose (probable) mild and currently
   uncomplicated vascular dementia. You properly recommend she consider which of the following?

   a. A trial of a cholinesterase inhibitor
   b. A trial of a N-methyl-D-aspartate (NMDA) receptor antagonist
   c. Review of her will and financial affairs, advance care directives,
      and arrangements
   d. Further diagnostic workup, including neuropsychological testing
      and functional brain studies
   e. Psychotherapy
   f. Advice that she should stop driving and disband her practice imme-
      diately
   g. Answers a and c
   h. Answers a, c, d, and e
   i. All of the above

6. An 82-year-old retired accountant comes with his wife for evaluation
   out of concern he may be developing Alzheimer's disease. On questioning, you learn that the suggestion for examination came from a highway patrolman, who realized the man could not follow directions that
   the officer had provided at the patient's request. You elicit the specific
   observation that the patient has lost the ability to distinguish right
   from left. In other areas of mental status, you are impressed that he
   functions at a high level, consistent with his professional accomplish-

ments. What features would you seek on the examination to substantiate your suspicions of the etiology of his syndrome?

a. Impaired arithmetical skills
b. Loss of the ability to spell reliably
c. History of sudden onset of symptoms following a cardiac arrest
d. Inability to identify his different fingers
e. All of the above

Chapter 18
Delirium

Choose the best response to the following questions:

1. A 75-year-old man with Parkinson's disease treated with carbidopa/levodopa has minimal cognitive impairment. He has a long history of bipolar disorder treated with lithium carbonate despite mild chronic renal failure. He is hospitalized for a transurethral resection of the prostate, and an indwelling catheter is placed postoperatively. He is eating and drinking poorly. The next day, he is somnolent and grossly confused with an ataxic gait. The most likely cause of his confusion is

a. Urinary tract infection
b. Dehydration
c. Worsening renal failure
d. Lithium toxicity
e. Worsening Parkinson's disease

2. An 80-year-old man presents to the emergency room with a cough and fever. His wife reports that he has been showing progressive memory problems for several years. In addition, for many years he has had two to three cocktails with dinner every night. Chest x-ray shows pneumonia, and he is admitted and given intravenous antibiotics. On his third day in the hospital, he is disoriented and inattentive and complains of seeing bugs on the wall; he becomes agitated, sweaty, and tachycardic. The most likely diagnosis is

a. Delirium caused by pneumonia
b. Delirium caused by alcohol withdrawal
c. Delirium caused by an allergy to antibiotics
d. New onset of late-life schizophrenia
e. Worsening dementia

3. For a delirious 80-year-old man who is in the intensive care unit and showing signs of alcohol withdrawal, what would be the most appropriate specific treatment for his delirium?

    a. Intravenous haloperidol
    b. Intravenous lorazepam
    c. Reassurance
    d. Intravenous carbamazepine
    e. Intravenous hydration

4. An 89-year-old woman presents to an emergency room after slipping on the ice outside her apartment. X-rays show swelling but no fracture. She has difficulty walking, is weak and hypotensive, and is admitted to the hospital. She is given acetaminophen with codeine for her pain. Electrocardiogram shows new atrial fibrillation, and she is started on digoxin. She complains that she cannot fall asleep and is given 5 mg zolpidem. The next morning, her nephew comes in to see her and finds her somnolent and quite confused. He tells the doctor that for the last year he has been paying her bills because she was forgetting to do so, and her electricity was almost shut off. The most important predisposing factor in the development of her delirium is

    a. Preexisting cognitive impairment
    b. Vision impairment
    c. Severe illness
    d. Age

5. Considering the vignette in question 4 and putting aside the importance of preexisting cognitive impairment as a predisposing factor, the most important *precipitating* factor associated with the development of her delirium is

    a. Atrial fibrillation
    b. Soft-tissue injury
    c. Sleep deprivation
    d. Addition of three new medications

Chapter 19
Other Dementias and Mental Disorders
Due to General Medical Conditions

Choose the best response to the following questions:

1. A 64-year-old married lawyer was assessed at a psychiatric outpatient clinic. He was referred by his family doctor because of a "personality change." He had always been perfectionistic, hardworking, and highly professional, but over the previous 12 months, he had become less motivated and less interested in his practice. He had become overly familiar with his clients and was noted to make inappropriate comments, often with a sexual connotation. He was much less careful with his appearance and was somewhat disheveled. He voiced no concerns. He had become unreliable and had begun to drink excessive amounts of alcohol. He had experienced one episode of depression a year and a half earlier, which had lasted for a period of about 2 months. He scored 27/30 on the Mini-Mental State Examination, losing 2 points for attention and 1 point for recall. He was able to recall the forgotten word with cuing. Neurological examination was normal except for the presence of palmomental and snout reflexes. Laboratory tests were unremarkable, and a computerized tomographic (CT) scan showed mild nonspecific cerebral atrophy. A single-photon emission computed tomographic scan of the brain showed decreased perfusion in frontal regions. The most likely diagnosis in the case is

   a. Major depressive episode
   b. Vascular dementia
   c. Mixed dementia
   d. Frontotemporal dementia (FTD)
   e. Dementia with Lewy bodies (DLB)

2. A patient who has a frontotemporal dementia has recently begun to display more behavioral problems. He had become increasingly disinhibited and intrusive. He was very inappropriate, asking strangers for money and was highly agitated on occasion, swearing and making hostile gestures. There is conclusive evidence that the best medication for first-line treatment is

   a. An atypical antipsychotic
   b. A serotonergic antidepressant
   c. A benzodiazepine
   d. A cholinesterase inhibitor
   e. None of the above

3. A 72-year-old married retired seamstress was referred to a memory clinic because of increasing forgetfulness with significant symptoms of anxiety and distress. She complained that she saw "mites" flying around her apartment. She noted that these mites would sometimes talk to her, and she believed that they were "dead souls" who had come back to life. She also described seeing children running around her sofa. Her family reported that at times she seemed reasonably alert and oriented, but at other times she appeared to be totally confused. On examination, there was evidence of a mild pill-rolling tremor and some bradykinesia, which had been present for about 6 months. She was anxious but denied significant depression. She scored 24/30 on the Mini-Mental State Examination, losing points for attention, short-term memory, and visuospatial function. She had great difficulty drawing the face of a clock, in particular having difficulty spacing the numbers. Her family doctor had started her on low-dose loxapine because of the hallucinations. Shortly thereafter, she had developed an acute dystonic reaction, especially a very stiff neck. The most likely diagnosis in this case is

a. Alzheimer's disease
b. Mixed dementia
c. Frontotemporal dementia
d. Late-onset schizophrenia
e. Dementia with Lewy bodies

4. You are asked for a treatment recommendation for a patient with DLB who is experiencing vivid visual hallucinations accompanied by significant distress and agitation. Her family doctor had started her on low-dose haloperidol because of the hallucinations. Shortly thereafter, she developed marked parkinsonism. Which of the following class of medication would you initially recommend to her family physician?

a. An atypical antipsychotic
b. A serotonergic antidepressant
c. A mood stabilizer
d. A benzodiazepine
e. A cholinesterase inhibitor

5. A 54-year-old engineer was referred to a psychiatric outpatient clinic because of apathy and irritability. He also complained of some mild memory loss. In recent months, he had developed some unusual movements of his arms and legs, which were nonrepetitive, jerky, and abrupt. He admitted to feelings of depression. On examination, he had mild word-finding difficulty, and there was evidence of mild memory loss with delayed responses to questions. He also demonstrated diffi-

culty with frontal systems tasks, including visual pattern completion tests, tests of alternating motor patterns, and the go/no go test. There was a family history of mood disorders, suicide, and presenile dementia. His father developed dementia in his late 40s and died in a nursing home at age 60. The most likely diagnosis is

a. Parkinson disease
b. Frontotemporal dementia
c. Amyotrophic lateral sclerosis
d. Huntington disease
e. Toxic encephalopathy

Chapter 20
Grief and Bereavement

Choose the best response to the following questions:

1. The duration of "normal" grief is

   a. 4–8 weeks
   b. 2–12 months
   c. 12–24 months
   d. >2 years

2. The percentage of bereaved individuals meeting symptomatic criteria for major depression 2 months after the death of their spouse is

   a. 5%–10%
   b. 10%–30%
   c. 30%–50%
   d. >50%

3. The best clue for differentiating normal bereavement from major depression are

   a. Time since death
   b. Feelings of worthlessness, psychomotor retardation, and suicidal ideation
   c. A positive dexamethone suppression test
   d. The nature of the relationship with the deceased

4. Which of the following is most likely to be associated with grief complications?

   a. Looking for the deceased in crowds more than 2 months after the death
   b. Visual images of the deceased
   c. Dreams of the deceased
   d. A past history of recurrent major depression

5. For bereaved persons who develop a bereavement-related depression,

   a. Pharmacological treatment alone is ineffective
   b. Psychotherapy interferes with the grief work
   c. Antidepressant medication plus psychotherapy is a preferred treatment
   d. Treatment may prolong grief reaction

6. Posttraumatic stress disorder (PTSD) following bereavement

   a. By definition does not exist; bereavement does not fulfill the A (stressor) criterion
   b. Occurs only after an unnatural death (e.g., suicide, homicide, or accident)
   c. Is the most frequently seen form of PTSD in Detroit, Michigan
   d. Is benign

7. After the death of a spouse

   a. Many (>20%) men develop a new intimate relationship or remarry within 2 years
   b. Most (>50%) women develop a new intimate relationship or remarry within 2 years
   c. Widows should be discouraged from getting involved in new relationships for at least 1 year after the death of a spouse
   d. Widowers who remarry have higher rates of depression than widowers who do not

8. The strongest predictors of making a good adjustment to bereavement include

   a. Gender and age
   b. Positive self-esteem and personal competencies
   c. An ambivalent relationship with the deceased
   d. Intense early grief reactions

9. Among women aged 65 years or older, what percentage have been widowed one or more times?

   a. 10%
   b. 20%
   c. 30%
   d. 40%
   e. 50%

10. All of the following are risk factors for bereavement-related depression *except*

    a. Early intense reactions soon after the loss
    b. Female gender
    c. Family history of depression
    d. Increased alcohol use soon after the loss
    e. Poor physical health

Chapter 21
Late-Life Mood Disorders

Choose the best response to the following questions:

1. Which of the following statements about pseudodementia in geriatric patients is correct?

   a. It is common in depressed elderly patients with histrionic personality disorder
   b. It represents a catastrophic reaction
   c. It has a benign long-term outcome
   d. After the initial cognitive improvement, a considerable number of patients progress to dementia over a period of a few years
   e. It occurs principally in patients with recurrent depression

2. Which of the following statements about the medical burden of depression in elderly patients is correct?

   a. Geriatric depression occurs in the context of multiple medical illnesses
   b. Depression increases mortality
   c. Depression increases medical morbidity

d. Depression worsens the outcomes of medical disorders

e. All of the above

3. Which of the following statements about disability is correct?

   a. Depression is the ninth leading cause of disability in the United States

   b. Deficits in initiation and perseveration seem to have a stronger relationship to instrumental activities of daily living (IADL) impairment than other cognitive impairments in depressed elderly patients

   c. Although disability compromises quality of life, it does not increase the risk for specific medical disorders

   d. Once disability develops, improvement of depressive symptoms rarely leads to a substantial reduction of disability

   e. In most depressed elders, disability can be fully explained by the severity of depression, medical burden, and cognitive impairment

4. Which of the following statements about suicide and suicidal ideation in the elderly is correct?

   a. Female suicide rates continue to increase slightly during late life

   b. The rate of suicide for elderly individuals steadily decreased from the 1930s until today

   c. Suicide attempts and suicidal ideation decrease with aging

   d. Depression is the most common psychiatric diagnosis of suicide victims across the life span

   e. None of the above

5. Which of the following statements about geriatric bipolar disorder is correct?

   a. Unlike early-onset mania, late-onset mania is associated with medical disorders or drug treatment

   b. Bipolar disorder is extremely uncommon in geriatric populations because of selective mortality

   c. Late-onset bipolar patients have an equal rate of mood disorders among relatives as those with early-onset mania

   d. Bipolar disorder increases mortality but not to the level of unipolar depressive disorder

   e. None of the above

Chapter 22
Psychoses

Choose the best response to the following questions:

1. Compared to patients with early-onset schizophrenia, those with late-onset schizophrenia

   a. Are more refractory to treatment with antipsychotic medications
   b. Are more likely to be diagnosed with the disorganized subtype of schizophrenia
   c. Are less likely to have held a job and have children
   d. Show less-severe negative symptoms
   e. Have a higher risk of suicide

2. Late-onset schizophrenia is characterized by all of the following statements *except*

   a. Higher incidence in women than men
   b. Association with premorbid antisocial personality
   c. Response to low doses of antipsychotic medications
   d. Stable cognitive deficits in most patients
   e. None of the above

3. Patients with very-late-onset schizophrenia-like psychosis (onset after age 60 years)

   a. Are more likely than patients with younger onset schizophrenia to have an underlying medical or neurological illness
   b. Usually have a history of poor premorbid social functioning
   c. Are difficult to treat with conventional or atypical antipsychotic medications
   d. Tend to have a family history of schizophrenia
   e. Show prominent negative symptoms

4. Psychosocial therapies for schizophrenia

   a. Include cognitive behavioral therapy but not family interventions
   b. Should only be utilized in patients with good insight
   c. Are less effective in combination with antipsychotic drug therapy
   d. May help reduce relapse and improve coping skills
   e. None of the above

5. Psychosis of Alzheimer's disease (AD) is a distinct syndrome character-ized most commonly by

    a. Reduced risk of aggressive behaviors
    b. Greater severity in the late stages of AD
    c. Olfactory hallucinations
    d. Delusions or visual or auditory hallucinations
    e. Signs of delirium

6. Delusional disorder

    a. Usually begins in patients' teens to early 20s
    b. Is often associated with prominent auditory hallucinations
    c. Is characterized by the presence of nonbizarre delusions
    d. Has a somewhat earlier age of onset in women than in men
    e. Occurs in about 5%–8% of the elderly population

7. For the older patient with schizophrenia or other psychotic disorders, atypical antipsychotic medications

    a. Are as likely as conventional neuroleptics to cause acute extrapyra-midal symptoms (EPS)
    b. Should be considered second-line agents after high-potency antipsy-chotic agents such as haloperidol
    c. Should be prescribed in doses equivalent to those prescribed for younger patients with schizophrenia
    d. Are unlikely to cause sedation and orthostasis
    e. Are less likely to carry a risk of causing tardive dyskinesia

8. Prominent visual hallucinations and non-drug-induced EPS are most commonly associated with which of the following late-life disorders?

    a. Delusional disorder
    b. Dementia with Lewy bodies (DLB)
    c. Brief psychotic reaction
    d. Late-onset schizophrenia
    e. Bipolar disorder

9. A patient with AD develops the delusion that his caregiver daughter is stealing from him. He has become increasingly difficult to manage at home, destroying papers around the home. He once wandered from the house and was found several blocks away, disoriented to his loca-tion. There is no evidence from the physical examination and labora-tory workup of an underlying medical illness such as an infection. Which of the following interventions would be most useful initially?

    a. Use of a low-potency antipsychotic agent such as chlorpromazine
    b. Supportive psychotherapy for the patient
    c. Prescribing 100 mg trazodone tid
    d. A low dose of an atypical antipsychotic agent
    e. Reassurance to the daughter that the symptoms are transient

10. As patients with early-onset schizophrenia age, the most common pattern is one of

    a. Stability or even improvement in symptoms
    b. Increased severity of positive symptoms
    c. Complete "burnout" of symptoms
    d. Appearance of visual hallucinations
    e. Development of new types of delusions

Chapter 23
Anxiety Disorders

Choose the best response to the following questions:

1. A 75-year-old woman in generally good health reports that she fell on the sidewalk 6 months ago. She was not injured, but since then she has feared having another fall and has restricted her level of activity. Because of her fear of falling, she no longer goes for walks by herself and will only leave her house when absolutely necessary. As a result, she has less social contact than previously. What is the most likely diagnosis?

    a. Posttraumatic stress disorder
    b. Panic disorder with agoraphobia
    c. Agoraphobia without history of panic disorder
    d. Social phobia
    e. Major depressive disorder

2. For the person described in question 1, what is the most appropriate treatment?

    a. Lorazepam
    b. Sertraline
    c. Relaxation therapy
    d. Exposure therapy

3. A 72-year-old man suffers a left hemispheric stroke. Several months after the stroke, he starts to feel anxious, worried, keyed up, and on edge. In addition, he becomes preoccupied with physical sensations in his body and reports light-headedness, hot flashes, pressure in his head, and nausea. He is referred to a psychiatrist, who establishes that the patient also has depressed mood, anhedonia, initial and middle insomnia, anergia, anorexia, and feelings of hopelessness. The most likely diagnosis is

   a. Major depressive disorder with associated generalized anxiety
   b. Panic disorder
   c. Hypochondriasis
   d. Somatization disorder
   e. Adjustment disorder

4. A 67-year-old man has a 45-year history of obsessive-compulsive disorder (OCD), which is treated with clomipramine. He is referred to a urologist for evaluation and management of symptoms of prostatic hypertrophy. The urologist prescribes tamsulosin hydrochloride and questions whether the patient's OCD could be treated with a medication that is less likely to aggravate symptoms of prostatic hypertrophy. Given the circumstances, what medication would be the most appropriate alternative treatment of this patient's OCD?

   a. Sertraline
   b. Paroxetine
   c. Venlafaxine
   d. Buspirone
   e. Lorazepam

5. Which of the following anxiety disorders is most prevalent in people aged 65 years or older?

   a. Panic disorder
   b. Social phobia
   c. Agoraphobia
   d. Obsessive-compulsive disorder

6. An 82-year-old woman, living independently at home, is admitted to the hospital after she falls and fractures her hip. The day after surgical repair of her hip, she suddenly becomes anxious, fearful, and agitated. She reports that during the night she heard the nurses laughing about her, and she believes they are planning to harm her. On examination, she is inattentive and distractible and is temporally disoriented. What is the most likely cause of this woman's anxiety?

a. Dementia
b. Delirium
c. Major depressive disorder
d. Delusional disorder
e. Adjustment disorder

7. A 65-year-old man presents with mixed symptoms of major depression and generalized anxiety. His physician prescribes nefazodone, starting with a dose of 50 mg bid. Because of the patient's high level of anxiety and disturbing insomnia, the physician also initiates treatment with a benzodiazepine, to be given on a short-term basis until the antidepressant becomes effective. Which of the following benzodiazepines is most suitable?

a. Alprazolam
b. Clonazepam
c. Diazepam
d. Lorazepam

8. A 70-year-old widow with a long-standing history of generalized anxiety disorder is brought by her daughter to a new primary care physician. The patient recently relocated after the death of her husband 6 months earlier. The woman asks the physician for a prescription for 10 mg qd diazepam, a medication that she has taken for the past 30 years. The physician is concerned about her taking diazepam because it can contribute to cognitive impairment, falls, and hip fractures in older people. What is the physician's most appropriate course of action at this point?

a. Stop the diazepam
b. Continue the diazepam
c. Substitute buspirone for the diazepam
d. Substitute paroxetine for the diazepam

Chapter 24
Personality Disorders

Choose the best response to the following questions:

1. Which of the following personality disorders has been the most prevalent in patients over the age of 50 years?

a. Avoidant

    b. Obsessive-compulsive
    c. Schizoid
    d. Paranoid
    e. Dependent

2. An 81-year-old man with no prior history of depression or clinically significant personality dysfunction suffered a cerebrovascular accident, resulting in an infarct in the right frontotemporal region. He subsequently experienced a major depressive episode, for which he was successfully treated with venlafaxine and psychotherapy. However, he then developed occasional irritability (unusual for him) and louder than normal speech and began to tell jokes with inappropriate sexual content to his school-aged grandchildren. Sleep and appetite remained normal. Score on the Mini-Mental State Examination was 30/30. The disinhibited behavior continued after lowering the venlafaxine dose and adding a mood stabilizer but was somewhat moderated after 4 months by the use of 1 mg risperidone qd. The clinical picture would best be characterized as

    a. Late-onset bipolar disorder (mania)
    b. Residual depressive symptomatology
    c. Posttraumatic stress disorder
    d. Narcissistic personality disorder
    e. Personality change caused by a general medical condition

3. Individuals with late-onset schizophrenia or delusional disorder are likely to have had which of the following personality disorders premorbidly?

    a. Borderline with "minipsychotic" episodes
    b. Narcissistic
    c. Histrionic
    d. Antisocial
    e. Paranoid or schizotypal

4. Which of the following statements about personality traits in normal aging is *incorrect*?

    a. A quiet, inner-directed attitude can be found in many individuals
    b. In cross-sectional studies, older persons score lower on scales assessing impulsivity and hostility
    c. In cross-sectional studies, criminality and sociopathy decline with age
    d. With respect to personality traits, individuals develop more exaggerated manifestations of their adult personalities

e. In longitudinal studies of personality traits, individuals tend to show overall stability as they age

5. Based on clinical data and theoretical constructs, which of the following statements best characterizes the relationship between geriatric personality disorders and depressive disorders?

a. Personality and depressive disorders may coexist but otherwise are clinically independent of one another
b. Personality and depressive disorders are synergistic
c. Personality disorders represent a *form fruste* of depressive disorders
d. There is a scarring relationship; that is, repeated depressive episodes alter or scar the personality
e. All of the above

6. A 69-year-old man developed rapid onset of decreased interest, poor concentration, impaired appetite, and mild weight loss. His sleep and energy are undisturbed, and he denied suicidal ideation and substance abuse. However, he strongly endorsed feelings of tension, shortness of breath, stomach tightness, nausea, and leg weakness. Cognitive abilities and activities of daily living were unimpaired, and there were no other symptoms of anxiety or psychosis. There was a prior history of similar feelings when he was left by his wife many years before. Medical history was unremarkable. There was no family history of depression. Preoccupations focused on concerns that, because of business problems, he would not be able to maintain his income, and that this would cause him to lose his girlfriend, who he thought was most interested in his money and business. In the initial exploratory sessions in treatment, he would rock back and forth in his chair, moaning like a child, and focus on abdominal complaints. Past history revealed a cold, distant, and unavailable mother and few emotional supports. He had strong feelings of betrayal and abandonment throughout his life. Formal assessment of personality revealed strong dependency characteristics as well as some dramatic cluster B characteristics. The therapist diagnosed major depression with personality disorder not otherwise specified. Antidepressant medication produced some remission of the major affective symptoms but left significant residual anxiety. Regarding this case, which of the following statements is most true?

a. Despite the poor emotional support, life stress, and frequent separations in this patient's history, there is no specific evidence to link these factors with personality disorder in someone of his age
b. This patient demonstrates depression comorbid with a personality disorder, but it is an atypical presentation because this association is less typical in elderly patients compared to younger adult patients

c. Compared to younger adults, this patient's depressive symptoms are likely to be chronic despite adequate antidepressant therapy and concurrent psychotherapy

d. The presence of residual symptoms following antidepressant therapy is unusual in patients with this type of clinical profile.

Chapter 25
Substance Abuse

Choose the best response to the following questions:

1. A 68-year-old man is referred because of persistently troubling bereavement 6 months after his spouse's death. He does not meet criteria for a depressive disorder and experiences relief after several psychotherapy sessions focusing on the marriage relationship and his loss. In the initial workup, he indicated that for years he has regularly consumed a 750-cc bottle of table wine in the evening, five or six evenings per week (about 25 to 30 standard drinks a week) but never more than this per occasion. He suffers no hangovers or other perceived ill effects. He exercises and is in good physical health according to his referring primary physician, has never had any obvious alcohol-related problems, and is CAGE negative. He seems surprised and interested when you inform him that his level of drinking is much higher than recommended safe levels and could eventually result in health problems. What step in management is indicated next regarding this patient's use of alcohol?

   a. Refer back to primary physician
   b. Advise reduction in alcohol use
   c. Prescribe naltrexone
   d. Refer for alcoholism assessment

2. A 72-year-old man is referred because of depression for the past several months. Evaluation shows that he clearly meets criteria for current major depression, with moderately severe symptoms but no evidence of suicidal intent, agitation, or psychotic features. This appears to be the first episode. In the past 2 years, there have been no adverse life events. Further history reveals that he was treated for alcohol dependence 20 years earlier, remained abstinent for 10 years, but resumed drinking after retirement. For the past 2 years, he has consumed about a pint of vodka on drinking days (about 10 standard drinks), but the

number of drinking days per week has increased from three or four to nearly daily, up to and including the evening before this evaluation. He says that his father and a paternal uncle were "alcoholic" and also suffered from depression, although neither was ever treated for these conditions. What is the most likely diagnosis of this patient's mood disorder?

a. Alcohol-induced depression
b. Major depression
c. Major depression complicated by alcohol effects
d. Diagnosis cannot yet be determined

3. A 69-year-old woman is referred because of memory loss for the past 2 years. Mental examination shows that she suffers from dementia, with significant deficits in memory, object recognition, and executive functioning; there is no evidence of anomia. Neurological examination reveals coarse horizontal nystagmus, gait ataxia, and peripheral neuropathy with a stocking distribution in the lower extremities. Computerized tomographic scan of the brain shows generalized moderate cortical atrophy. What new information will be most useful as an aid to diagnosis?

a. Family history of neurological disorder
b. Personal history of alcohol use
c. Neuropsychological evaluation
d. Imaging study of the cerebellum

4. Several studies have demonstrated that moderate alcohol consumption is associated with reduced overall mortality compared to both heavy drinking and abstention. What is the most important explanation of this finding?

a. Abstainers include persons who are ill
b. Abstainers include former alcoholics
c. Moderate drinking benefits cognitive status
d. Moderate drinking reduces coronary heart disease
e. Heavy drinkers have more accidents

5. Several pharmacological variables increase the risk of benzodiazepine dependence, including long duration of treatment, higher daily dose level, shorter elimination half-life, and higher milligram potency. Several patient variables also increase this risk, including prior history of substance abuse, personality disorder, and major presenting symptoms that require treatment. Which chronic disorder is most highly associated with risk of dependence when a benzodiazepine is prescribed?

a. Social anxiety disorder
b. Generalized anxiety disorder
c. Sleep disorder
d. Panic disorder

6. Compared to typical clinical presentations of benzodiazepine withdrawal in younger adults, which one of the following is probably more likely to occur in an older patient?

a. Delirium
b. Psychosis
c. Depression
d. Anxiety

7. A 75-year-old woman has taken 5 mg diazepam tid for 8 years for generalized anxiety symptoms that occur in conjunction with her chronic obstructive pulmonary disease. The medication effectively controls her anxiety and aids her sleep. You are asked to consult about whether to continue this regimen by her primary physician, who you know provides close medical supervision to his patients. What is the most important issue requiring assessment?

a. Prior alcohol or substance dependence
b. Prior response to alternative treatments
c. Current evidence of diazepam toxicity
d. Patient's reliability and adherence

8. Beliefs about smoking influence readiness to quit. Older adult smokers share in common with younger adult smokers certain attitudes and beliefs about smoking and quitting, but in other important respects, smokers differ in beliefs by age. For example, older smokers are *more* likely than younger smokers to perceive smoking as a positive habit to enhance coping, reduce stress, and control weight. What other important belief is *less* characteristic of older smokers when compared to younger smokers?

a. Smoking influences children
b. Smoking impairs health
c. Smoking reduces irritability
d. Smoking improves concentration

9. In 1981, it was first proposed that smoking (nicotine dependence) might protect against AD. Since then, more than 30 studies have examined the relationship between smoking and dementia. How can the findings to date best be summarized?

a. Population-based prospective studies and most case–control studies demonstrate no protective effect of smoking against AD
b. At least two recent case–control studies affirmed a protective effect of smoking against AD
c. In prospective studies, the risk of AD is lower in smokers who possess the E [APOE]-ε4 allele than in those who lack this allele
d. Senile plaque formation is less prominent in the brains of patients with AD who were smokers than in those who were nonsmokers

Chapter 26
Sleep Disorders in Geriatric Psychiatry

Choose the best response to the following questions:

1. All of the following statements are true *except*

   a. Some of the change in sleep patterns of older people is caused by alteration in the circadian rhythm
   b. Older people may live in settings that are not conducive to uninterrupted sleep
   c. Caregiving roles may require older people to be up all night
   d. One of the best predictors of future depression in older people who are not currently depressed is current sleep disturbance
   e. In older people, there is usually only one significant cause of insomnia

Use the following list to answer questions 2 through 4.

   a. Decreased amounts of stage 3 and 4 sleep
   b. Significant medical morbidity if untreated
   c. Daytime sleepiness usually present and may be present early in the course of the illness
   d. Associated with sundowning
   e. Decreased rapid eye movement (REM) latency
   f. Paradoxical daytime alertness

2. Which of the features are most often associated with dementia?

   a. Answers a and e
   b. Answers a, b, and c
   c. Answers a and d
   d. Answers a, b, c, d

e. Answer f
f. None
g. All are true

3. Which of the features are most often associated with depression?

   a. Answers a and e
   b. Answers a, b, and c
   c. Answers a and d
   d. Answers a, b, c, d
   e. Answer f
   f. None
   g. All are true

4. Which of the features are most often associated with sleep apnea?

   a. Answers a and e
   b. Answers a, b, and c
   c. Answers a and d
   d. Answers a, b, c, d
   e. Answer f
   f. None
   g. All are true

5. All of the following statements are false *except*

   a. Caregivers rarely report that nocturnal difficulties played an important role in their decision to institutionalize their elderly relative
   b. In most patients who are placed in a nursing home, the first sign of sleep disorder occurs after placement
   c. The nursing home environment is usually conducive to good sleep
   d. Nursing practices related to incontinence are particularly helpful
   e. On average, nursing home residents only get 40 minutes of sleep for every hour spent in bed

6. All of the following are true *except*

   a. Transient, situational insomnia may respond to sedatives
   b. An elderly person who has trouble with maintaining sleep should try a small amount of alcohol before bed
   c. Sedative/hypnotics cause falls both at night and during the day
   d. Sedative/hypnotic use in elderly patients may cause cognitive problems, performance problems, and irritability
   e. A trial of improved sleep hygiene is often the best initial approach

Chapter 27
Sexuality and Aging

Choose the best response to the following questions:

1. Mr. S is a 76-year-old man with a history of coronary artery disease and hypertension, for which he is currently taking atenolol, isosorbide dinitrate, and verapamil. He visits his doctor seeking treatment for erectile dysfunction. He reports no previous history of sexual dysfunction prior to the last 6 months. He denies that he is experiencing any marital discord. What would be the most appropriate treatment for his sexual dysfunction?

   a. Sildenafil
   b. Sex therapy
   c. Penile prosthesis
   d. Penile injection therapy

2. Mr. R is a 70-year-old man complaining of delayed orgasm and erectile dysfunction. Which of the following medications is a likely cause?

   a. Sildenafil
   b. Papaverine
   c. Imipramine
   d. Bupropion
   e. Buspirone

3. A 90-year-old man who is a resident at a nursing home was described by nurses as "sexually aggressive" because he grabbed at a nurse's chest and appeared to have a lewd facial expression. What would be the most appropriate initial step to address the situation?

   a. Treat with estrogen to decrease sexual aggression
   b. Treat with 0.5 mg risperidone qd to reduce agitated, aggressive behaviors
   c. Interview staff to determine whether behavior actually represented sexual aggression
   d. Develop a behavioral plan to prevent further episodes of sexual aggression
   e. Treat with 10 mg fluoxetine to reduce libido

4. Mr. and Mrs. P live together in a nursing home. Mr. P suffers from Parkinson disease and mild cognitive impairment; Mrs. P suffers from

Alzheimer's disease and has a history of depression. A nursing aide walked in on the couple engaged in sexual activity. She was upset by seeing this and reported it to the charge nurse, who then brought up the issue with the couple's physician. How should staff respond to the situation?

a. Contact the children of the couple to discuss the situation
b. Move the couple into separate rooms
c. Nothing; leave them alone
d. Maintain privacy for the couple and consider having the social worker or physician initiate a discussion with them regarding their sexual needs
e. Discipline the nursing aid for invading their privacy

5. Normal age-associated changes in male sexual functioning include

a. Erectile dysfunction and anorgasmia
b. Decreased libido and decreased refractory period
c. Decreased erectile durability and increased refractory period
d. Increased libido and increased duration of plateau stage
e. Decline in sexual pleasure associated with reduced penile sensitivity

6. Which of the following statements best characterizes sexuality in late life?

a. Predictors of sexual activity include physical health and partner availability
b. The rates of sexual intercourse decrease equally for married and single individuals
c. Sex therapy is usually unsuccessful in late life
d. A major problem is the lack of available partners for men

7. Surveys of sexual activity in late life have indicated that

a. Rates of sexual activity increase from ages 65 to 75 years, but taper off thereafter
b. In general, men are more sexually active than women in late life
c. Despite high levels of sexual activity, most individuals are not fully satisfied with their sexual performance
d. Compared to younger individuals, older cohorts are equally approving of sex between unmarried partners

8. Mr. F is a 78-year-old man with a history of chronic obstructive pulmonary disease, coronary artery disease, diabetes mellitus, and morbid obesity. He wants to continue a sexual relationship with his wife but

describes sex as physically difficult and exhausting. What would be the most appropriate suggestions to improve his situation?

a. Attempt sexual foreplay only and cease sexual intercourse
b. Focus on foreplay and choose a more comfortable sexual position
c. Start taking sildenafil to increase erectile strength and endurance
d. Start a rigorous exercise program to build up endurance and strength

IV Treatment

Chapter 28
The Practice of Evidence-Based Geriatric Psychiatry

Choose the best response to the following questions:

1. A primary characteristic that distinguishes evidence-based medicine from traditional medical paradigms is the use of
   a. Local opinion on preferred practice
   b. A hierarchy of evidence to aid decision making
   c. Internal clinical skills, judgment, and experience
   d. Clinical wisdom and opinion of experts

2. The use of evidence-based practices specific to older adults is important because
   a. Cognitive changes of aging can affect response to psychotherapy
   b. There is substantial variation in competence and practice
   c. Changes associated with aging can alter pharmacological response
   d. Older adults are generally more susceptible to medication side effects
   e. All of the above

3. Meta-analyses find support for the effectiveness of the following treatment(s) of cognitive impairment in dementia of the Alzheimer type
   a. Atypical antipsychotics
   b. Cholinesterase inhibitors
   c. Cognitive remediation therapy
   d. Estrogen

4. Based on meta-analyses and evidence-based reviews of the literature, the following show comparable efficacy and tolerability in the treatment of older adults with major depression *except*
   a. Tricyclic antidepressants (TCAs)
   b. Non-selective serotonin reuptake inhibitor norepinephrine reuptake inhibitors (NSSRIs)
   c. Benzodiazepines
   d. Selective serotonin reuptake inhibitors (SSRIs)

5. Based on meta-analyses and evidence-based reviews the use of cognitive-behavioral therapy (CBT) has empirical support for individuals with all of the following *except*

   a. Depression
   b. Alcohol abuse
   c. Anxiety
   d. Schizophrenia

6. Which of the following has empirical support from multiple studies as an effective geriatric mental health service?

   a. Geropsychiatric inpatient units
   b. Community-based, multidisciplinary, geriatric mental health treatment teams
   c. Geriatric psychiatry consultation services to nursing homes
   d. Hospital-based geriatric psychiatry consultation-liaison services

7. Meta-analytic procedures can be negatively affected by

   a. Differences in the duration of studies
   b. Ignoring important differences between studies
   c. Lack of interchangeable instruments
   d. Excluding informative studies
   e. All of the above

8. For the busy, practicing geriatric clinician, which source provides the most objective summarized information on empirically tested, effective interventions?

   a. Clinical guidelines from professional societies
   b. Treatment algorithms from expert consensus panels
   c. Prefiltered databases (e.g., Cochrane Data Base, Best Evidence, Evidence-Based Mental Health)
   d. MEDLINE or PubMed

9. In the hierarchy of evidence, the highest level of evidence is

   a. Case reports
   b. A single well-designed RCT
   c. A meta-analysis or evidence-based systematic review
   d. Quasi-experimental designed studies
   e. Pre–post or matched case–control studies

10. In general, treatment guidelines

    a. Are unlikely to be biased when produced by professional societies
    b. Have been shown to be effective in changing clinical practice

    c. Are an objective and reliable summary of the evidence base

    d. Should be critically evaluated for sources of supporting evidence

11. All of the following have been associated with interactions between physicians and representatives from the pharmaceutical industry *except*

    a. Requests to add medications to formularies

    b. Decreased prescribing of generic drugs

    c. Higher prescribing costs

    d. Underpublication of unfavorable research findings

    e. Greater use of an evidence-based approach to clinical decision making

12. Which of the following are accurate statements with respect to potential conflicts of interest associated with published clinical guidelines?

    a. Most of the time, authors of guidelines report existing or potential conflicts of interest

    b. More than 4/5 authors of clinical guidelines have a financial relationship with at least one pharmaceutical manufacturer

    c. Published guidelines frequently list potential conflicts of interest with pharmaceutical manufacturers by the authors or participating experts

    d. Users of published guidelines can generally assume that major conflicts of interest are uniformly disclosed

Chapter 29
Electroconvulsive Therapy

Choose the best response to the following questions:

1. A 68-year-old man with a history of recurrent psychotic depression is referred for electroconvulsive therapy (ECT) after failing four adequate medication trials, including a tricyclic antidepressant and antipsychotic combination. Which of the following statements is true regarding his likelihood of response to ECT?

    a. His age makes him less likely to respond than a younger patient

    b. The presence of psychosis indicates a severe illness that is less likely to respond

    c. Medication resistance may decrease the likelihood of ECT response

    d. Multiple prior depressive episodes increase the likelihood of ECT response

    e. He has greater than a 90% chance of complete response to ECT regardless of prior treatment history

2. A 68-year-old man with a history of recurrent psychotic depression is referred for ECT after failing four adequate medication trials, including a tricyclic antidepressant and antipsychotic combination. Which of the following factors is associated with a lower risk of relapse following ECT?

    a. Bilateral electrode placement

    b. Final Hamilton Depression Rating Scale (HAM-D) scores less than 7

    c. Lack of postictal confusion

    d. Lowered seizure threshold over the course of treatment

    e. Seizure durations of at least 60 seconds

3. A 70-year-old man with a history of recurrent depression shows a rapid response to ECT, with complete remission of depressive symptoms following his sixth treatment. The best next step would be

    a. Immediately initiate continuation/maintenance treatment (pharmacotherapy and/or ECT)

    b. Stop ECT because such a rapid improvement indicates a likely placebo response

    c. Stop ECT only if he has reached his lifetime maximum of 100 treatments

    d. Continue the ECT series for a total of at least eight treatments because this is the average number of treatments needed for full response

    e. Continue ECT until he shows evidence of cognitive impairment

4. A 67-year-old man with depression is taking propranolol for hypertension and ischemic heart disease. Stimulus dosage titration is performed at the first ECT treatment to estimate initial seizure threshold. The first stimulus results in a missed seizure, and within seconds the patient develops sinus bradycardia with a heart rate of 20 beats per minute. Which of the following is the most likely explanation for this arrhythmia?

    a. Relative increased activity of the sympathetic and parasympathetic nervous systems

    b. Relative increased activity of the sympathetic nervous system

    c. Relative increased activity of the parasympathetic nervous system

    d. Relative increased activity of the sympathetic nervous system and decreased activity of the parasympathetic nervous system

    e. Relative decreased activity of the sympathetic and parasympathetic nervous systems

5. With increasing patient age, ECT seizure threshold can be expected to

    a. Decrease, with associated longer seizure duration
    b. Decrease, with associated shorter seizure duration
    c. Increase, with associated longer seizure duration
    d. Increase, with associated shorter seizure duration
    e. Show no change

6. An 80-year-old man, 2 months after coronary artery bypass surgery with significantly impaired left ventricular function and severe major depression with psychotic features, is referred for ECT. On further cardiac testing, ejection fraction is 15%. To decrease cardiac risk, which of the following anesthetic medications might be considered?

    a. Droperidol
    b. Fentanyl
    c. Lidocaine
    d. Etomidate
    e. Nitrous oxide

7. In combining maintenance lithium therapy with outpatient maintenance ECT

    a. Lasix should be given as pretreatment to clear the lithium
    b. Patients should receive an additional 300 to 600 mg of lithium on the day of ECT to prevent drug washout
    c. Lithium must be tapered off (to a level of 0 Meq) before each ECT
    d. Lithium should be held for at least 24 hours before each ECT
    e. Intravenous fluids should be minimized to prevent causing a subtherapeutic lithium level

8. Which of the following statements generally characterizes right unilateral ECT compared to bilateral ECT?

    a. Decreased efficacy in all patients
    b. Increased seizure threshold
    c. Decreased cognitive impairment
    d. Increased prolactin release
    e. Increased ECT course length in all patients

9. A computerized tomographic (CT) scan of the brain prior to ECT

   a. Is indicated as part of the routine work-up
   b. Should not be obtained because magnetic resonance imaging (MRI) scans are more sensitive
   c. Should be obtained every 6 months during maintenance ECT
   d. Should be performed if other data suggest the presence of a central nervous system (CNS) abnormality
   e. Is never indicated because electroencephalograms (EEGs) are cheaper and equally useful

10. Which nonpsychiatric conditions listed below may benefit from a course of ECT?

   a. Pheochromocytoma
   b. Hyperthyroidism
   c. Parkinson disease
   d. Asthma
   e. Hypertension

Chapter 30
Psychopharmacology

Choose the best response to the following questions:

1. Which of the following physiological changes associated with aging influences the pharmacodynamic responses to psychiatric medications?

   a. Decreased renal plasma flow
   b. Decreased hepatic blood flow
   c. Decreased plasma albumin
   d. Decreased striatal dopamine neurons
   e. Decreased activity of the P450 2D6 isoenzyme system

2. Which side effect of selective serotonin reuptake inhibitors (SSRIs) is thought to occur more frequently in older patients than young adults?

   a. Diarrhea
   b. Syndrome of inappropriate antidiuretic hormone secretion (SIADH)
   c. Insomnia
   d. Diminished memory
   e. Akathisia

3. Based on randomized, controlled studies, which of the following statements about the treatment of psychiatric symptoms associated with dementia of the Alzheimer type with atypical antipsychotic medications is correct?

   a. Efficacy for psychosis is greater than for behavioral symptoms
   b. The minimum efficacious dose of risperidone is generally 0.5 mg/ day
   c. The minimum efficacious dose of olanzapine is 5 mg/day
   d. Efficacious doses are also associated with a significantly greater incidence of worsening of cognition than occurs in association with placebo
   e. Are more efficacious than conventional antipsychotic medications

4. Which of the following medications will most likely cause increased alprazolam levels?

   a. Nefazodone
   b. Fluoxetine
   c. Nortriptyline
   d. Buproprion
   e. Venlafaxine

5. Which of the following factors confounds treatment studies of the depression associated with Alzheimer disease?

   a. High placebo response rates
   b. High rates of treatment resistance
   c. High incidence of somatic side effects
   d. Low prevalence of syndrome
   e. Worsening of cognition during antidepressant treatment

6. The maxim to "start low and go slow" when treating geriatric patients with psychotropic medication is based on

   a. Evidence that older patients require lower doses to respond
   b. Evidence that older patients require a longer time to respond
   c. The increased incidence of idiopathic sensitivity to side effects among older patients
   d. The assumption that older patients will tolerate and adhere to medications better if doses are increased gradually
   e. The assumption that identifying side effects early in treatment will decrease the risk of aging-related serious adverse drug reactions

7. Which of the following is the strongest risk factor for the development of torsades de pointes (TdP)?

a. PR interval greater than 0.2
b. History of myocardial infarction
c. QTc interval above 450 ms
d. History of hypertension
e. Electrocardiographic evidence of left ventricular hypertrophy

8. Elevation of lithium levels is most likely to occur in association with daily treatment with which of the following medications?

a. Furosemide
b. Theophylline
c. Nifedipine
d. Potassium hydrochloride
e. Ibuprofen

For questions 9–13, match each of the P450 enzymes listed with the atypical antipsychotic medication for which it is the primary metabolic pathway. An answer may be used once, more than once, or not at all.

9. 1A2   a. Olanzapine
10. 2D6   b. Risperidone
11. 3A4   c. Ziprasidone
12. 2C9   d. Quetiapine
13. 2C19   e. Clozapine

14. Which statement regarding venlafaxine-associated hypertension is true?

a. Occurs despite concomitant treatment with antihypertensives
b. Increased risk occurs at doses of greater than 200 mg/day
c. Risk is greatest among patients with hypertension preceding venlafaxine
d. Primarily involves elevation of diastolic blood pressure
e. Occurs more commonly with increased age

15. Which of the following characterizes secondary amine tricyclic antidepressants (TCAs) as contrasted with tertiary amine TCAs?

a. Greater orthostatic hypotensive effects
b. Less anticholinergic effect
c. Higher plasma concentrations per milligram dose
d. Less efficacy in elderly patients
e. Greater efficacy for comorbid anxiety symptoms

16. Which of the following side effects of benzodiazepine use is greater in elderly patients than in young adults?

    a. Diminished recent memory
    b. Withdrawal seizures
    c. Psychological dependence
    d. Displacement of other medications from α-acid glycoprotein
    e. Bleeding caused by interactions with warfarin

17. Which of the following anticholinergic side effects is most likely to lead to discontinuation of a psychiatric medication in older patients?

    a. Constipation
    b. Bradycardia
    c. Delirium
    d. Decreased working memory
    e. Elevated intraocular pressure

18. Which of the following is the most practical method to enhance adherence to antidepressant treatment of elderly patients?

    a. Dividing the dose to be taken with meals
    b. Involving a visiting nurse service
    c. Simplifying the dosage to once daily
    d. Explaining the need not to miss doses
    e. Ensuring that the patient's primary care physician is aware of the rationale

19. The least frequent consequence of neuroleptic treatment in elderly patients is

    a. Dystonia
    b. Pseudoparkinsonism
    c. Tardive dyskinesia
    d. Akathisia
    e. Hip fracture

20. Regarding management of elderly patients with manic states, which of the following statements is true?

    a. Sodium valproate increases the hepatic metabolism of concomitant psychotropic agents
    b. Plasma lithium levels should be targeted routinely at less than 0.4 mEq/L
    c. Divalproex sodium should be dosed to achieve target levels that are 50% lower than those used to treat young adults

    d. Dosage should be reduced gradually following remission of symptoms

    e. Continuation pharmacotherapy should be provided routinely

21. What is the most common side effect associated with cholinesterase inhibitors?

    a. Nausea

    b. Insomnia

    c. Dizziness

    d. Muscle cramps

    e. Elevated transaminase levels

22. Which of the following best describes the role of memantine in the treatment of Alzheimer's disease?

    a. Memantine is most effective in slowing the rate of decline of Alzheimer's disease in mildly impaired patients

    b. Memantine is contraindicated in patients who are receiving donepezil

    c. The action of memantine is related to cholinesterase inhibition

    d. Among patients with severe impairment, improvement is greater than that of placebo on global measures of functioning, activities of daily living, and cognition

    e. Memantine is thought to act by stimulating nerve growth factor

23. Based on placebo-controlled studies, which of the following statements about the efficacy of maintenance treatment for late-life depression is correct?

    a. Patients between ages 60 and 70 years have a greater recurrence rate than those older than 70 years of age

    b. Long-term SSRI treatment is more efficacious than maintenance nortriptyline

    c. Monthly maintenance psychotherapy does not affect recurrence rates

    d. Impaired memory is associated with a higher likelihood of recurrence

    e. Impaired executive functioning is associated with an increased risk of recurrence

Chapter 31
Individual Psychotherapy

Choose the best response to the following questions:

1. An 83-year-old woman of Chinese descent who emigrated to New York in 1963 presents to her general practitioner with symptoms of grief following the death of her husband of 52 years. It is most likely that this patient

   a. Prefers to see a mental health professional
   b. Will be referred by her general practitioner for psychotherapeutic treatment
   c. Is too old to benefit from insight-oriented therapy
   d. Will preferentially respond to cognitive-behavioral therapy (CBT)
   e. Will at first complain of physical problems

2. An 81-year-old woman presents with a 6-month history of depressed mood, sleeplessness, new-onset anxiety, and suicidal ideation. She also reports diurnal variation of mood, apparently unrealistic ruminations about being abandoned by her children, and a history of unstable and chaotic interpersonal relationships through her adult life. Her family doctor diagnosed depressive disorder and referred her to a psychiatrist. Based on the best evidence available on therapeutic efficacy for this condition, the most effective recommendation would be

   a. CBT alone
   b. Selective serotonin reuptake inhibitor (SSRI) medication with intermittent monitoring follow-up
   c. SSRI medication with psychotherapy
   d. Interpersonal therapy (IPT) alone

3. A 68-year-old woman is referred to a therapy clinic by her family doctor; at the clinic, she sees a psychiatric resident. She comes to therapy about 6 months after the sudden, unexpected death of her husband. Her family doctor had treated her for many years, during which time she spoke to him frequently about the angry conflicts she had with her husband and her mixed feelings for him. The physician correctly judged that she was at higher risk for complicated grief because of her agitation, anxiety, and failure to return to her usual activities 6 months following the death of her husband, together with her history of trauma and loss in her childhood. She had always relied on her husband to look after the problems of their home and rarely had taken the lead in

solving problems. This pattern of deferring to others was present in all her relationships. During long-term therapy, her psychiatrist notes that their relationship is characterized by behaviors that he found annoying and difficult, such as calling between sessions and expressions of clinging and obvious distress when each session ended. The most accurate way for him to understand his patient's behavior is that

a. It is most likely an enactment of a realistic reaction to the therapist's failure to provide the patient with appropriate support
b. It is most likely an enactment of feelings deriving from childhood abandonment by her parents and now her husband
c. It is most likely an enactment of a fear that she will be institutionalized because she cannot look after herself
d. It is most likely an enactment of a disguised form of anger caused by her belief that the therapist is too young to understand her problems.

4. Psychotherapy with patients from a culture different from that of the therapist can be a challenging process calling on the therapist to use a variety of skills and techniques. Recommended therapeutic approaches in these cases include

a. Actively encouraging the patient to integrate with the dominant culture
b. Using background information from seminars on cross-cultural therapy to provide the main basis for understanding the patient's struggles
c. Beginning a brief, structured form of psychotherapy early on, after educating the patient about the biological and social basis of their problem
d. Exploring the patient's relationship to the dominant culture, including racism

5. Cognitively impaired elders in institutions are often depressed, anxious, lonely, unconnected, and abandoned. In these situations,

a. Reminiscence therapy generally provokes increased feelings of loss
b. Psychodynamic understanding adds little to the management of problems
c. Touch and attending to nonverbal cues are important to treatment
d. The patient is calmed and reassured by the structure of cognitive mental status questions at the beginning of each meeting with the therapist

Chapter 32
Group Therapy

Choose the best response to the following questions:

1. In considering the recommendation of group psychotherapy for an 82-year-old man under treatment for a major depressive episode, the most important factor to consider regarding group composition is

   a. Age of other members
   b. Level of physical functioning
   c. Marital status
   d. Level of cognitive functioning
   e. Gender

2. Cognitive-behavioral group approaches with elderly patients generally do not emphasize

   a. Role playing
   b. Relaxation exercises
   c. Log book and homework assignments
   d. Psychoeducation
   e. Interpretation of conflict

3. In developing a group psychotherapeutic approach that is aimed at improving cognitive and behavioral functioning in patients who suffer from cognitive impairment, it is essential to

   a. Provide frequent opportunities for unstructured social interaction
   b. Discourage reminiscing in the group
   c. Examine group process and the group dynamics within the group
   d. Coordinate a compatible, ongoing reality orientation approach on the ward

4. Therapist interventions that make use of the concept of "prizing" is frequently associated with

   a. Increasing undue dependence in patients
   b. Enhancing patient self-concept
   c. Therapist countertransference
   d. Impeding group cohesion
   e. Increased idealization of the therapist

5. Psychosocial interventions for burdened caregivers, including the provision of structured group experiences have demonstrated

   a. No improvement in measures of caregiver burden despite high subjective valuation of the group experience
   b. Some improvement in measures of caregiver burden and a 1-year reduction in rates of institutionalization of the identified patient of up to 50%
   c. Little impact on rates of institutionalization
   d. Improved psychosocial functioning in the identified care receiver

6. Two men, both in their late 70s and bereaved, participating in a partial hospitalization program for depression are noted to be spending a great deal of time together outside the treatment groups. Concern is raised by a staff member that a subgrouping phenomenon is taking place that could have a deleterious impact on the rest of the patients in group therapy. A first consideration to employ in response to this concern is

   a. Restrict extragroup contact
   b. Do not address it because it is benign
   c. Interpret other group members' envy of the closeness achieved by these two men
   d. Interpret it as it reflects a self-object transference
   e. Explore in the group the meaning and experience of this special relatedness

7. In establishing a group therapy program within an institutional setting, an often-neglected but important consideration within the system in which treatment is provided relates to

   a. The therapist-to-patient relationship
   b. The patient-to-patient relationship
   c. The relationship between the patient and group
   d. The relationship between the cotherapists
   e. The relationship between the group and the institution

8. Effects of pregroup preparation for patients entering group therapy include

   a. Reducing patient anxiety
   b. Increasing patient hopefulness
   c. Facilitating the therapeutic alliance
   d. Improving patient adherence to the group task
   e. All of the above

Chapter 33
Family Issues in Mental Disorders of Late Life

Choose the best response to the following questions:

1. Which of the following *less consistently* influences whether an elderly person is likely to live with his or her family?

   a. Race and ethnicity
   b. Sex
   c. Age
   d. Chronic health conditions

2. Which groups of relatives are most likely to be involved in caring for a demented, elderly person?

   a. Siblings
   b. Aunts and uncles
   c. Sons and daughters-in-law
   d. Spouse and daughters

3. Family caregiving for an elderly chronically mentally ill patient can produce serious subjective burden on caregivers, such as medical (e.g., immune function disturbance) and psychosocial morbidity (e.g., depression) and deterioration in family relations and work-related performance. All of these factors have been shown to predict subjective burden except

   a. Presence of behavioral disturbances
   b. Lack of availability of informal social support
   c. Cognitive or functional status of the patient
   d. Cultural and ethnic background

4. When confronted with family units that hold opposing points of view, the clinician should

   a. Ally him- or herself with the main caregiver to ensure the patient gets appropriate care
   b. Remain neutral and facilitate the family in resolving their issues
   c. Take a clear position on the issues and encourage the family to unite and debate the conflict with the clinician
   d. Develop a strong alliance with the most influential member of the family to ensure a therapeutic decision

5. In-home respite care has been shown in one study to have

   a. Little effect on "upset" in caregiver spouses
   b. Little effect on self-efficacy of caregivers managing difficult behaviors
   c. Little effect on self-efficacy in managing functional dependency
   d. All of the above
   e. None of the above

Chapter 34
Psychiatric Aspects of Long-Term Care

Choose the best response to the following questions:

1. Epidemiological studies reveal that the prevalence of psychiatric disorders in nursing homes is

   a. Less than 50%
   b. Between 50% and 60%
   c. Between 65% and 75%
   d. Greater than 80%

2. Most psychiatric consultations requested in the nursing home are for evaluation and treatment of

   a. Depression
   b. Psychosis
   c. Behavioral disturbances
   d. Anxiety
   e. Insomnia

3. Evidence from research conducted in nursing home residents indicates that depression in this setting is associated with

   a. Poor nutrition
   b. Increased pain complaints
   c. Disability
   d. Increased mortality
   e. All of the above

4. Among the many factors that prompted Congress to pass the Nursing Home Reform Act as part of the Omnibus Budget Reconciliation Act in 1987 was pressure from various consumer groups. The greatest concern of patient advocacy groups was

    a. Inadequate recognition and undertreatment of depression
    b. Inappropriate admission of acutely psychotic patients to nursing homes
    c. Attempts to shift the cost of nursing home care from the states to the federal government
    d. Inappropriate use of physical and chemical restraints

5. Federal guidelines permit the use of physical restraints in nursing homes if

    a. The patient has severe motor restlessness from any cause
    b. There is documentation that the use of restraints is necessary to enhance body positioning
    c. The patient has a history of falls when trying to get out of bed
    d. The nursing home is not staffed to provide 1:1 supervision for an agitated patient

6. After implementation of federal regulations in the early 1990s,

    a. The use of antipsychotic medications declined, then plateaued
    b. The use of antidepressant drugs increased
    c. Anxiolytic prescriptions increased to replace antipsychotic agents
    d. There was no change in psychotropic prescribing until 1995, when the use of atypical antipsychotics increased dramatically

7. Randomized, placebo-controlled trials of which of the following drugs have demonstrated efficacy for treatment of psychosis specifically in nursing home patients with dementia?

    a. Clozapine and olanzapine
    b. Risperidone and olanzapine
    c. Risperidone and quetiapine
    d. Carbamazepine and divalproex

8. Which of the following statements is true regarding serotonin reuptake inhibitors (SRIs) in nursing home patients?

    a. A large-scale, randomized, controlled nursing home trial demonstrated efficacy for treatment of depression
    b. They are equally effective in depressed patients with dementia and those who are cognitively intact

    c. They are consistently tolerated without significant adverse effects, even in the oldest, most frail residents

    d. They are associated with a nearly two-fold increase in risk of falls in nursing home residents

9. Low agitation levels on special care units (SCUs) in nursing homes are correlated with

    a. Low rate of physical restraint use
    b. Greater functional dependency among residents
    c. A high proportion of residents who are out of bed during the day
    d. High comorbid illness burden among residents
    e. Large unit size

Chapter 35
Psychogeriatric Programs: Inpatient Hospital Units and Partial Hospital Programs

Choose the best response to the following questions:

1. The characteristics of patients admitted to geriatric psychiatry inpatient units have changed over the past 10 years. Which of the following characteristics of hospitalized patients have become more common?

    a. They are older
    b. They are more likely to be demented
    c. They are more likely to have psychotic symptoms
    d. They are more likely to have severe medical problems
    e. All of the above

2. An 85-year-old woman with a progressive dementia syndrome is admitted to a geriatric psychiatry inpatient unit because of combativeness. Which of the following factors will determine how long she is hospitalized?

    a. Her comorbid medical problems
    b. Her personal financial resources
    c. Her caregiver's level of stress
    d. Her compliance with medications
    e. All of the above.

3. Patients admitted to a geriatric psychiatry unit for the treatment of major depression vary in their long-term affective outcomes. Which admission characteristic best predicts continued depressive symptoms after discharge?

   a. Being introverted
   b. Being unable to walk
   c. Having a urinary catheter
   d. Having pain complaints
   e. Being widowed

4. A substantial proportion of older patients admitted to geriatric psychiatry inpatient units have a personality disorder (PD). The most frequently diagnosed PD among older psychiatrically hospitalized patients is

   a. Dependent
   b. Narcissistic
   c. Hysterical
   d. Borderline
   e. Schizoid

5. Among older patients with major depression admitted to a geriatric psychiatry inpatient unit, patients with comorbid PDs are more likely to have which of the following characteristics compared with patients without PDs?

   a. Later age of onset of depression
   b. Comorbid psychotic symptoms
   c. History of mania
   d. Previous suicide attempts
   e. Longer length of stay

Chapter 36
Geriatric Consultation-Liaison Psychiatry

Choose the best response to the following questions:

1. The evaluation of competency in a medical setting must

   a. Be completed at the time of admission
   b. Determine if a patient is legally competent to make all decisions

    c. Include evaluation of the patient's financial status

    d. Assess a patient's ability to understand the choices and the consequences of a decision.

2. Psychiatric consultation for geriatric inpatients requires special geriatric skills because

    a. About 40% of elderly inpatients have some psychiatric disorder

    b. Elderly patients are more likely to have drug interactions than younger patients

    c. Elderly patients with medical illness are at high risk for suicide

    d. All of the above

3. Consultation always includes

    a. Examining the patient

    b. Discussing findings with family

    c. Teaching the nursing staff

    d. Comprehensive evaluation of the patient

4. When an elderly patient suddenly becomes delirious in a medical setting, the first thing that should be done is

    a. A complete medical and pharmacological assessment

    b. Give haloperidol to reduce the agitation

    c. Leave the lights on to prevent "sundowning"

    d. Have the family bring in familiar objects from home

5. Which of the following are risk factors for persistent depression following hospital discharge?

    a. History of dysthymia or depression

    b. Stressful life events in the year prior to the index admission

    c. Greater number of active medical diagnoses

    d. Patient's perception of severity of depression

    e. All of the above

    f. None of the above

Chapter 37
Integrated Community Services

Choose the best response to the following questions:

1. Which of the following would be an appropriate service for an older person with a moderate level of functional impairment?

   a. Foster grandparent program
   b. Skilled nursing facility
   c. Assisted living
   d. Retired Seniors Volunteer Program

2. Congregate meal programs are provided under which governmental program?

   a. Title XVIII of the Social Security Act
   b. Title V of the Older American Act
   c. Title III of the Older American Act
   d. Title XIX of the Social Security Act

3. Area agencies on aging

   a. Primarily provide information and referral
   b. Generally provide direct services
   c. Were created under Title V of the OAA
   d. All of the above

4. The three case management approaches that are commonly used to secure and coordinate services are

   a. Social, benefits, and educational models
   b. Brokering, service management, and managed-care models
   c. Quality-of-life, utilization, and screening models
   d. Mobility, seedling, and developmental models

5. In most states, adult protective services (APS) serve persons who may have all the following problems *except*

   a. Incapable of performing functions necessary to meet basic physical requirements
   b. Incapable of managing finances
   c. Exhibiting behavior that brings them into conflict with society
   d. Neglect and abuse occurring in nursing homes

6. All of the following governmental programs provide specifically for in-home services *except*

    a. Medicaid
    b. Title III of the OAA
    c. Social Services Block Grant
    d. Supplemental Security Income

7. Of the various respite programs, which of the following has been found to most consistently achieve its goals for relieving the distress and improving the mood of caregivers?

    a. In-home services
    b. Adult day programs
    c. Overnight respite
    d. Adult homes

8. Which of the following is true about mental health services for older adults?

    a. The 1981 federal block grant mandated that treatment of elderly persons be a required psychiatric service for mental health centers
    b. Outreach services have not been very effective in addressing mental health needs of older persons
    c. The existence of a specialized outpatient unit for older adults does not seem to enhance utilization of services
    d. The two basic types of vocational rehabilitation programs are sheltered employment and transitional employment

9. All of the following are true about senior centers *except*

    a. About one third of seniors attend senior centers
    b. Race is not associated with participation
    c. Centers are used by "less-advantaged" seniors
    d. Title III of the OAA provides support for centers

10. Which of the following is true about housing for older adults?

    a. About one fifth of older adults live in planned housing (i.e., housing specifically for the aging)
    b. Funding levels for senior housing under Section 202 has remained stable over the past 20 years
    c. Assisted living is designed to accommodate frail elderly
    d. Congregate housing typically does not provide any health services or other support services

11. Which is true about Natural Occurring Retirement Communities (NORCs)?

    a. They include any building or neighborhood where more than one third of residents are over age 60 years
    b. About two fifths of elderly persons live in NORCs
    c. NORCs typically include social and health supports
    d. They are the most common form of retirement community in the United States

V Medical-Legal, Ethical, and Financial Issues

Chapter 38
Legal and Ethical Issues

Choose the best response to the following questions:

1. Which of the following statements about incompetency is not correct?

   a. It can be used interchangeably with "impaired decisional capacity"
   b. It requires evaluation of functional abilities
   c. It may be partial and apply only to specific areas of functioning
   d. It can indicate that the patient is at risk for harm

2. Which of the following is not true regarding decisional capacity?

   a. It can fluctuate
   b. It can be evaluated using the MacArthur Competence Assessment Tool (MacCAT)
   c. It has clearly defined standards depending on the jurisdiction
   d. It can be enhanced by therapeutic interventions

3. Proxy decision making for decisionally incapacitated persons

   a. Only can be performed after a court finding of incompetence
   b. Has been found to correlate inadequately with decisions the impaired person would make for himself
   c. Should follow the "best interests" standard
   d. Serves as an adequate safeguard for research participation

4. The Patient Self Determination Act (PSDA) requires that

   a. A standard advance directive format be used nationally
   b. The facility to which a person is being admitted is responsible to inform the person about its policy concerning which directives it will and will not honor
   c. The primary care doctors familiarize patients with advance directives in office and nursing home settings
   d. Incompetent patients have guardians assigned

5. Disclosure of the diagnosis of probable Alzheimer's disease (AD)

    a. Enables advance directives regarding future research participation to be formulated

    b. Is recommended by the Alzheimer's Disease and Related Disorders Association (ADRDA)

    c. Can both enhance and disrupt family dynamics

    d. All of the above

6. The following is true regarding the guardianship process:

    a. It is often expensive and time consuming

    b. It is required before any significant surgical procedure is performed on an incapacitated person

    c. It ensures that the ward will not be subject to abuse

    d. It can be arranged by psychiatrists working in conjunction with attorneys

7. Which of the following statements is not true regarding research with older subjects?

    a. It usually does not differ from research with younger subjects

    b. It requires special safeguards for cognitively impaired subjects

    c. When it involves nursing home residents, it is best conducted by nursing home staff familiar to them

    d. Incapacitated patients who refuse should not be included even if their proxy decision makers have given permission

8. Which of the following is *not true* of older drivers?

    a. They often compensate for changes by reducing mileage and refraining from night driving

    b. Compared with other seniors, drivers with mild AD generally do not yet show declines in their driving skills

    c. They experience significantly more crashes, more severe injuries, and more fatalities after age 65 years

    d. They often react with profound feelings of loss if driving privileges are revoked

Chapter 39
Financial Issues

Choose the best response to the following questions:

1. A 78-year-old man with hypertension, hypercholesterolemia, and diabetes developed severe depression after having right knee surgery 4
weeks earlier. A trial of an antidepressant was initiated, but the patient
continued to deteriorate. The patient was hospitalized on a geropsychiatric unit and improved but continued to have significant anxiety, depression, and anhedonia. The patient also needed encouragement to
dress and groom himself, go to the dining room for meals, and engage
in activities during the day rather than retreating to his bed. Nursing
expressed concerns that he was so apathetic that he would not take all
of his medications correctly. The dietician had developed an American
Diabetes Association diet for the patient to which he could adhere in
the hospital because his meals were prepared for him, but the dietician
expressed grave reservations about whether the patient would be able
to maintain a proper diet at home. The physical therapist believed that
the patient would benefit from additional physical therapy for his right
knee, but that he needed extra encouragement to participate. The patient insisted that he wanted to get well but lacked the confidence to
"make it" at home.

   Following his knee surgery, the patient had spent 20 days on a rehabilitation unit. The patient has Medicare Parts A and B and Medicare
supplemental insurance that would cover skilled nursing facility copay-
ments. Which of the discharge aftercare plan options would best serve
the patient and be covered by his insurance plans?

   a. Subacute rehabilitation
   b. Transitional care unit
   c. Discharge home with referral to the local visiting nurse association
   d. Acute rehabilitation hospitalization

2. An 81-year-old female nursing home long-term care resident with dementia, recurrent delirium, and associated behavioral difficulties has
required three geropsychiatric hospitalizations totaling 110 days in the
past year. During this time, there has been no continuous out-of-hospital period longer than 60 days. The patient has Medicare and Medicaid insurance. The patient is again admitted to a geropsychiatric unit
because she developed behavior problems that the nursing home staff
could not manage safely. Which of the following are true?

   a. Medicare will cover the patient's hospital costs indefinitely

b. Medicare and Medicaid will cover the full cost of the patient's hospitalization
c. The patient would have all her Medicare lifetime reserve days available for use in the future
d. Medicare will not cover hospital services costs beyond hospitalization day 150

3. Which of the following statements about entitlement to Medicare health benefits is correct?

a. Recent legislation ensures that the payment of full Social Security benefits and Medicare coverage will continue to begin at age 65 years for future retirees
b. Individuals who are younger than age 65 years are not be eligible for Social Security or Medicare benefits
c. Part B benefits are reimbursed only for treatments delivered in a licensed facility
d. Benefits for mental health treatment are limited to covered services
e. Medicare coverage is limited to patients who are entitled to Social Security benefits

4. Which of the following statements about reimbursement paid to providers under Medicare is correct?

a. Billing by providers who have not signed Medicare contracts is also subject to Medicare regulations
b. Participating Medicare providers are prohibited from billing Medicare recipients for copayment of covered services
c. Limiting charges for participating providers are lower than those for providers who do not participate
d. Nonparticipating providers may accept assignment for Medicare-covered services
e. Nonparticipating providers are not required to accept assignment for patients who have both Medicare and Medicaid coverage

5. Which of the following statements about reimbursement to institutions for Part A Medicare services is correct?

a. Prospective payment systems (PPSs) are customarily used to specify the Medicare limits of hospital coverage for the treatment of patients in psychiatric hospitals
b. Reimbursement for inpatient stays at psychiatric hospitals are determined by the patient's diagnosis related group (DRG)
c. Capitation rates determined under the Tax Equity and Fiscal Responsibility Act (TEFRA) limit reimbursement for the hospital stay

of individual patients to costs anticipated for the treatment of the patient's diagnosis

d. Capitation of institutional payments has been shown to improve the quality of care rendered to psychiatric patients

e. Medicare reimbursement rates for psychiatric treatments rendered to patients in freestanding psychiatric hospitals, psychiatric units in general hospitals, and general hospital scatter beds are all subject to federally mandated limitations

6. Which of the following statements about possible local variations in Part B reimbursement under Medicare is correct?

a. Federal legislation determines the details of the allowed frequency at which specific provider services may be reimbursed

b. States are required to follow federally mandated Medicare fee schedules

c. Medicare reimbursement rates to providers are always higher than those provided through coverage available to Medicaid recipients

d. Local carriers interpret federal guidelines in determining which services are allowable for reimbursement under the "medical necessity" provision of Medicare regulations

7. Which of the following statements about Medicare Part B coverage for provider services is correct?

a. The Omnibus Budget Reconciliation Acts (OBRA) refers to legislation passed to regulate provider reimbursement under Medicare

b. OBRA legislation limits the annual dollar amount of reimbursement of outpatient mental health treatment

c. Psychiatrists are prohibited from billing under the evaluation and management (E and M) codes utilized by most primary care physicians

d. Psychiatrists, psychologists, and social workers are eligible to become participating Medicare providers

e. Psychotherapy provided by psychologists and social workers in inpatient and nursing home settings is covered by Medicare

Chapter 40
Private Practice Issues

Choose the best response to the following questions:

1. The average net annual income for psychiatrists

   a. Has risen faster than the average increase for all physicians in the decade 1989–1999
   b. Was about $126,000 in 1999
   c. Is approximately in the middle for the top 20 medical specialties
   d. Has risen faster than the inflation rate for the decade 1989–1999

2. All of the following statements about psychiatrists in the United States are true *except*

   a. Over 2,500 have subspecialty certification in geriatric psychiatry
   b. Of American psychiatrists, 18% have geriatric caseloads exceeding 20% of their practices
   c. Psychiatrists with larger geriatric caseloads spend proportionately more time in their offices seeing patients than those seeing fewer geriatric patients
   d. Psychiatrists with larger geriatric caseloads average more patient visits per week and a longer average work week than those seeing fewer geriatric patients

3. Medicare billing for psychiatric services requires the exclusive use of

   a. The 908xx psychiatric services coding system
   b. The *Diagnostic and Statistical Manual of Mental Disorders, Fourth Edition* (DSM-IV; American Psychiatric Association, 1994) diagnostic coding system
   c. The *International Classification of Diseases, Ninth Revision—Clinical Modification*(ICD-9-CM; 2000) coding system
   d. The American Medical Association's evaluation and management (E and M) coding system

4. Billing for services under "incident to" provisions

   a. Is paid at 85% of the physician's fee schedule
   b. Requires a physician to be available by telephone
   c. Can be performed by nurse practitioners and physician assistants (PAs) but not psychologists or social workers
   d. Can only be provided by the physician's employees

5. Medicare

   a. Pays 62.5% of fees for psychotherapy performed during nursing home visits
   b. Was created in 1959
   c. Requires acceptance of Medicare assignment from patients who are also Medicaid recipients and those below the federal poverty level
   d. Pays only 50% of the fee for office-based consultation services even if you send a report back to the referring physician

6. Which of the following is true?

   a. Participating providers have their claims sent automatically to the patient's Medigap provider
   b. Participating providers may bill up to 115% of the Medicare fee schedule
   c. Nonparticipating providers are not required to submit Medicare insurance claims for their services
   d. Nonparticipating providers may not accept Medicare assignment because of the "limiting charge"

7. E and M service codes

   a. May be used to code initial psychiatric office visits
   b. May not be coded in combination with psychiatric diagnosis codes
   c. Are dependent on the time spent providing them
   d. Are documented according to rules that are updated annually

8. All of the following are important steps to take in setting up a geriatric practice *except*

   a. Creating a practice brochure and other written materials using large fonts
   b. Have comfortable, deep, soft chairs in your office to make your older patients feel at ease because many will be unfamiliar with psychiatric treatment and may be anxious
   c. Deciding whether to register as a participating physician with Medicare
   d. Evaluating transportation issues; stairs, ramps, and elevators; proximity to senior housing, activity centers, and to other doctors

Chapter 41
Psychiatry at the End of Life

Choose the best response to the following questions:

1. Mrs. B is an 83-year-old woman with advanced gastrointestinal cancer and extensive liver metastases who was admitted to home hospice 3 weeks ago. She is bed bound because of her illness, and the hospice medical director estimates that her survival is less than 2 weeks. She has been steadily less interested in activities such as reading and watching TV, which she found pleasurable even 2 weeks ago. She is more listless and tired, and her sleep is very poor. This morning she is tearful, agitated, and distraught and complains of vivid dreams of her late husband in which he seemed to be touching her. What should you do first?

   a. Start 5 mg methylphenidate bid
   b. Test her attention, concentration, and memory
   c. Explain to the family that these are normal symptoms that are part of the letting go process at the end of life
   d. Send her to the emergency room for further evaluation, including neuroimaging
   e. Start 1 mg lorazepam tid

2. Mr. R is a 65-year-old man with advanced lung cancer who has been in home hospice for 4 weeks. Within the last 2 days, he has been increasingly fearful, confused, agitated, and paranoid. He denies pain and is receiving only very low doses of morphine. He is still drinking fluids well and is able to take oral medications. His family caregivers are distressed by these changes but are coping well, able to get breaks from his care, and able to sleep at night. His favorite brother is expected to arrive by plane tomorrow to say his goodbyes. Which approach would you advise?

   a. Counsel the family that death is imminent and the risks and burdens of any treatment outweigh the benefits
   b. Start 25–50 mg diphenhydramine po bid/tid
   c. Start 0.5–1.0 mg clonazepam po bid/tid
   d. Start 1.0–3.0 mg haloperidol po bid/tid
   e. Start 2.5–5.0 mg olanzapine qhs

3. Mr. R is a 76-year-old widowed man with advanced colon cancer and difficulties with pain control in hospice. He is bed bound, and his internist estimates less than a month of survival. His mood has been

increasingly low for several weeks, he has lost interest in other activities, his appetite is poor, and he is hopeless and apathetic. On examination, he scores 28/30 on the Mini-Mental State Examination. He refuses some of his oral morphine because he does not like the sedation. Medications you might consider to treat him include

a. 20 mg citalopram qd
b. 1 mg lorazepam tid
c. 7.5 mg mirtazapine qhs
d. 20 mg fluoxetine qd
e. 5 mg methylphenidate at 8:00 AM and noon

4. In the United States, what percentage of people who die receive hospice service before death?

a. 7%
b. 17%
c. 29%
d. 42%

5. Which of the following is *not* associated with interest in assisted suicide or hastened death in cancer patients?

a. Hopelessness
b. Low religiousness
c. Sense of burden to others
d. Female gender

6. Based on qualitative studies of dying patients, which one of the following is among the most important goals for patients at the end of life?

a. To die quickly without warning
b. To achieve transcendence
c. To separate from loved ones
d. To obtain good pain and symptom control

7. Which one of the following is *not* covered under the Medicare hospice benefit?

a. Bereavement services for the family after the patient's death
b. Home health aide services
c. Medications for pain
d. Respite care
e. Emergency services for life-threatening medical events

8. Mr. X is a 65-year-old patient you have treated for depression with psychotherapy and 100 mg sertraline qd. He is now in hospice care, terminally ill with multiple myeloma. You have not seen him for 4 months because of his worsening medical status. His hospice nurse calls you with the following information. His pain is well controlled, his cognition is unimpaired, he continues to take the sertraline, but he is very weak from anemia and illness. He has been tearful several times when talking about missing his grandson's growing up. His appetite is poor, and his sleep impaired. He was formerly an active gardener and feels bad about not being able to help his wife in the garden. He worries that his care is a burden to her. He denies feeling depressed but has mentioned your name several times. He still takes pleasure in seeing family and has been actively working toward closure in many of his relationships. His nurse asks you what should be done. What is the best recommendation?

   a. Increase sertraline to 150 mg
   b. Start 5 mg methylphenidate bid
   c. Tell your secretary to arrange for him to come to your office within the next 2 weeks
   d. Arrange to visit the patient at home

9. Which of the following is *not* true about hospice care in the United States?

   a. The median stay in community hospice in the United States is less than 6 weeks
   b. Experts believe patients and families benefit from hospice stays of greater than 3 months
   c. Physicians are more likely to underestimate than overestimate survival of hospice patients
   d. In the United States, most hospice care is delivered in patients' residences

10. All but one of the following support the use of psychostimulants such as methylphenidate for the treatment of depressive syndromes in terminally ill cancer patients:

   a. Augmentation of opioid analgesia
   b. Diminished opioid sedation
   c. Response within 1 to 3 days
   d. Support of efficacy demonstrated in several randomized clinical trials among terminally ill patients

11. Among patients with Alzheimer's disease who have lost function in an ordinal fashion on the Functional Assessment Strategy Scale (FAST), median life expectancy of 3 months is associated with the presence of which characteristic?

    a. Patient has one word or less of speech
    b. Psychosis
    c. Hypoalbuminemia
    d. Aggressive behavior

12. Which one of the following statements regarding patients with Alzheimer's disease in hospice is true?

    a. Approximately 15% of all patients in hospice have Alzheimer's disease as the terminal diagnosis
    b. Most geriatricians do not support the concept of hospice in end-stage Alzheimer's disease
    c. Difficulties in predicting survival in Alzheimer's disease have constituted a major impediment to enrollment if Alzheimer's patients are in hospice

13. Which one of the following is true about delirium in terminally ill patients?

    a. Delirium is the third most common psychiatric disorder in dying patients
    b. With expert management, sedation is rarely required to treat delirium in terminally ill patients
    c. Delirium improves pain control
    d. Delirium improves about half the time in the final weeks of life, sometimes even without intervention

14. Which of the following is a good treatment recommendation for major depressive disorder in terminally ill cancer patients in hospice?

    a. Consider using a psychostimulant if the patient has less than 2 months to live
    b. Because of the risks of medications, give a trial of psychotherapy before a trial of antidepressants
    c. Psychotherapeutic approaches that focus on psychological understanding and developmental issues are recommended
    d. Because of the high risk of brain metastasis, neuroimaging should be a routine part of the evaluation of depression in hospice patients

ANSWERS

I The Aging Process

Chapter 1
Epidemiology of Psychiatric Disorders

1. The risk of a depressive syndrome is *increased* by
   a. Poor quality of social supports
   b. Increase in number of medications
   c. Recent bereavement
   d. Caregiver burden
   e. All of the above
   f. None of the above

The correct answer is e.

Risk of depression is increased by bereavement, medications, living alone, weak social supports, and caregiver burden. Female gender is also a risk factor, and females, because of their longer life span, are more likely than males to suffer bereavement and be caregivers to male spouses with dementia, stroke, and other causes of dependency. Bereavement and caregiving can be viewed as acute and chronic life stressors and as such add to the probability of depression. For older persons, death of a spouse is often more depressing than death of a parent or child. Medications, which obviously increase in chronic medical conditions, are also likely to induce depression both because of depressogenic pharmacological properties and because of associated pain, discomfort, limitations of activities, and life-threatening aspects. Poor quality of social supports is often a consequence of the isolating effects of caring for persons with advancing dementia, particularly if respite care is not available. The effect of social patterns on depression may work through the sense of control persons have over their lives, interaction with negative personality traits, their perception of support, and on the nature of problem-solving communication at times of crisis.

References

Jorm AF. The epidemiology of depressive states in the elderly: implications for recognition, intervention and prevention. *Soc Psychiatry Psychiatr Epidemiol.* 1995;30:53–59.
Norris FH, Murrell SA. Social support, life events, and stress as modifiers of

adjustment to bereavement by older adults. *Psychol Aging.* 1990;5:429–436.

Schoevers RA, Beekman AT, Deeg DJ, Geerlings MI, Jonker C, Van Tilburg W. Risk factors for depression in later life; results of a prospective community-based study (AMSTEL). *J Affect Disord.* 2000;59:127–137.

Ustun TB. Cross-national epidemiology of depression and gender. *J Gender-Specific Med.* 2000;3:54–58.

2. Which of the following disorders may begin in late life?

   a. Anxiety symptoms
   b. Agoraphobia
   c. Major depression
   d. Schizophrenia
   e. Only a and c
   f. All of the above

The correct answer is f.

Anxiety disorders in elders are reported to decrease (although this has been questioned); however, anxiety symptoms such as those associated with depression and dementia may emerge in late life and remain at a level frequency until an advanced age. Agoraphobia is commonly of late onset and is often precipitated by comorbid physical illness or other traumatic incidents. It is true that if risk factors are controlled, rates of major depression may fall with age. Nevertheless, the risk for all types of depression in the physically ill older patient is increased up to threefold. A substantial minority of patients with schizophrenia have an onset after 40 years of age (late-onset schizophrenia) or after 60 years of age (very late onset schizophrenia-like psychosis).

References

Fuentes K, Cox BJ. Prevalence of anxiety disorders in elderly adults: a critical analysis. *J Behav Ther Exp Psychiatry.* 1997;28:269–279.

Howard R, Rabins PV, Seeman MV, Jeste DV. Late-onset schizophrenia and very-late-onset schizophrenia-like psychosis: an international consensus. The International Late-Onset Schizophrenia Group. *Am J Psychiatry.* 2000; 157:172–178.

Lindesay J. Phobic disorders in the elderly. *Br J Psychiatry.* 1991;159:531–541.

3. Risk for dementia of the Alzheimer or vascular types is *increased* by

   a. The presence of the APOE ε4 allele
   b. Down syndrome
   c. Stroke
   d. Cigarette smoking

e. a, b, and c only
f. All of the above

The correct answer is f.

Reported risk factors for Alzheimer's disease and vascular dementias include APOE ε4 allele, Down syndrome, stroke, hypertension, and heart disease. The last three are increased by cigarette smoking, which becomes an indirect risk factor. About a quarter of patients who have had a stroke are noted to be demented. Untreated hypertension is a particular risk for vascular dementia; conversely, rates of vascular dementia are declining, probably because of preventive treatment of hypertension.

References

Dartigues JF. Dementia: epidemiology, intervention and concept of care. *Gerontol Geriatr.* 1999;32:407–411.

Folin M, Baiguera S, Conconi MT, et al. The impact of risk factors of Alzheimer's disease in the Down syndrome. *Int J Mol Med.* 2003;11:267–270.

Leys D, Pasquier F, Parnetti L. Epidemiology of vascular dementia. *Haemostasis.* 1998;28:134–150.

Tzourio C, Dufouil C, Ducimetiere P, Alperovitch A. Cognitive decline in individuals with high blood pressure: a longitudinal study in the elderly. EVA Study Group. Epidemiology of Vascular Aging. *Neurology.* 1999;53:1948–1952.

Van Kooten F, Koudstaal PJ. Epidemiology of post stroke dementia. *Haemostasis.* 1998;28:124–133.

4. Dementia of the Alzheimer type often leads to

a. Death
b. Dependency
c. Hip fractures
d. Weight loss
e. Only b and d
f. All of the above

The correct answer is f.

Characteristic consequences of dementia include premature death; dependency; physical deterioration, including weight loss (in the later stages of Alzheimer's disease); fractures; and falls.

Reference

Rose S, Maffulli N. Hip fractures. An epidemiological review. *Bull Hospital Joint Dis.* 1999;58:197–201.

5. Compared to early-onset forms of schizophrenia, late-onset schizophrenia is characterized by

   a. Increased thought disorder
   b. A negative history of lifelong isolation
   c. Increased levels of negative symptoms
   d. Relatively impaired premorbid levels of independent functioning
   e. All of the above
   f. None of the above

The correct answer is f.

Late-onset schizophrenia is characterized by relatively good premorbid
functioning, milder negative symptoms, and a less prominent disorder.
Lifelong isolation, lower rates of marriage, and fewer children further
characterize this population. However, premorbid independent life is
the norm overall.

Reference

Wynn O, Castle D. Late onset schizophrenia: epidemiology, diagnosis, man-
    agement and outcomes. *Drugs Aging.* 1999;15:81–89.

6. Patients with schizophrenia who have grown old in long-term mental
   hospitals have high rates of

   a. Auditory hallucinations
   b. Visual hallucinations
   c. Negative symptoms
   d. Severe aggressivity
   e. All of the above
   f. None of the above

The correct answer is c.

Patients over age 65 years who have aged in long-stay public institutions are characterized by deficit states with negative symptoms. A
subset who have not been able to be discharged have more severe behavioral problems, such as aggression, impulsivity, agitation, and sus-
piciousness.

Reference

White L, Parella M, McCrystal-Simon J, et al. Characteristics of elderly psy-
    chiatric patients retained in a state hospital during down-sizing: a prospec-
    tive study with replication. *Int J Geriatr Psychiatry.* 1997;12:474–480.

7. In patients over 60 years of age admitted to psychiatry units, rates of alcohol abuse and related problems can be as high as

a. 5%
b. 40%
c. 60%
d. 85%

The correct answer is b.

Rates of excess alcohol consumption and associated problems for samples aged over 60 years admitted to psychiatry units can be as high as 44% and can be about 5% in primary medical care settings.

Reference

Liberto J, Oslin D, Ruskin P. Alcoholism in older persons: a review of the literature. *Hosp Community Psychiatry*. 1992:43:975–984.

Chapter 2
Genetics of Dementia

1. Males and females are equally likely to inherit a disease through all of the following transmission patterns *except*

a. Autosomal recessive
b. X-linked recessive
c. Autosomal dominant
d. None of the above

The correct answer is b.

This pattern of transmission involves genes on the X chromosome. Females inherit two X chromosomes from their parents; males inherit one X and one Y chromosome. Therefore, phenotypes determined by genes on the X chromosome have a characteristic sex distribution and pattern of inheritance. On the other hand, in autosomal recessive and autosomal dominant inheritance, disease transmission does not involve the sex chromosomes, and offspring of both sexes are equally likely to inherit the disease gene.

Reference

Gelehrter TD, Collins FS. *Principles of Medical Genetics*. Baltimore, MD: Williams and Wilkins; 1990:29–45.

2. Which of the following is *not* an established risk factor for Alzheimer's disease (AD)?

   a. Positive family history
   b. Advancing age
   c. History of head trauma
   d. *Apolipoprotein E ε4 (APOE ε4)* allele
   e. Genetic mutations in the tau gene

   The correct answer is e.

   Although a modified product of the tau gene is a major component of the neurofibrillary tangles (NFTs) seen in AD, mutations in the tau gene have been associated with frontotemporal dementia (FTD). Over 20 tau mutations have been identified in FTDP-17 families. However, positive family history, advancing age, history of head trauma, and presence of the *APOE ε4* allele have all been identified as factors that increase the risk of AD.

   Reference

   Levy-Lahad E, Tsuang D, Bird TD. Recent advances in the genetics of Alzheimer's disease. *J Geriatr Psychiatry Neurol.* 1998;11:42–54.

3. A mature messenger ribonucleic acid (mRNA)

   a. Consists of exons
   b. Consists of introns
   c. Is derived from transfer RNA
   d. Is a large part of the human genome

   The correct answer is a.

   Genomic DNA undergoes transcription, yielding mRNA. Small parts of the genome form mRNA transcripts, which in turn form sequences called exons. Interspersed, noncoding DNA sequences called introns are spliced out when the mature mRNA is formed. Only a small proportion of the genome consists of exons, which are then transcribed into mRNA.

   Reference

   McConkey EH. *Human Genetics: The Molecular Revolution.* Sudbury, UK: Jones and Bartlett; 1993:24–26

4. Characteristics of polygenic traits include all of the following *except*

   a. Usually quantitative
   b. Indicate an interplay between multiple genes

c. Traits typically follow the normal distribution curve
d. Traits typically follow a mitochondrial inheritance pattern

The correct answer is d.

Polygenic inheritance refers to inheritance of disease through a large number of genes with small, equal, and additive effects. This type of inheritance therefore is quantitative, involves interplay between multiple genes, and causes traits to follow a normal distribution curve. Conversely, mitochondrial inheritance involves only a single mitochondrial gene and causes transmission only through the maternal line, such that all offspring are affected.

Reference

Gelehrter TD, Collins FS. *Principles of Medical Genetics.* Baltimore, MD: Williams and Wilkins; 1990:57–58

5. Direct DNA testing is currently available for all of the following *except*

a. Early-onset familial AD
b. Huntington's disease (HD)
c. Cerebral autosomal dominant arteriopathy with subcortical infarcts and leukoencephalopathy (CADASIL)
d. Vascular dementia
e. Familial Creutzfeldt-Jakob (CJD) disease

The correct answer is d.

No direct DNA testing is currently available for vascular dementia, a disorder that typically does not have a distinct genetic risk factor. Rather, the genetics of this disease are likely multifactorial; as a result, assessing the genetic contributions of each of the risk factors is extremely complicated. There are commercially available genetic tests for all of the other disorders.

Reference

Tsuang DW, Bird TD. Genetics of dementia. In: Sadavoy J, Jarvik L, Grossberg G, Meyers B, eds. *Comprehensive Textbook of Geriatric Psychiatry*, 3rd ed. New York, NY: Norton; 2004:39–84.

6. All of the following should take place *prior* to genetic testing for asymptomatic persons at risk for HD *except*

a. Obtain informed consent from the individual undergoing testing
b. Establish the diagnosis of HD in a family member

   c. Determine that the individual has adequate health and disability insurance

   d. Offer psychiatric assessment for at-risk individuals

   e. Discuss the implications of genetic testing to other family members

   f. Avoid formal genetic counseling by a genetics professional

The correct answer is f.

Ethical genetics research requires obtaining informed consent from the individual undergoing genetic testing. Once a diagnosis of disease has been confirmed in an affected family member, genetic counseling involves educating the consultee and and his or her family members about the clinical and genetic aspects of the disease, the implications of genetic testing, as well as recurrence risk estimates. It is often critical to assess and reassess the psychological state of the consultee prior to and after genetic testing. Because the use of genetic information by insurance companies is currently under debate, based on their genetic test results individuals undergoing genetic testing may become vulnerable to discrimination by such companies. Formal genetic counseling prior to genetic testing should always be provided by a genetics professional.

Reference

Bird TD, Bennett RL. Why do DNA testing? Practical and ethical implications of new neurogenetic tests. *Ann Neurol.* 1995;38:141–146.

7. Tau mutations have been identified in which disease?

   a. Alzheimer's disease

   b. Frontotemporal dementia

   c. Huntington's disease

   d. Cerebral autosomal dominant arteriopathy with subcortical infarcts and leukoencephalopathy

   e. Familial Creutzfeldt-Jacob's disease

The correct answer is b.

Although a modified product of the tau gene is a major component of the neurofibrillary tangles (NFTs) seen in AD, mutations in the tau gene were discovered to be associated with frontotemporal dementia (FTD). Over 20 tau mutations have been identified in FTDP-17 families. Mutations in the *amyloid precursor protein (APP)*, *presenelin 1 (PS1)*, and *presenelin 2 (PS2)* genes as well as the presence of the $\varepsilon 4$ allele in the *APOE* gene are known to be associated with AD. Mutations in the *NOTCH3* gene have been associated with CADASIL; HD is associated with a gene containing an expanded cytosine-adenine-guanine (CAG) trinucleotide repeat. Finally, CJD results from a mutation in the human *PRNP* gene located on the short arm of chromosome 20.

Reference

Wilhelmsen K, Lynch T, Pavlou E, et al. Localization of disinhibition-dementia-parkinsonism-amyotrophy complex to 17q21–22. *Am J Hum Genet.* 1994;55:1159–1165.

8. All of the following chromosomes harbor susceptibility genes for AD *except*

   a. 20
   b. 14
   c. 1
   d. 21

The correct answer is a.

The human *PRNP* gene, known to be associated with CJD, is located on the short arm of chromosome 20. Chromosome 14 contains the *PS1* gene, causative for early-onset AD. Chromosome 1 harbors the *PS2* gene, also causative for early-onset AD. The long arm of chromosome 21 contains the *APP* gene causative for AD.

Reference

Levy-Lahad E, Tsuang D, Bird TD. Recent advances in the genetics of Alzheimer's disease. *J Geriatr Psychiatry Neurol.* 1998;11:42–.

9. The prion gene (*PRNP*) that harbors mutations associated with CJD is on chromosome

   a. 19
   b. 20
   c. 21
   d. 1
   e. 10

The correct answer is b.

The human *PRNP* gene, known to be associated with CJD, is located on the short arm of chromosome 20. Chromosome 19 contains the *APOE* gene, a susceptibility gene for AD. The long arm of chromosome 21 contains the *APP* gene causative for AD. Chromosome 1 harbors the *PS2* gene causative for AD. Linkage analyses suggest that chromosome 10 harbors susceptibility genes believed to be associated with late-onset AD.

Reference

Prusiner S, Molecular biology and genetics of prion diseases. *Cold Spring Harbor Symp Quant Biol.* 1996;61:473–493.

For questions 10–14, match the following genetic findings with their specific disease(s):

    a. Valine-to-isoleucine amino acid substitution, codon 717
    b. CAG trinucleotide repeats
    c. Glutamic acid-to-lysine amino acid substitution, codon 200
    d. *APOE ε4* allele
    e. Trisomy 21

    10. Creutzfeldt-Jakob prion disease
    11. Early-onset AD (*APP* gene)
    12. HD
    13. Late-onset AD
    14. Down syndrome

10. The correct answer is c.

The most common prion protein (PrP) mutation associated with familial Creutzfeldt-Jakob prion disease is the E200K glutamic acid (GAG)–to-lysine (AAG) mutation.

Reference

Mastrianni JA. The prion diseases: Creutzfeldt-Jakob, Gerstmann-Straussler-Scheinker, and related disorders. *J Geriatr Psychiatry Neurol.* 1998;11:78–97.

11. The correct answer is a.

The *APP* gene mutation associated with early-onset AD is a valine-to-isoleucine substitution at codon 717.

Reference

Levy-Lahad E, Tsuang D, Bird TD. Recent advances in the genetics of Alzheimer's disease. *J Geriatr Psychiatry Neurol.* 1998;11:42–54.

12. The correct answer is b.

A novel gene containing a trinucleotide repeat of the three nucleotides cytosine-adenine-guanine (CAG) that is repeated beyond the normal range is associated with HD.

Reference

Nance MA. Huntington disease: clinical, genetic, and social aspects. *J Geriatr Psychiatry Neurol.* 1998;11:61–70.

13. The correct answer is d.

A strong allelic association between *APOE ε4* and AD was established and rapidly confirmed in autopsy-proven sporadic and late-onset AD cases.

Reference

Levy-Lahad E, Tsuang D, Bird TD. Recent advances in the genetics of Alzheimer's disease. *J Geriatr Psychiatry Neurol.* 1998;11:42–54.

14. The correct answer is e.

An extra copy of chromosome 21 is genetically responsible for the most common form of Down syndrome.

Reference

Levy-Lahad E, Tsuang D, Bird TD. Recent advances in the genetics of Alzheimer's disease. *J Geriatr Psychiatry Neurol.* 1998;11:42–54.

Chapter 3
Genetics of Mood Disorders and Associated Psychopathology

1. The single best study design for demonstrating the genetic basis of a human disease is

   a. Twin study
   b. Family study
   c. Linkage study
   d. Adoption study
   e. None of the above

The correct answer is d.

Twin studies measure relative contributions of genes and environment, but cannot always separate shared environmental from genetic factors. Family studies measure the ways in which illnesses run in families, but familial traits are not necessarily genetic. Linkage studies are not powerful under many circumstances, so that an illness with a strong genetic basis may still reveal no linkage throughout the genome. Adoption studies are the best way to separate genetic and environmental effects in humans.

References

McMahon FJ, DePaulo JR. Affective disorders. In: Jamison JL, ed. *Principles of Molecular Medicine*. Totowa, NJ: Humana; 1998.

Risch N. Linkage strategies for genetically complex traits. *Am J Hum Genet.* 1990;46:229–241.

2. Which statement best describes the current understanding of the etiology of mood disorders in the elderly?

   a. Mood disorders primarily result from adverse life events
   b. The same genetic factors are equally important in younger and older people
   c. Genetic diseases seen mostly in the elderly are sometimes important factors
   d. Mood disorders are primarily complications of degenerative brain diseases
   e. None of the above

   The correct answer is c.

   Mood disorders in the elderly are thought to be a mixture of persistent, early-onset diseases and incident, late-onset diseases. The former are related to the same genetic factors thought to operate in younger people, and the latter result from genetic, degenerative, and other diseases that occur primarily in the older population. Adverse life events are an important contributor as well.

References

Childs B, Scriver C. Age at onset and causes of disease. *Perspect Biol Med.* 1986;29:437–460.

McMahon FJ, DePaulo JR. Genetics and age at onset. In: Shulman KI, Tohen M, Kutcher S, eds. *Mood Disorders Throughout the Lifespan*. New York, NY: Wiley-Liss; 1996.

3. Single-nucleotide polymorphisms (SNPs)

   a. Are rare genetic mutations that may lead to disease
   b. May have no impact on gene function
   c. Are widely used as genetic markers in linkage studies
   d. Can be used for case–control but not family-based association studies
   e. All of the above

   The correct answer is b.

   SNPs are an abundant form of genetic variation that encompass both nonfunctional marker SNPs and functional SNPs that can play a direct role in determining disease susceptibility. They are not widely used for linkage studies because more informative markers, known as microsatellites, are available for this purpose. SNPs can be used for both case–control and family-based association studies.

References

Chakravarti A. It's raining SNPs, hallelujah? *Nat Genet.* 1998;19:216–217.
Morton NE, Collins A. Toward positional cloning with SNPs. *Curr Opin Mol Ther.* 2002;4:259–264.

4. Family studies show that, in relatives of probands with unipolar disorder, the risk is

   a. Not increased for unipolar or bipolar disorder
   b. Increased 2-fold for unipolar or bipolar disorder
   c. Increased 10-fold for unipolar or bipolar disorder
   d. Increased 15-fold for unipolar or bipolar disorder
   e. Increased for schizophrenia

Correct answer is b.

Affective disorder in a proband increases the risk of either unipolar or bipolar disorder about 2-fold. It does not seem to increase the risk of schizophrenia. Similarly, relatives of probands with bipolar disorder have about a 4-fold risk of unipolar disorder and 10- to 15-fold increased risk of bipolar disorder.

Reference

McMahon F, DePaulo J. Affective disorders. In: Jamison JL, ed. *Principles of Molecular Medicine.* Totowa, NJ: Humana; 1998.

5. Family studies show that the proportion of relatives with mood disorder

   a. Increases with increasing age of onset of affective disorder in the proband
   b. Increases with decreasing age of onset of affective disorder in the proband
   c. Decreases with decreasing age of onset of affective disorder in the proband
   d. Is unchanged by the age of onset of affective disorder in the proband

Correct answer is b.

Family studies usually show that the proportion of relatives affected with a mood disorder increases with decreasing age at onset in the proband. This has generally been interpreted as a sign of the greater burden of susceptibility genes in families with early-onset mood disorders.

References

Loranger A, Levine P. Age at onset of bipolar affective illness. *Arch Gen Psychiatry.* 1978;35:1345–1348.

Weissman M, Wickramarante P. Age of onset and familial risk in major depression. *Arch Gen Psychiatry.* 2000; 57:513–514.

6. Compared to mood disorders at younger ages, late-onset mood disorders are characterized by

   a. Increased genetic loading
   b. Decreased genetic loading
   c. Decreased medical/neurological comorbidities
   d. Mutations on chromosome 11

The correct answer is b.

Family studies generally show smaller proportions of affected relatives in late-onset mood disorder compared to early onset. Therefore, answer a is false, and answer b is true. Neurological and medical comorbidities (especially cardiovascular disease) are more, not less, frequent in geriatric compared to younger adult patients; therefore, answer c is false. Even though over 100 linkage studies of mood disorder have been reported, no specific gene mutation has as yet been identified; therefore, answer d is false.

References

Alessi C, Cassel CK. Medical evaluation and common medical problems. In: Sadavoy J, Jarvik L, Grossberg G, Meyers B, eds. *Comprehensive Textbook of Geriatric Psychiatry,* 3rd ed., New York, NY: Norton; 2004:281–313.

Tsuang DW, Bird TD. Genetics of dementia. In: Sadavoy J, Jarvik L, Grossberg G, Meyers B, eds. *Comprehensive Textbook of Geriatric Psychiatry,* 3rd ed. New York, NY: Norton; 2004:39–84.

Victoroff J. The neurological evaluation in geriatric psychiatry. In: *Comprehensive Textbook of Geriatric Psychiatry,* 3rd ed. New York, NY: Norton; 2004:315–370.

Weissman MM, Wickramaratne P. Age of onset and familial risk in major depression [Comment. Letter. Twin Study]. *Arch Gen Psychiatry.* 2000;57: 513–514.

For questions 7–10, the diseases listed below may present with symptoms of mood disorder. Match the abnormality with the disease.

7. Notch3 mutations
8. Amyloid precursor protein (APP)
9. Chromosome 20 prion protein (PrP)
10. Presenilins

a. Frontotemporal dementia
b. Alzheimer's disease
c. Hereditary multiinfarct dementia (cerebral autosomal dominant arteriopathy with subcortical infarcts and leukoencephalopathy, CADASIL)
d. Creutzfeldt-Jakob disease (CJD)

The correct answers are 7c, 8b, 9d, and 10b.

7. Notch3 mutations on chromosome 19 have been found in hereditary multiinfarct dementia, a rare disorder also known as CADASIL.

References

Joutel A, Dodick DD, Parisi JE, et al. De novo mutation in the Notch3 gene causing CADASIL. *Ann Neurol.* 2000;47:388–391.

Salloway S, Hong J. CADASIL syndrome: a genetic form of vascular dementia. *J Geriatr Psychiatry Neurol.* 1998;11:71–77.

8. APP gene on chromosome 21 was the first genetic mutation identified in Alzheimer families (Goate et al., 1991). Families with this mutation are very rare, with some 20 families identified worldwide. APP mutations also occur in another disorder, cerebral hemorrhagic amyloidosis of the Dutch type.

Reference

Goate A, Chartier-Harlin MC, Mullan M, et al. Segregation of a missense mutation in the amyloid precursor protein gene with familial Alzheimer's disease. *Nature.* 1991;349:704–706.

9. PrP mutations (chromosome 20) have been identified in the transmissible prion disorders, CJD, and Gerstmann-Sträussler-Scheinker syndrome (GSS) in humans, as well as bovine spongiform encephalopathy in cattle (mad cow disease).

Reference

Hedge RS, Tremblay P, Groth D, et al. Transmissible and genetic prion disease share a common pathway of neurodegeneration. *Nature.* 1999;402;822–826.

10. *Presenilin 1* and *2* (chromosome 1) are the other two "Alzheimer genes" identified in familial Alzheimer's disease (after *APP*).

References

Cruts M, Van Broeckhoven C. Presenilin mutations in Alzheimer's disease. *Hum Mutat.* 1998;11:183–190.

Levy-Lahad E, Tsuang D, Bird TD. Recent advances in the genetics of Alzheimer's disease. *J Geriatr Psychiatry Neurol.* 1998;11:42–54.

Selkoe DJ. Alzheimer's disease: genes, proteins, and therapy. *Physiol Rev.* 2001;81:741–766.

Chapter 4
The Biology of Aging

1. A 72-year-old woman has an average blood pressure of 164/91 measured on three different occasions without orthostatic changes. She eats an unrestricted diet and has a weight appropriate for her height. Fundoscopic examination reveals arteriovenous nicking without hemorrhages. Vibration sensation is decreased at the ankles, but pulses are normal. Random serum urea nitrogen, glucose, and electrolytes are normal, and serum creatinine is 1.2 mg/dL. What are the next steps in her evaluation?

   a. None, these are normal findings for her age
   b. Do a 24-hour urine collection for creatinine clearance
   c. Check fasting serum lipids and glucose level
   d. Exercise stress testing

   The correct answer is c.

   Blood pressure increases over the lifespan in a linear fashion, although diastolic pressure tends to level off after the eighth decade. A blood pressure greater than 140/80 is considered pathological and greatly increases the risk for morbidity and mortality from cerebrovascular and cardiovascular events. Although a high-normal creatinine may overestimate the true level of renal function, a 24-hour creatinine clearance would not change the approach to management or be helpful in revealing another cause of declining renal function other than hypertension. Exercise stress testing is not warranted in an asymptomatic individual. In addition to beginning treatment with an antihypertensive agent, fasting serum lipids and fasting glucose levels may reveal other serious but treatable conditions that confer additional risk for heart disease and strokes.

References

Asmar R. Benefits of blood pressure reduction in elderly patients. *J Hypertens.* 2003;21(suppl 6):S25–S30.

Clark B. Biology of renal aging in humans. *Adv Ren Replace Ther.* 2000;7: 11–21.

Lakatta EG. Cardiovascular function and age. *Geriatrics.* 1987;42;84–94.

Lindeman RD, Romero LJ, Yau CL, Baumgartner RN, Garry PJ. Prevalence of mild impairment in renal function in a random sample of elders from a biethnic community survey. *Int Urol Nephrol.* 2001;33:553–557.

2. Which of the following statements concerning changes in the aging skeleton is *not true*?

   a. Men do not lose significant bone mineral density with increasing age
   b. Women experience an accelerated rate of bone mineral density loss following menopause
   c. Gonadal hormones have an important role in maintaining trabecular bone mineral density
   d. Calcium and vitamin D are critical in maintaining bone integrity of cortical bone
   e. The increased rate of long-bone fractures with age occurs 10 years earlier in women compared to men

The correct answer is a.

Men display progressive and significant loss in bone mineral density with aging, at a rate similar to that of postmenopausal women. Because they achieve a greater peak bone density than women early in life, this loss leads to an increased risk of fracture only at a greater age unless other comorbid conditions predisposing to osteoporosis are present (i.e., smoking, exogenous steroid use, etc.). The accelerated bone loss experienced by women at menopause is caused by the abrupt decline in circulating estrogen levels and is often manifested by compression fractures of the vertebral trabecular bones. Cortical long-bone fractures are associated with calcium and vitamin D deficiency and lack of weight-bearing activity.

References

Kenny AM. Osteoporosis. *Pathogenesis Rheum Dis Clin North Am.* 2000;26: 569–591

Raiz LG. The osteoporosis revolution. *Ann Intern Med.* 1997;126:458–462.

3. Dosing of psychotropic medications in the elderly must often be adjusted. Which of the following statements is *not* a correct explanation of why?

a. Total body water declines with age, leaving a smaller volume of distribution for many medications
b. Hepatic metabolism of phase I pathway drugs declines with age and may result in higher levels of some agents for a longer period of time
c. Increase in central adipose tissue enhances the distribution of these highly lipid-soluble molecules and leads to prolonged elimination of many agents
d. Older adults are less sensitive to some of these medicines and so often require higher doses

The correct answer is d.

Although some drugs are metabolized to less-active compounds, in general older adults are more sensitive to the pharmacological effects of most medications and are more likely to experience adverse effects. The effect of lipid solubility on the duration of action of drugs such as the benzodiazepines is confounded by hepatic biotransformation to active metabolites, greatly increasing the drug effects on the central nervous system (e.g., diazepam has three active metabolites, and clonazepam has five via biotransformation by oxidative hydroxylation and reduction). The tricyclics are also highly lipid soluble. Decrements in renal and hepatic function that occur with normal aging and the presence of other comorbid conditions often result in prolonged half-lives of major tranquilizers and sedative–hypnotic agents. In addition, pharmacological treatments prescribed for other chronic conditions result in an increased incidence or risk for drug–drug interactions in older adults. For example, β-blockers can slow the elimination of benzodiazepines that compete for hepatic oxidative reactions. The plasma concentration of trazodone is significantly increased when a concurrent cytochrome P450 3A4 inhibitor such as ritonavir is administered. The antipsychotics undergo extensive biotransformation in the liver; one half of the excretion of these agents occurs via the kidneys, and the other half is through the enterohepatic circulation. The function of both of these organ systems is compromised by age.

References

Altman DF. Changes in gastrointestinal, pancreatic, biliary and hepatic function with aging. *Gastroenterol Clin North Am.* 1990;19:227–234
Clark B. Biology of renal aging in humans. *Adv Ren Replace Ther.* 2000;7: 11–21.
Varanasi RV, Varanasi SG, Howell CD. Liver diseases. *Clin Geriatr Med.* 1999;5:559–561.

4. Choose which of the following statements about age-related changes in skin is false:

   a. Skin atrophies with loss of the subcutaneous fat cushion
   b. Cool temperatures and low humidity ameliorate the effects of reduced sebaceous and eccrine glands
   c. Elastin fragments with age
   d. Sun exposure encourages increased collagen deposition
   e. Age-related changes in elastin and collagen lead to skin wrinkling

The correct answer is b.

Aging of the skin is a reflection not only of physical changes, but also of environmental exposure. The skin as a whole atrophies, and the subcutaneous fat cushion is lost. Loss of sebaceous and eccrine glands causes skin to become dry or xerotic. Cold and low humidity exacerbate the condition and produce itchiness and sometimes cracking of the skin. The stretch in skin is impaired by fragmentation of elastin. Excessive tanning and sun exposure produce pathology because of loss of skin melanocytes, leading to decreased pigmentation, accelerated loss of elastin, and encouragement of the deposition of collagen. Hence, people with prolonged tanning exposure have more wrinkles at an earlier age.

Reference

Yaar M. Cellular and molecular mechanisms of cutaneous aging. *J Dermatol Surg Oncol.* 1990;16:915–922.

5. Choose the incorrect statement regarding thyroid function in old age:

   a. Thyroxine (T_4) gradually declines
   b. 3,5,3'-Triiodothyronine (T_3) gradually declines
   c. Thyroid-stimulating hormone (TSH) is inconsistently elevated in some studies
   d. All of the above
   e. None of the above

Correct answer is a.

T_4 does not appear to change with aging; T_3 concentrations gradually decline, especially in late old age. Elevated TSH levels have been reported in some studies, but the data are not consistent.

Reference

Mooradian A, Wong N. Age-related changes in thyroid hormone action. *Eur J Endocrinol.* 1994;131:451–461.

Chapter 5
Normal Aging: Changes in Cognitive Abilities

1. Functional abilities in the normal older adult are

   a. Impaired for their instrumental activities of daily living by age 70 years, but their ability to perform their activities of daily living is not impaired
   b. Are unrelated to risk of nursing home placement
   c. Typically not impaired, although the speed of performance declines
   d. Impaired because of age-related changes in cognitive abilities

   The correct answer is c.

   Older adults may have trouble with their instrumental activities of daily living, but the rates of impairment remain fairly low by age 70 years. However, the speed of performance is likely to decline. They are critically important to evaluate because declines in functional abilities are associated with death and nursing home placement. Functional abilities are not likely to be impaired by normal age-related changes in cognitive abilities.

   References

   Messinger-Rapport B, Snader C, Blackdtone E, et al. Value of exercise capacity and heart rate recovery in older people. *J Am Geriatr Soc.* 2003;51: 63–68.
   Myers AM, Holliday PJ, Harvey KA, Hutchinson KS. Functional performance measures: are they superior to self-assessments? *J Gerontol Med Sci.* 1993; 48:M196–M206.
   Ribbon D, Si A, Kimpau S. The predictive validity of self-report and performance-based measures of function and health. *J Gerontol Med Sci.* 1992; 47:M106–M110

2. A 75-year-old Spanish-speaking woman who is a recent refugee from a South American country seeks consultation because of difficulty with her memory. Which of the following is true regarding assessment of her cognitive function?

   a. Results of intelligence tests will not be influenced by cultural background
   b. Administering the usual tests in Spanish ensures adequate assessment of verbal fluency
   c. As a Hispanic, she is likely to perform as well as English speakers on test of digit span
   d. The norms developed for Spanish versions of cognitive tests will likely be applicable to her
   e. None of the above

The correct answer is e.

Many investigators have shown that the results of intelligence tests are influenced by the cultural background of the individual tested. Measures of semantic memory and language measures may be biased against those individuals for whom English is a second language. Healthy Spanish-speaking elderly living in the community in the United States tend to evidence lower performance on certain tests of verbal fluency, such as the Controlled Word Association Test, even when the test was administered in the patient's native language. Digit Span of the Wechsler Adult Intelligence Scale–Revised is biased against normal elderly Cuban-American Spanish speakers, but this bias can be greatly minimized by employing a paradigm in which digits are presented as groups rather than as single digits. Even with normative data for a given measure that appears to be adequate, the measure may still not be valid. Different cultural and language groups may be unwilling to participate in normative studies, and even when they do, it is often extremely difficult to account adequately for the impact of the immigration experience and sociopolitical influences such as discriminatory laws and practices. Although it is best to present tests in the older adult's primary language and to use only those tests that have normative data for Spanish-speaking older adults, the correct answer remains none of the above. Even with these appropriate precautions, it is possible that bias can remain. A test must be rigorously tested with the appropriate population before concluding that poor performance on the test is meaningful.

References

Argüelles T, Loewenstein DA. Research says "sí" to the development of culturally appropriate cognitive assessment tools. *Generations*. 1997;21: 30–31.

Argüelles T, Loewenstein DA., Argüelles S. The impact of the native language of Alzheimer's disease and normal elderly individuals on their ability to recall digits. *Aging Mental Health*. 2001;5:358–365.

Loewenstein D, Quiroga M. Neuropsychological assessment of Alzheimer's disease: an examination of the important issues underlying current practice. In: Kumar V, Eisdorfer C, eds. *Advances in the Diagnosis and Treatment of Alzheimer's Disease*. New York, NY: Springer; 1998:152–169.

Loewenstein DA, Argüelles T, Argüelles S, Linn-Fuentes P. Potential cultural bias in the neuropsychological assessment of the older adult. *J Clin Exp Neuropsychol*. 1994;16:623–629.

Loewenstein DA, Rubert MP. The NINCDS-ADRDA neuropsychological criteria for the assessment of dementia: limitations of current diagnostic guidelines. *Behav Health Aging* 1992;2:113–121

Pick AD. Cognition: psychological perspectives. In: Trandis HC, Lonner W, eds. *Handbook of Cross-Cultural Psychology: Basic Processes*, Vol. 3. Boston, MA: Allyn and Bacon; 1980:117–153.

3. Although there can be several ways to define "successful aging," data indicate that the preservation of mental functioning is important because

   a. It is necessary to health and overall ability to function
   b. It is associated with greater wisdom
   c. It ensures adequate performance of instrumental activities of daily living
   d. All of the above

   The correct answer is a.

   The preservation of mental functioning does not mean that you can perform your instrumental activities of daily living, which can be impaired by many other factors, as is so obviously shown by Dr. Stephen Hawking. Wisdom has not been associated with preservation of mental functioning. However, health and overall ability to function have been associated with preservation of mental functioning.

   References

   Poon LW, Martin P, Clayton GM, Messner SA, Noble CA, Johnson MA. The influence of cognitive resources on adaptation and old age. In Poon LW, ed. *The Georgia Centenarian Study.* Amityville, NY: Baywood; 1992.

   Rowe JW, Kahn RL. *Successful Aging.* New York, NY: Pantheon Books; 1998.

4. Exercise has been shown to

   a. Preserve cognitive function
   b. Improve cardiovascular fitness even in the very old
   c. Improve attentional capacity
   d. Improve memory in depressed elders
   e. All of the above

   The correct answer is e.

   Cardiovascular function and musculoskeletal fitness can be improved by regular exercise, perhaps even into the 80s. Exercise has been shown to improve memory in depressed older adults, although current data do not clarify whether there is a general beneficial effect on memory in all elders. There is some data that indicate that aerobic exercise has beneficial effects on attentional capacity, presumably because of the improvement in cardiovascular efficiency. Aerobic exercise has similarly been shown to have beneficial effects on performance of certain cognitive tasks, such as performance on simple and choice reaction times.

References

Barnes D, Yaffe K, Satariano W, et al. A longitudinal study of cardiorespiratory fitness and cognitive function in healthy older adults. *J Am Geriatr Soc.* 2003;51:459–465.

Bashore T. Age, physical fitness and mental processing speed. In: Lawton MP, ed. *Annual Review of Gerontology and Geriatrics.* New York, NY: Springer; 1989:120–144.

Evans WJ, Campbell WW. Sarcopenia and age-related changes in body composition and functional capacity. *J Nutrition* 1993;123:465–468.

Khatri P, Blumenthal J, Babyak M, et al. effects of exercise training on cognitive functioning among depressed older men and women. *J Aging Phys Activ.* 2001;9:43–57.

Vaitkevicius P, Ebersold C, Shah M, et al. Effects of aerobic exercise training in community-based subjects aged 80 and older: a pilot study. *J Am Geriatr Soc.* 2002;50:2009–2013.

Warren BJ, Nieman DC, Dotson RG, et al. Cardiorespiratory responses to exercise training in septuagenarian women. *Int J Sports Med.* 1993;14:60–65.

Chapter 6
Sociodemographic Aspects of Aging

1. Which statement most accurately describes the current demographic landscape of aging in the United States?

   a. The population in the United States older than age 65 will both grow and age during the next 40 years because of the aging of the baby boomers
   b. Men and women are about equally represented in the older population
   c. Increases in life expectancy during the past 100 years have been caused primarily by life extension after 40 years of age
   d. The United States has the highest life expectancy in the world today
   e. All of the above

The correct answer is a.

Contrary to answer b, women outlive men, thereby increasing their proportion in the older population. Increases in life expectancy have been caused primarily by reduced infant mortality. Several countries have higher life expectancy rates than the United States.

Reference

Weeks J. *Population.* 7th ed. New York, NY: Wadsworth; 1998.

2. Which of the following statements about work and retirement is *false*?

   a. Labor force and retirement patterns were different for men and women during the 20th century
   b. Corporation workers who seek early retirement are more frequently motivated by health problems
   c. There is a correlation between a person's age at retirement and their propensity to work after their retirement
   d. Workers employed by businesses and corporations have greater variation in their age at retirement than workers who are self-employed

The correct answer is d.

The greatest variation in retirement age is found among the self-employed. Business owners, for example, who are able to amass enough wealth for a comfortable retirement tend to retire earlier, whereas farm owners and independent professionals tend to cut down the amount of work and retire much later than others.

References

Hobbs FB. *65+ in the United States*. Bureau of the Census, Washington, DC: US Government Printing Office; 1994.

Mulvey J. Retirement behavior and retirement plan designs: strategies to retain an aging workforce. *Benefits Q*. 2003;19:25–35.

3. Which of the following statements concerning the economic and educational resources of persons over 65 is *true*?

   a. A higher proportion of older persons (than working-aged persons) feels that their income is inadequate
   b. Older adults are slightly less likely than younger adults to live in households with an income below the poverty level
   c. Older persons in the United States tend to have higher incomes than those younger than 65 years
   d. Fewer than half of recent retirees have as much as a high school education

The correct answer is b.

The highest poverty rates are associated with minority women living alone. The overall poverty rate was 10.2% in 2000. A sense of income adequacy is high among the elderly even though they have lower incomes than adults in general. Income levels drop after retirement. There has been a surge in the educational level of recent retirees. Two-thirds of those aged 65–74 years have a high school education. These are important facts because they do not support traditional images of social aging.

References

Himes C. *Elderly Americans*. Washington, DC: Population Reference Bureau; 2001.

Hobbs FB. *65+ in the United States*. Bureau of the Census, Washington, DC: US Government Printing Office; 1994.

Hungerford T, Rassette M, Iams H, Koenig M. Trends in the economic status of the elderly, 1976–2000. *Soc Secur Bull.* 2001–2002;64:12–22.

4. Concerning family and housing issues, which of the following statements is *not true?*

   a. Most older people own their own homes
   b. Over a third of persons over age 85 years are living alone
   c. Men and women over 65 years are living in family settings in about equal proportions
   d. Only about 5% of persons over age 60 years have moved across state lines in any 5-year period in recent decades according to US census data

The correct answer is c.

Of seniors, 80% own their own homes; 75% of men live in family settings in old age compared to 44% of women because men tend to die first and leave their wives widows, many of whom live alone after that event.

References

Himes C. *Elderly Americans*. Washington, DC: Population Reference Bureau; 2001.

Hobbs FB. *65+ in the United States*. Bureau of the Census, Washington, DC: US Government Printing Office; 1994

5. Which of the statements about religion and older adults is *false*: Religion is important to the health of older adults . . .

   a. Despite the fact that a minority of older adults are affiliated with a church
   b. Because churches can promote social integration
   c. Particularly in rural communities
   d. Because of the tangible support churches provide older adults

The correct answer is a.

Current cohorts of older adults have a much higher rate of religious participation than younger adults. This is linked to a variety of measures of morbidity and mortality. Delineating the mechanisms by which religion affects health is currently the focus of considerable research.

It is most likely that health is affected by social and psychological support of older adults: Church congregations frequently provide their older members with companionship, food, and transportation. There are suggestive research findings that religious participation and faith also affect immune function and other physiological parameters.

References

Koenig HG. Religion and health in later life. In: Kimble MA, McFadden SH, Ellor JW, Seeber JJ, eds. *Aging, Spirituality, and Religion: A Handbook.* Minneapolis, MN: Fortress Press; 1995:9–29.

Levin JS, Taylor RJ, Chatters LM. Race and gender differences in religiosity among older adults: findings from four national surveys. *J Gerontol Soc Sci.* 1994;49:S137–S145.

Princeton Religious Research Center. Importance of religion climbing again. *Emerg Trends.* 1994;16:1–4.

6. The high rates of diabetes complications among minority elders reflect

   a. Greater rates of screening for complications among minority groups
   b. Refusal of minority elders to seek medical treatment for diabetes
   c. Less utilization of preventive services among minority elders
   d. The tendency for minority elders to be fatalistic about their health

The correct answer is c.

Diabetes is a major health focus for older adults, particularly for minority elders, who experience excess rates of diabetes-related morbidity and mortality. Diabetes is chronic, requiring lifelong self-management and medical care to prevent neurological and cardiovascular complications. Limited access to care is a major barrier for minority and disadvantaged elders. The area of diabetes complications among minority adults is under study as an area in which genetic variability and environmental factors may interact to produce the ethnic disparities observed.

Reference

Centers for Disease Control and Prevention. Levels of diabetes-related preventive-care practices—United States, 1997–1999. *MMWR Morb Mortal Wkly Rep.* 2000;49:954–958.

7. The rates of health risk behaviors such as smoking and physical inactivity in the elderly population

   a. Are relatively unchanged over the past several decades
   b. Are equally characteristic of men and women
   c. Are lower in the old-old than the young-old
   d. Should improve over the next several decades

The correct answer is d.

Rates of smoking have decreased in the general population. Leisure time physical activity was not a usual activity for most of today's oldest adults during their preretirement years. Thus, we can expect that future cohorts may arrive at old age with lower rates of some health risk behaviors. Nevertheless, because health risk behaviors like access to health care and many other determinants of health are patterned by gender, ethnicity, and socioeconomic status, the disparities in the practice of risk behaviors may well be marked between different segments of the population.

Reference

National Center for Health Statistics. *Health, United States, 1999 with Health and Aging Chartbook.* Hyattsville, MD: US Dept of Health and Human Services; 1999.

8. The cumulative health effects of lack of resources over the life course are shown by

   a. Higher rates of disability among blacks than whites
   b. Higher prevalence of diabetes complications among minority elders
   c. Tendency for elders of low socioeconomic status to rate their health as poorer than elders of high socioeconomic status
   d. All of the above

The correct answer is d.

There are considerable disparities in health between those advantaged and disadvantaged by economics, education, and ethnicity. In general, research demonstrates that socioeconomic status confounds ethnicity. Because health conditions in old age reflect lifetime accumulation of health behaviors, health care, and access to health resources, ethnic differences in health widen.

References

Centers for Disease Control and Prevention. CDC surveillance summaries, December 17, 1999. *MMWR Morb Mortal Wkly Rep.* 1999;48(SS-8):51–88.
Centers for Disease Control and Prevention. Levels of diabetes-related preventive-care practices—United States, 1997–1999. *MMWR Morb Mortal Wkly Rep.* 2000;49:954–958.
National Center for Health Statistics. *Health, United States, 1999 with Health and Aging Chartbook.* Hyattsville, MD: US Dept of Health and Human Services; 1999.

Chapter 7
Self, Morale, and the Social World of Older Adults

1. A 70-year-old man, a successful lawyer with a love of ancient history, decides to return to graduate school for an advanced degree in classics. He reports this decision to his primary care physician, who determines that the patient appears to be well adjusted and aging successfully. However, despite the patient's enthusiasm and vigor, the physician questions the wisdom of the patient's decision to begin a new course of study so late in life and consults a colleague who is a geriatric psychiatrist. The psychiatrist is most likely to conclude

   a. The patient is trying to put off recognition of his own mortality
   b. The patient's goal reflects enhanced self-efficacy
   c. The patient is denying his own aging
   d. The patient is trying to find younger persons in order to feel younger

   The correct answer is b.

   The concept of self-efficacy has been significant in the study of "successful aging." This man's decision probably reflects a view of aging as development rather than decline and fosters enhanced morale and self-regard in light of the fact that he is apparently adapting to aging well and aging successfully in other ways. The geriatric psychiatrist should review the patient's perceptions of his future, mortality, and his ability to accept the aging process . It is likely that a highly educated man who has enjoyed the challenges of his career may seek additional challenges later in life and personal vitality as a result of this decision to return to school.

   Reference

   Seeman T, Unger J, McAvay G, Mendes de Leon C. Self-efficacy and perceived decline in functional ability: the McArthur studies on of successful aging. *J Gerontol.* 1999;54B:P214–P222.

2. A scientist in his late 60s loves his work but wonders if he should retire because he is not sure he will ever match his earlier achievements. He is reassured to learn that

   a. Creative productivity continues into advanced old age for some scientists
   b. Creative productivity plateaus, but it does not decline with age on average
   c. Creative productivity shows no clear relationship to age on average

  d. Creative productivity does not diminish with age for career scientists

The correct answer is a.

Although research data are still few, a study of career artists and scientists suggests that, on average, creative productivity does peak and then decline with age. However, the peak may be very late in some seniors, and the decline may be very gradual, depending on the domain of activity. Simonton (1998) showed that there is evidence for adopting a more optimistic portrayal of the relationship between creativity and age because of the number of major creative achievements that individuals have made in advanced old age.

Reference

Simonton DK. Career paths and creative lives: a theoretical perspective on late life potential. In: Adams-Price C, ed. *Creativity and Successful Aging.* New York, NY: Springer; 1998:3–18.

3. Well-being in later life has been associated in longitudinal studies with voluntary pursuit of creative activities such as painting or writing

  a. For men, but not for women
  b. For women, but not for men
  c. For neither men nor women
  d. For both men and women

The correct answer is d.

Research shows that health and well-being in old age are associated with participation in creative activities when the activities are pursued voluntarily. Vaillant (2001) analyzed data from two major longitudinal studies and found that the most creative individuals were more likely to "age well" than those who were less creative. In particular, they sustained greater physical vigor in later life. Importantly, this finding held for both men and women.

Reference
Vaillant GE. *Aging Well.* New York, NY: Little, Brown; 2001.

4. Regarding relations with family and friends, older adults

  a. Become less concerned with the quality of social ties
  b. Prefer friends and confidants rather than offspring for social support

c. Seem to tolerate restrictions on their own time posed by contact with adult children
d. All of the above
e. None of the above

The correct answer is b.

The 2000 meta-analysis of Pinquart and Sorenson, reporting on almost 300 studies, showed that elders continue to be concerned with the quality of their social ties and gain important sources of satisfaction from adult children as long as contact does not impinge too much on their personal time and resources. Elders seem to prefer friends and confidantes rather than offspring for social support.

Reference

Pinquart M, Sorensen S. Influences of socioeconomic status, social network and competence on subjective well-being in later life: a meta-analysis. *Psychol Aging*. 2000;15:187–224.

Chapter 8
The Role of Religion/Spirituality in the Mental Health of Older Adults

1. Choose the correct answer that describes how *most* older persons view themselves in terms of religion and spirituality.

   a. As spiritual but not religious
   b. As religious but not spiritual
   c. As neither religious nor spiritual
   d. As both religious and spiritual

The correct answer is d.

According to surveys, most older adults see themselves as both religious and spiritual and do not make distinctions between these terms as educators and academics typically do.

References

Koenig HG. *Impact of Religion and Spirituality on Health Service Use (1998–2002): Preliminary Results*. Durham, NC: Center for the Study of Religion/Spirituality and Health; 2000a.

Zinnbauer B, Pargament KI, Cowell B, et al. Religion and spirituality: unfuzzying the fuzzy. *J Scientific Study Religion*. 1997;36:549–564.

2. What proportion of older adults in America indicate that religion is "very important" to them?

    a. 10%–20%
    b. 30%–40%
    c. 50%–60%
    d. 70%–80%
    e. 90%–100%

The correct answer is d.

Gallup surveys between 1995 and 2000 consistently found that about 75% of persons over age 65 years reported that religion is very important in their lives.

References

Princeton Religion Research Center. *Religion in America*. Princeton, NJ: Gallup Poll; 1996.

Princeton Religion Research Center. *America Remains Predominantly Christian*. Poll release. Princeton, NJ: Gallup Organization; April 21, 2000. Available at: www.gallup.com/poll/indicators/indreligion.asp.

3. Regarding trends between 1980 and 2000 in the importance of religion to older adults and in religious attendance, choose the answer that best describes this trend.

    a. Religious attendance and religious importance have been steadily decreasing during this time
    b. Religious attendance and religious importance have remained about the same
    c. Religious attendance has been increasing and religious importance decreasing
    d. Religious attendance has been significantly decreasing and religious importance increasing
    e. Religious attendance and religious importance have been steadily increasing

The correct answer is b.

Religious attendance and importance between 1980 and 2000 among older adults have remained about the same. Weekly religious attendance among persons aged 65 years or older in 1981 was 49%, whereas it was 53% in 1995; religion was very important among 74% of older adults in 1981 compared to 75% in 2000 (both figures indicating stability).

References

Princeton Religion Research Center. *Religion in America*. Princeton, NJ: Gallup Poll; 1976.

Princeton Religion Research Center. *Religion in America*. Princeton, NJ: Gallup Poll; 1982.

Princeton Religion Research Center. *America Remains Predominantly Christian*. Poll release. Princeton, NJ: Gallup Organization; April 21, 2000. Available at: http://www.gallup.com/poll/indicators/indreligion.asp. Accessed February 1, 2005.

4. Choose the correct answer about the role religion played in psychiatry in 19th century America.

   a. Religion played little or no part in psychiatric care in America during the mid-1800s
   b. Religion was seen as having a neurotic influence on patients and was discouraged
   c. Attending religious services was used to reward good behavior
   d. Chaplains played little role in the psychiatric care of institutionalized patients
   e. Chaplains were not allowed to see patients without an order from the psychiatrist

The correct answer is c.

According to Taubes (1998), superintendents of some of America's earliest psychiatric institutions rewarded patients for good behavior by allowing them to attend chapel services. Chaplains often lived right on the grounds of these institutions and played an important role in the treatment that patients received. It was not until Freud that religion began to be viewed as neurotic and became excluded from psychiatric treatment.

Reference

Taubes T. "Healthy avenues of the mind": psychological theory building and the influence of religion during the era of moral treatment. *Am J Psychiatry*. 1998;155:1001–1008.

5. Among older medical patients in the southeastern United States, what percentage use religious beliefs or practices to help them cope with the stress of their illness?

   a. 5% or less
   b. 30%
   c. 50%
   d. 70%
   e. Up to 90%

The correct answer is e.

Studies in North Carolina have found that up to 90% of older patients use religion a moderate-to-large extent to help them cope with the stress of medical illness. Furthermore, national Gallup polls indicate that 87% of persons aged 65 years or older receive personal comfort and support from religion.

References

Koenig HG, Cohen H, Blazer D, et al. Religious coping and depression in elderly hospitalized medically ill men. *Am J Psychiatry.* 1992;149:1693–1700.

Koenig HG, George LK, Peterson BL. Religiosity and remission from depression in medically ill older patients. *Am J Psychiatry.* 1998;155:536–542.

Princeton Religion Research Center. *Religion in America.* Princeton, NJ: Gallup Poll; 1982.

6. Choose the correct statement about the relationship between religious beliefs and practices and depression in later life.

   a. Religious practices are associated with a greater prevalence of depression in older adults
   b. Intrinsic religiosity is unassociated with speed of recovery from depression
   c. Intrinsic religiosity is associated with more rapid remission of depression
   d. Religious activities are not associated with lower rates of depressive symptoms
   e. Religious attendance is not as strongly related to depression as private religious activities

The correct answer is c.

A variety of epidemiological community studies and studies in medically ill populations have shown that positive religious practices, especially attendance at religious services, are associated with fewer depressive symptoms in older adults. Based on some community studies and a prospective clinical study, intrinsic religiosity may be associated with a faster rate of remission from depression in older patients.

References

Idler EL. Religious involvement and the health of the elderly: some hypotheses and an initial test. *Soc Forces.* 1987;66:226–238.

Koenig HG, George LK, Peterson BL. Religiosity and remission from depression in medically ill older patients. *Am J Psychiatry.* 1998;155:536–542.

Koenig HG, Hays JC, George LK, Blazer DG, Larson DB, Landerman LR.

Modeling the cross-sectional relationships between religion, physical health, social support, and depressive symptoms. *Am J Geriatr Psychiatry*. 1997; 5:131–143.

7. Choose the *incorrect* statement about how religion influences depressive symptoms in later life.

   a. Religious beliefs and practices increase guilty preoccupations among older adults
   b. Religious involvement is associated with increased social support
   c. Religious involvement is associated with greater hope and optimism
   d. Religious activities are associated with lower rates of substance abuse
   e. Religious beliefs are associated with greater meaning and purpose

The correct answer is a.

There is no evidence that religious beliefs and practices increase guilty preoccupations among older adults. Of 20 studies that examined the relationship between religious involvement and social support, 19 found significant correlations. Most studies find that religious involvement is associated with greater hope, optimism, meaning, and purpose, particularly among older adults with physical illness. Substance abuse is less common among the more religiously involved at any age.

Reference

Koenig HG, McCullough M, Larson DB. *Handbook of Religion and Health: A Century of Research Reviewed*. New York, NY: Oxford University Press; 2001.

8. Choose the correct statement about the relationship between religion and schizophrenia.

   a. Religious involvement predisposes to the development of schizophrenia in older patients
   b. Traditional religious beliefs and practices have a stabilizing influence in chronic psychosis
   c. Exorcism has been successful in the treatment of schizophrenia
   d. Religious interventions worsen psychotic symptoms in schizophrenic patients
   e. Religious delusions are rare among schizophrenic older patients

The correct answer is b.

Adult studies in a therapy group for schizophrenia and a multicenter follow-up study in India suggest that traditional religious beliefs and practices appear to have a stabilizing influence on patients with chronic psychoses. Religious delusions are common among older psychiatric patients.

References

Kehoe NC. A therapy group on spiritual issues for patients with chronic mental illness. *Psychiatr Serv.* 1999;50:1081–1083.

Koenig HG, McCullough M, Larson DB. *Handbook of Religion and Health: A Century of Research Reviewed.* New York, NY: Oxford University Press; 2001.

Verghese A, John JK, Rajkumar S, Richard J, Sethi BB, Trivedi JK. Factors associated with the course and outcome of schizophrenia in India: results of a 2-year multicentre follow-up study. *Br J Psychiatry.* 1989;154:499–503.

9. Choose the correct statement about psychiatric interventions that involve religion.

   a. Psychiatrists should take a spiritual history when evaluating older patients
   b. Psychiatrists should routinely offer spiritual advice to their older patients
   c. Psychiatrists should pray with all older patients when experiencing severe crisis
   d. Psychiatrists should regularly share their own religious beliefs with older patients
   e. All older patients should be encouraged to attend religious services if not already doing so

The correct answer is a.

As part of their initial evaluation of older patients, it is appropriate for psychiatrists to inquire about the patient's religious beliefs and practices and the role that the patient perceives religion plays in their illness (as a supportive resource or exacerbating factor). Adult studies suggest that a trained therapist may benefit religious patients by using religious psychotherapy, but there are no data on use by untrained therapists. Sharing personal religious beliefs requires the same care as introducing other personal information into the therapeutic context, and there are few reliable data in support of this practice. Although data support widespread religious belief and practice among most seniors, they are far from universal, and there are no data to support the contention that religious practice in noncommitted individuals is helpful to them.

References

Accreditation Council on Graduate Medical Education. *Special Requirements for Residency Training in Psychiatry (March, 1994).* Chicago, IL: Accreditation Council on Graduate Medical Education; 1994.

Koenig HG. Religion, spirituality and medicine: application to clinical practice. *JAMA.* 2000b;284:1708.

Lo B, Quill T, Tulsky J. Discussing palliative care with patients. *Ann Intern Med.* 1999;130:744–749.

Chapter 9
Ethnocultural Aspects of Aging in Mental Health

1. Which Asian ethnic group has over 60% American-born minority elderly?

   a. Chinese
   b. Japanese
   c. Korean
   d. Vietnamese
   e. Filipino

   The correct answer is b.

   American born versus foreign born and distance from immigration are clinically important aspects of judging risk of depression and acculturation stress. Almost all Asian groups have less than 25% American born because of the Asian exclusion act of the 1920s.

   Reference
   US Census Bureau data. *Profiles of General Demographic Characteristics and Summary.* Washington, DC: US Census Bureau; 2000.

2. Which illness creates the highest risk of excess mortality for Native American elderly?

   a. Hypertension
   b. Alcoholism
   c. Tuberculosis
   d. Diabetes
   e. Stroke

   The correct answer is b.

   Native American elderly show the same types of health disabilities at age 45 years that Caucasian elderly show at age 65 years. For many, physical and mental health are not conceptually separable. The rate of death from alcoholism is 459% higher than for whites, which is almost double the rate of the next closest health condition listed above.

   References
   American Society on Aging. *Serving Elderly of Color: Challenges to Providers and the Aging Network.* San Francisco, CA: American Society on Aging; 1992.
   US Department of Health and Human Services. *Mental Health: Culture, Race,*

and Ethnicity, a Supplement to Mental Health: A Report of the Surgeon General. Rockville, MD: US Dept of Health and Human Services, Substance Abuse and Mental Health Services Administration, Center for Mental Health Services; 2001.

3. Compared to Caucasians, immigrant Mexican American elderly in the epidemiologic catchment area (ECA) study had

   a. One half the lifetime prevalence for a psychiatric disorder
   b. Double the lifetime prevalence for a psychiatric disorder
   c. The same lifetime prevalence for a psychiatric disorder
   d. Slightly higher lifetime prevalence for a psychiatric disorder
   e. Slightly lower lifetime prevalence for a psychiatric disorder

The correct answer is a.

This unexpected finding has fueled the fire of questions about the accuracy of epidemiological studies in elderly minorities (whether the scales, translations, or sampling are adequate) versus the possibility of unique buffers against mental illness.

References

Escobar JI. Psychiatric epidemiology. In: Gaw A, ed. *Culture, Ethnicity and Mental Illness.* Washington, DC: American Psychiatric Press; 1993:43–74.
US Department of Health and Human Services. *Mental Health: Culture, Race, and Ethnicity, a Supplement to Mental Health: A Report of the Surgeon General.* Rockville, MD: US Dept of Health and Human Services, Substance Abuse and Mental Health Services Administration, Center for Mental Health Services; 2001.

4. Of the groups below, the highest rate of suicide in the elderly is seen in

   a. African Americans
   b. Japanese Americans
   c. Chinese Americans
   d. Caucasians
   e. Native Americans

The correct answer is d.

The actual figures reflect a rise primarily in elderly white males. The rates of suicide overall are equal or lower for minority groups compared to the dominant reference group.

References

Group for the Advancement of Psychiatry, Committee on Cultural Psychiatry. *Suicide Among Ethnic Minorities in the United States.* New York, NY: Brunner/Mazel; 1989. Report 128.

US Department of Health and Human Services. *Mental Health: Culture, Race, and Ethnicity, a Supplement to Mental Health: A Report of the Surgeon General.* Rockville, MD: US Dept of Health and Human Services, Substance Abuse and Mental Health Services Administration, Center for Mental Health Services; 2001.

5. Slow metabolizers of medications using cytochrome 2D6 are most likely to be

   a. Asian
   b. African American
   c. Native American
   d. Caucasians
   e. Native Hawaiian and other Pacific Islanders

The correct answer is d.

This is based on early work from the Center for the Psychobiology of Ethnicity. Some of the slower genetic polymorphisms were reported in Scandinavians.

References

Lin K, Poland RE, Nakasaki G, eds. *Psychopharmacology and Psychobiology of Ethnicity.* Washington, DC: American Psychiatric Press; 1993.

Mendoza R, Smith MW, Poland RE, et al. Ethnic psychopharmacology: the Hispanic and Native American perspective. *Psychopharmacol Bull.* 1991; 27:449–461, 1991.

6. The American Society on Aging has suggested that when programs are developed for minority elderly, these programs require

   a. A mission statement
   b. Proportional representation of minority groups on governing bodies
   c. Special programs (meaningful)
   d. All of the above

The correct answer is d.

The main idea behind minority involvement is to reach the local community. The guidelines assume that the organization will make decisions based on its mission statement, and involvement of community leaders in the decision-making arm of a service organization will lead to special meaningful programs. This same idea has been stated in numerous places within the minority literature to bring about "mainstreaming."

Reference

American Society on Aging. *Serving Elderly of Color: Challenges to Providers and the Aging Network.* San Francisco, CA: American Society on Aging; 1992.

7. A key element in differentiating a culture-bound syndrome from a similar *Diagnostic and Statistical Manual of Mental Disorders, Fourth Edition (DSM-IV)* disorder in the elderly is

   a. Unusual symptoms
   b. Short duration of symptoms
   c. High frequency of occurrence (in the culture)
   d. Patient's explanatory model for symptoms
   e. Response to medication

The correct answer is d.

Culture-bound syndromes can appear similar to *DSM-IV* entities. For example, neurasthenia is similar to an affective disorder. Many disorders are not all that prevalent even in the countries of origin. The major differentiating feature is the pathway to the doctor via the explanatory model for the symptom.

References

American Psychiatric Association. *Diagnostic and Statistical Manual of Mental Disorders.* 4th ed. Washington, DC: American Psychiatric Association; 1994.
Kleinman A. *Rethinking Psychiatry: From Cultural Category to Personal Experience.* New York, NY: Free Press; 1988.
Littlewood R. From categories to contexts: a decade of the "new cross-cultural psychiatry." *Br J Psychiatry.* 1990;156:308–327.

8. A culture-fair dementia screening tool for non-English-speaking minority elderly is the

   a. MMSE (Mini-Mental State Examination)
   b. MSQ (Mental Status Questionnaire)
   c. MMPI (Minnesota Multiphasic Personality Inventory)
   d. CDT (Clock Drawing Test)
   e. CASI (Cognitive Abilities Screening Instrument)

The correct answer is d.

Approaches to culture-fair testing have utilized everyday memory items, validated translations of existing scales, and nonverbal test approaches (of universally known tasks). The Clock Drawing Test appears to be more sensitive and reliable than standard verbally based tests (in English) with non-English-speaking people.

References

Borson S, Brush M, Gil E, et al. The Clock Drawing Test: utility for dementia detection in multiethnic elders. *J Gerontol.* 1999;54A:M534–M540.

Borson S, Scanlan J, Brush M, Vitaliano P, Dokmak A. The Mini-Cog: a cognitive 'vital signs' measure for dementia screening in multi-lingual elderly. *Int J Geriatr Psychiatry.* 2000;15:1021–1027.

9. Early findings showed significantly lower prevalence rates of Alzheimer's dementia in their native countries than in the United States for which groups?

   a. Cree Indians
   b. Nigerians
   c. Japanese
   d. Chinese
   e. All of the above

The correct answer is e.

This question was meant to show that people of color were thought to have reduced risk. However, in the United States, rates of Alzheimer's dementia for African Americans are actually higher than for whites, suggesting gene–environment interactions are involved in the variability. This is currently under investigation in studies sponsored by the World Health Organization.

References

Chang L, Miller BL, Lin KM. Clinical and epidemiologic studies of dementia: cross-ethnic perspectives. In: Lin KM, Poland RE, Nakasaki G, eds. *Psychopharmacology and Psychobiology of Ethnicity.* Washington, DC: American Psychiatric Press; 1993:223–252.

Hendrie HC, Hall KS, Pillay N, et al. Alzheimer's disease is rare in Cree. *Int Psychogeriatr.* 1993;5:5–14.

II   Principles of Evaluation

Chapter 10
Comprehensive Psychiatric Evaluation

1. Which of the following is true about an assessment for competence?

    a. Competence is best viewed as a task-specific assessment
    b. Geriatric psychiatrists are seldom required to assess a patient's capacity to make decisions
    c. Competence to consent to treatment is generally judged by the same criteria as competence to appoint a power of attorney
    d. Presence of delusions is never a sufficient reason to declare a patient incompetent

    The correct answer is a.

    Competency assessments each have their own criteria, depending on the task. For example, although a mildly impaired individual may be able to understand what is involved in issuing a power of attorney, the individual may be incompetent to consent to treatment because the latter task is more complex, involving higher executive cognitive functioning.

    References
    Grisso T, Applebaum PS. *Assessing Competence to Consent to Treatment: A Guide for Physicians and Other Health Professionals.* New York, NY: Oxford University Press; 1998.
    Kim SYH, Karlawish JHT, Caine ED. Current state of research on decision-making competence of cognitively impaired elderly persons. *Am J Geriatr Psychiatry.* 2002;10:151–165.
    Lieff S, Maindonald K, Shulman K. Issues in determining financial competence in the elderly. *Can Med Assoc J.* 1984;130:1293–1296.

2. All of the following are true about an interview with a collateral source *except*

    a. The quality of the informant's relationship with the patient sometimes interferes with obtaining an accurate history
    b. Informants are usually best interviewed when seeing the patient for the first time

c. When the informant is the caregiver of a geriatric patient, the informant is at high risk of depression.

d. An interview with the informant is necessary when the patient has dementia

The correct answer is b.

With the consent of the patient, most geriatric psychiatry assessments will benefit from an interview with an informant, even if the patient is cognitively intact. The interview with the informant provides corroboration of the patient's history, an opportunity to understand the caregiver's possible burden, and an opportunity to develop a therapeutic alliance with the informant.

Reference

Tuokko H, Hadjistavropoulos T. The role of the caregiver in neuropsychological assessment. In: Tuokko H, Hadjistavraopoulos T, eds. *An Assessment Guide to Geriatric Neuropsychology.* Mahwah, NJ: Erlbaum; 1998:205–221.

3. On a mental status examination, an elderly person looking vacantly into space who is appropriately dressed but apparently uncaring about stained clothes and smelling of urine is least likely to be diagnosed with

a. Affective disorder
b. Anxiety disorder
c. Cognitive disorder
d. Paranoid disorder

The correct answer is b.

A cognitive disorder would most likely produce the above clinical picture. However, a severe depression with melancholia with or without psychosis or a severe psychosis could produce the same clinical picture. Severe depression can result in the patient losing complete interest in self-care and personal hygiene. Anxiety disorders usually do not present with this degree of disconnectedness and inattention to appearance.

Reference

Lockwood KA, Alexopoulos GS, Kakuma T, van Gorp WG. Subtypes of cognitive impairment in depressed older adults. *Am J Geriatr Psychiatry.* 2000; 8:201–208.

4. An interview of an elderly paranoid patient might effectively employ which following interview technique?

   a. Redirect the patient to the correct reality when delusions are expressed
   b. Sit close to the patient and touch the patient reassuringly to establish contact and a therapeutic alliance
   c. Always inquire about Schneider's criteria
   d. Acknowledge the patient's fears of others while inquiring about their feelings regarding those around them

The correct answer is d.

Paranoid patients will respond best to a gentle, empathic inquiry about what they feel about those around them and about ideas of danger. Responding to the affect (often fear or anger) associated with the delusions is often very effective. ("I can see why you are so frightened about this.") Sitting too close to the patient or initially challenging the delusions may be very counterproductive. Schneider's criteria can be seen in some elderly schizophrenic or mood-disordered patients and should be asked about, but are much less common phenomena than persecutory or stealing delusions.

References

Evans J, Paulsen J, Harris M, et al. A clinical and neuropsychological comparison of delusional disorder and schizophrenia. *J Neuropsychiatry Clin Neurosci.* 1996;8:281–286.

Howard R, Rabins P, Seeman M, et al Late-onset schizophrenia and very-late-onset schizophrenia-like psychosis: an international consensus. *Am J Psychiatry.* 2000;157:172–178.

5. All of the following statements regarding the cognitive assessment are false *except*

   a. The cognitive assessment is best conducted at the end of the examination as a discrete part of the assessment
   b. The cognitive assessment is always an active process characterized by systematic questioning
   c. The examiner tries to introduce the cognitive assessment in a noninvolved, objective manner to avoid influencing the patient
   d. Much of the basic cognitive assessment can be conducted informally throughout the initial interview.

The correct answer is d.

Even when the formal cognitive assessment is left for the end of the examination, it is hoped the examiner will have already informally assessed multiple cognitive functions during history taking, including memory, concentration, and language. The cognitive assessment is not necessarily left to the end of the examination. When cognitive impairment is obvious, performing the cognitive assessment early ensures the patient will not be too tired or uncooperative to complete the testing and may save the examiner time that would have been spent attempting to acquire detailed history from an unreliable historian. The assessment is best introduced in a sensitive, nonthreatening manner to avoid increasing the patient's anxiety about personal abilities to perform well.

6. All of the following are examples of frontal systems tests *except*

   a. Go/no go
   b. Similarities task
   c. Multiple loop copying
   d. Word list generation
   e. Ideomotor apraxia

The correct answer is e.

Ideomotor apraxia is the inability to perform skilled motor movements in the presence of normal comprehension and motor and sensory function. Impairment occurs with dysfunction of the dominant parietal lobe, and therefore it is not a frontal systems task.

Reference

Cummings JL. *Clinical Neuropsychiatry*. Orlando, FL: Grune and Stratton; 1985:5–16.

7. The Mini-Mental State Examination (MMSE)

   a. Is a diagnostic test for Alzheimer's disease
   b. Subtests are fairly universal and unaffected by culture, age, and education
   c. Will decline, on average, by 3 points per year in patients with Alzheimer's disease
   d. Often produces false-negative results in frontotemporal dementias

The correct answer is c.

Based on a large number of studies, the average decline in MMSE scores for patients with Alzheimer's disease is approximately 3 points per year. The MMSE cannot be used as a diagnostic test and does not test frontal systems, and its scores should be adjusted for age and education level with published norms.

References

Crum RM, Anthony JC, Bassett SS, et al. Population-based norms for the Mini-Mental State Examination by age and education level. *JAMA.* 1993; 269:2386–2391.

Ham L, Cole M, Bellavance F, et al. Tracking cognitive decline in Alzheimer's disease using the Mini-Mental State Examination: a meta-analysis. *Int Psychogeriatr.* 2000;12:231–247.

Chapter 11
Medical Evaluation and Common Medical Problems of the Geriatric Psychiatry Patient

1. A 77-year-old man reports difficulty hearing. He has the most difficulty hearing conversation in crowded places, such as at restaurants and large gatherings. He has no known exposure to loud noises, and he has not had any recent illnesses or medication changes. Current daily medications include 81 mg aspirin, 25 mg hydrochlorothiazide, and 100 mg sertraline. On examination, he seems to hear you only when you speak slowly and clearly. When you whisper softly in each ear, he has difficulty hearing in both ears. Examination of the ear canal is within normal limits. At this time, you should recommend

   a. No further testing
   b. Discontinuation of the aspirin
   c. Meclizine 25 mg po q 6 hours as needed
   d. Referral for audiological testing
   e. Magnetic resonance imaging (MRI) of the brain

   The correct answer is d.

   This patient most likely has presbycusis, which can be identified on audiological testing. Such testing will also help determine whether he might benefit from a hearing aid. Structured questionnaires (e.g., the Hearing Handicap Inventory for the Elderly, HHIE) can also be used to help quantify the level of difficulty the person is having related to the hearing impairment. Although the patient is able to hear when he is alone with you in the examining room and you speak slowly and clearly, he is describing significant difficulty in other situations in which background noise interferes with his hearing. Unfortunately, the hearing loss in older people (presbycusis) is usually in the high-frequency range, which is important in conversation.

   Aspirin, particularly at high doses, can cause tinnitus, but this does not explain his symptoms. Meclizine is sometimes used for dizziness, but this is not a complaint in this patient. Furthermore, the side effects of meclizine can be quite problematic in the older patient. An MRI of the brain is not indicated at this time. The patient's hearing loss was not sudden in onset and seems to be bilateral, making serious underlying pathology such as tumor or vascular disease less likely. Results of the audiological testing should help determine whether additional testing is indicated.

References

American Speech, Language, and Hearing Association. Guidelines for the identification of hearing impairment/handicap in adult/elderly persons. *Am Speech Lang Hearing Assoc J*. August 1989:59–63.

Lavizzo-Mourey RJ, Siegler EL. Hearing impairment in the elderly. *J Gen Intern Med*. 1992;7:191–198.

Mulrow CD, Aguilar C, Endicott JE, et al. Association between hearing impairment and the quality of life of elderly individuals. *J Am Geriatr Soc*. 1990;38:45–50.

2. A month ago, you began treating a 76-year-old man with depression. He has a history of hypertension for many years, for which he takes 25 mg hydrochlorothiazide each day. On review of symptoms at that time, he did mention that for 1 year he has had some difficulty initiating urination, and he reported needing to get up two to three times each night to urinate. He also reported two to three episodes of urinary incontinence each week. You begin treatment with 50 mg sertraline each day for his depression and order a urinalysis, which is normal. After discussion with his primary care doctor, you also begin 5 mg oxybutinin po bid for the urinary incontinence.

   Now, 1 month later, the patient reports that his mood is improving. However, he has decreased many of his social activities, remaining home most days. After much questioning, he admits that his urinary incontinence has worsened, to the point that he is afraid to leave the house because he may have an accident in public. He reports often feeling a sensation of bladder fullness. What should you do next?

   a. Increase the oxybutinin to 5 mg po tid
   b. Discontinue oxybutinin and begin treatment with 2 mg tolterodine bid
   c. Discontinue the oxybutinin and refer for further urological evaluation
   d. Discontinue the sertraline and refer for further urological evaluation
   e. Order a prostate-specific antigen test and intravenous pyelogram

The correct answer is c.

This patient should have the oxybutinin discontinued and needs referral for further evaluation of his urinary symptoms. Loss of small amounts of urine and symptoms of difficulty initiating urination and nocturia in an older man are suggestive of prostatic enlargement with urinary retention as the underlying etiology of his (overflow) incontinence. Overflow incontinence typically presents as the loss of small amounts of urine associated with an overdistended bladder. The urinary retention commonly is related to obstruction (e.g., from an enlarged prostate) or a hypocontractile bladder (e.g., related to a neurological abnormality). This patient should have had an evaluation (by bladder ultrasound or straight catheterization) to rule out urinary retention prior to initiating the bladder relaxant oxybutinin. Prescribing a bladder relaxant may worsen symptoms in a patient with overflow incontinence.

It would not be appropriate to increase the oxybutinin given the symptoms suggestive of urinary retention. Changing his medication to tolterodine, a newer bladder relaxant with fewer occurrences of orthostatis, would not be indicated in this situation. He has had improvement in his mood with the sertraline, and it is unlikely that his worsened incontinence is related to this medication. Although additional testing, including prostate-specific antigen and selected imaging of his urinary tract, may be needed at some point in his evaluation, these are not indicated at this time.

Referral to a specialist is recommended for patients with chronic urinary incontinence that is difficult to diagnose or is present in a patient with other findings, such as severe pelvic prolapse in women, an enlarged prostate in men, or hematuria or prior urological procedure in either gender.

References

Klausner AP, Vapnek JM. Urinary incontinence in the geriatric population. *Mount Sinai J Med.* 2003;70:54–61.

Ouslander JG. Illness and psychopathology in the elderly. *Psychiatr Clin North Am.* 1982;5:145–157.

Ouslander JG, ed. Urinary incontinence. *Clin Geriatr Med.* 1986;2:715–730.

3. An 85-year-old woman with Alzheimer's disease comes to your office with her daughter for a routine follow-up visit. The patient appears well groomed and is pleasant and cooperative during the interview. She was started on donepezil 1 month ago, with 0.5 mg clonazepam each night for sleep. On further questioning, the daughter reports her mother has had four falls over the last month. The falls occur at various times during the day and do not seem to be associated with changes in body position or with environmental hazards in the home.

The last fall resulted in a visit to the emergency room, but there were no serious injuries.

On physical examination, the patient has a blood pressure of 136/72 and pulse of 72 while lying. On standing, her blood pressure is 132/70 and pulse is 80. She has an ecchymosis over her left flank, which the patient and daughter both report occurred with the last fall. There are no other ecchymoses. Her gait is normal. During mental status testing, you note that the patient seems to have difficulty with her vision. What should you do next?

a. Report the patient and daughter to Adult Protective Services
b. Discontinue the clonazepam, request vision testing, and refer the patient back to her primary care provider for further evaluation of her falls
c. Discontinue the clonazepam and encourage the patient to decrease her physical activity
d. Begin 0.1 mg fludrocortisone po three times per week
e. Refer the patient to physical therapy for gait training

The correct answer is b.

Falls are a serious and common problem in older people. The incidence of falls increases with age, and up to 10% of falls result in other serious injury. There is a wide range of etiologies for falls in older persons, including neurological disorders, environmental hazards, drugs that cause orthostatic hypotension, and mental status changes. The psychiatrist should question the older person about falls, particularly when medications are added or dosage changes are made. Falls may be a marker for serious underlying illnesses and disabilities that can be identified and potentially treated. The majority of these underlying problems can be identified from a careful history and physical examination.

This patient began to have falls coinciding with new treatment with a benzodiazepine. Benzodiazepines (and antipsychotics and certain other medications with central nervous system effects) have been associated with falls. Benzodiazepines, with a long half-life, are particularly problematic. In addition, vision impairment is an important and potentially correctable factor related to falls. In most cases, falls have multiple causes, so the older patient with falls needs a comprehensive evaluation.

The clinician should always look for evidence of elder abuse and neglect. Cognitive impairment may increase the risk, but in this patient, the ecchymosis clearly seems related to the most recent fall, and there is no evidence suggesting the daughter is harming the patient. It would not be appropriate to instruct the patient to decrease her physical activity. Despite some evidence of greater risk of falls among older people who are more physically active, the broad range of benefits related to physical activity and exercise far outweigh this possible risk. It would not be appropriate to begin treatment with the mineralocorticoid fludrocortisone. The patient does not have significant orthostasis, and the falls have not occurred with changes from a supine to upright position. Although physical therapy can be beneficial in many patients, this patient does not have evidence of gait impairment, and referral for gait training would not be your first intervention.

References

Hogan D, Maxwell C, Fung T, et al. Prevalence and potential consequences of benzodiazepine use in senior citizens: results from the Canadian study of health and aging. *Can J Clin Pharmacol.* 2003;10:72–77.

Neutel C, Hirdes J, Maxwell C, et al. New evidence on benzodiazepine use and falls: the time factor. *Age Aging.* 1996;25:273–278.

Rubenstein LZ, Josephson KR, Schulman BL, Osterweil D. The value of assessing falls in an elderly population. A randomized clinical trial. *Ann Intern Med.* 1990;113:308–316.

Tinetti ME, Coucette JT, Claus EB. The contribution of predisposing and situational risk factors to serious fall injuries. *J Am Geriatr Soc.* 1995;43: 1207–1213.

4. A 65-year-old woman who is a long-term resident at a psychiatric residential facility is noted to have an elevated thyroid-stimulating hormone (TSH) level of 8.2 µU/mL (normal 0.5–4.0) on routine laboratory testing. Her vital signs are within normal limits, and she is without physical complaints. Physical examination is within normal limits. Additional testing is ordered, with the following results:

Serum thyroxine (total)	6.4 µg/dL (normal 5–12)
Free thyroxine index (FTI)	10 (normal 5–12)
Antimicrosomal antibody	Negative

What is the best approach to these laboratory findings?

a. Begin 0.5 mg levothyroxine po each day and increase dose weekly by 0.25 mg until the TSH level is within normal limits
b. Begin intravenous levothyroxine therapy immediately
c. Order thyroid nuclear medicine scan
d. Order thyroid ultrasound
e. No therapy indicated; recheck thyroid function studies in 6 months

The correct answer is e.

This patient's elevated serum TSH, with other thyroid function testing (TFT) within normal limits, is suggestive of subclinical (or sometimes referred to as "compensated") hypothyroidism. The most appropriate approach at this time would be to recheck the TFTs at a future date. Beginning thyroid hormone replacement therapy is not indicated at this time. Subclinical (compensated) hypothyroidism is a very common pattern of abnormal TFTs in older patients and is characterized by elevated TSH with normal levorotatory thyroxine (T_4) and FTI. It may progress to overt hypothyroidism, particularly in patients with TSH values greater than 20 μU/mL or high titer-positive thyroid microsomal antibodies. Neither a thyroid nuclear medicine scan nor an ultrasound would be useful at this time.

References

Robuschi G, Safran M, Braverman LE, et al. Hypothyroidism in the elderly. *Endocr Rev.* 1987;8:142–153.

Samuels MH. Subclinical thyroid disease in the elderly. *Thyroid.* 1998;8:803–813.

Simons RJ, Simon JM, Demers LM, Santen RJ. Thyroid dysfunction in elderly hospitalized patients. Effect of age and severity of illness. *Arch Intern Med.* 1990;150:1249–1253.

5. A 70-year-old woman is being treated in your clinic for depression. During a routine visit, she reports that she has had gradually worsening discomfort of her hips, hands, and knees over the past 2 years. She has had no treatment for this condition in the past. Recent screening laboratory testing was all within normal limits, including a complete blood count, erythrocyte sedimentation rate, and kidney and liver panel testing. She recently began use of an over-the-counter pain reliever containing ibuprofen, with some relief of her symptoms. What medication change(s) would you recommend to this patient?

   a. Discontinue the ibuprofen and begin a trial of 1000 mg acetaminophen po tid
   b. Discontinue the ibuprofen and begin trial of 5 mg prednisone po qd
   c. Discontinue the ibuprofen and begin the cyclooxygenase-2 (COX-2) inhibitor celecoxib at 100 mg po bid
   d. Continue the ibuprofen and prescribe 100 mg misoprostol μg po bid
   e. Continue the ibuprofen and prescribe 20 mg omeprazole po qd

The correct answer is a.

This patient presents with symptoms consistent with osteoarthritis. Because of its safety and effectiveness in many patients, the initial drug of choice would be acetaminophen. In this patient, there is no evidence of an arthritic condition that would be responsive to steroid therapy. Although treatment with a combination of a nonsteroidal antiinflammatory drug (NSAID) and misoprostol or omeprazole might be considered if the patient's symptoms do not improve with acetaminophen, these would not be the initial recommended medications for this patient. Recent safety concerns about COX-2 inhibitors makes them an inappropriate recommendation.

Painful or stiff joints in older patients are usually caused by osteoarthritis. The joints usually involved include the hands, hips, knees, feet, and the spine. The diagnosis is suggested by symptoms in one or more of these joints combined with evidence of degenerative changes on plain x-rays. An elevated erythrocyte sedimentation rate, weight loss, or constitutional symptoms suggest another disease process besides osteoarthritis. Acetaminophen can be quite effective and safe in many patients, particularly when combined with measures to improve physical activity and lose weight (if overweight). If these measures are inadequate, aspirin or NSAIDs can be helpful, but these agents can cause severe gastric mucosal injury and renal insufficiency. The elderly, particularly women, are at increased risk of major gastrointestinal complications from NSAIDs; the majority of these individuals are asymptomatic on these drugs prior to the complication.

The prostaglandin analog misoprostol is effective in the prevention of NSAID-induced gastric and duodenal ulcers. Proton pump inhibitors (e.g., omeprazole) are equivalent or superior to misoprostol for the prevention of recurrent ulcers and are better tolerated than misoprostol, but their impact on NSAID-induced ulcer complications is not firmly established. Alternative analgesics, such as nonacetylated salicylates (e.g., salsalate) should be considered in older patients who do not have adequate relief with acetaminophen.

References

Ausiello JC, Stafford RS. Trends in medication use for osteoarthritis treatment. *J Rheumatol.* 2002;29:999–1005.

Moskowitz RW. Primary osteoarthritis: epidemiology, clinical aspects, and general management. *Am J Med.* 1987;83:5–10.

Sorenson LB. Rheumatology. In Cassel CK, Reisenberg D, Sorenson LB, et al., eds. *Geriatric Medicine,* 2nd ed. New York, NY: Springer-Verlag; 1989: 184–211.

6. You are asked to evaluate a 65-year-old woman with dementia. As part of your evaluation for potentially reversible causes of her illness, you find the patient has positive Venereal Disease Research Laboratory (VDRL) test and antitreponemal antibody testing. There is no record of prior syphilis treatment. She has no other health problems and is not on medications. On mental status testing, the patient has abnormalities in language, memory, and executive functioning. Physi-

cal examination is notable for generalized weakness and brisk reflexes. What would you do next?

a. Lumbar puncture with cerebrospinal fluid evaluation for evidence of neurosyphilis
b. Therapeutic trial of 2.4 million units benzathine penicillin im as a single dose, with repeat mental status testing in 6 months
c. Hospitalization and 10-day course of intravenous penicillin followed by three weekly doses of benzathine penicillin
d. Repeat antitreponemal antibody testing every 3 months for 1 year
e. Repeat VDRL testing every 3 months for 1 year

The correct answer is a.

This patient has dementia, positive syphilis serology, and neurological findings that are suggestive of neurosyphilis. A lumbar puncture is indicated. If neurosyphilis is present, 10 days of intravenous penicillin is the treatment of choice. This may be followed by intramuscular benzathine penicillin. Empiric single-dose benzathine penicillin therapy is inadequate for the treatment of neurosyphilis, and empiric hospitalization for intravenous penicillin is not warranted unless the diagnosis is documented by cerebrospinal fluid analysis. It would be inappropriate simply to follow syphilis serology over time in this patient. After therapy for syphilis, the VDRL test should be followed for evidence of decline in titer or conversion to seronegative status (which may take months). The fluorescent treponemal antibody absorption (FTA-ABS) test remains positive with or without therapy.

References

Berinstein D, DeHertogh D. Recently acquired syphilis in the elderly population. *Arch Intern Med.* 1992;152:330–332.

Naughton BJ, Moran MB. Patterns of syphilis testing in the elderly. *J Gen Intern Med.* 1992;7:273–275.

Ward TT, Szebenyi SE. Sexually transmitted diseases: syphilis. In: Reese RE, Douglas RG, eds. *A Practical Guide to Infectious Diseases*, 2nd ed. Toronto, ON: Little, Brown; 1986.

7. A 75-year-old man is referred to you for treatment of depression. Several trials of different antidepressant medications have been unsuccessful. The patient remains depressed and has lost 20 pounds over the past 6 months. He has a long history of hypertension and diabetes mellitus. He had a myocardial infarction 2 years ago, permanent pacemaker placement 1 year ago for symptomatic bradycardia, and an ischemic stroke 6 months ago with a residual mild hemiparesis. During evaluation by his primary care doctor for medical causes of weight

loss, he was noted to have mild anemia, but other testing was (chemistry panel, liver panel, and thyroid function tests) within normal limits. Which of the following would be a contraindication to electroconvulsive therapy (ECT) in this patient?

a. Permanent pacemaker
b. Symptomatic ischemic stroke within the past year
c. Myocardial infarction within the past 3 years
d. Anemia
e. None of the above

The correct answer is e.

This patient does not have any noted contraindications to ECT. Pretreatment evaluation of the older patient prior to ECT should focus on neurological and cardiovascular status. A relative contraindication to ECT is the presence of increased intracranial pressure. ECT can be safely given in stroke patients after neurological status has stabilized or even in patients with brain tumors who are carefully monitored during treatments.

Cardiac events are the major cause of mortality reported from ECT. Although patients with cardiac disease have a higher rate of cardiac complications during ECT, with close monitoring (for arrhythmias and ischemic episodes) ECT can be given with relative safety even to patients with severe cardiovascular disease. Pretreatment evaluation of cardiac status should focus on the presence of hypertension, angina, heart failure, and arrhythmias. If these problems are controlled, the patient may have ECT. All older patients should have cardiac monitoring during the ECT treatments. Patients with a pacemaker can receive ECT after pacer function has been documented. Demand pacemakers should be converted to fixed mode with an external magnet immediately prior to ECT, and the patient should be appropriately grounded. ECT is relatively contraindicated in patients with recent myocardial infarction because of an increased risk of cardiac arrhythmias with treatment. However, ECT has been done in the immediate postmyocardial infarction period in severe cases of depression, generally with a resuscitation team present. However, if possible, it is recommended to wait at least 6 weeks after myocardial infarction to allow cardiac status to stabilize.

References

Cattan R, Barry PP, Mead G, Reefe WE, Gay A, Silverman M. Electroconvulsive therapy in octogenarians. *J Am Geriatr Soc.* 1990;38:753–758.
Elliot DL, Linz DH, Kane JA. Electroconvulsive therapy: pretreatment medical evaluation. *Arch Intern Med.* 1982;142:979–981.

Van der Wurff FB, Stek ML, Hoogendijk WL, Beekman AT. Electroconvulsive therapy for the depressed elderly. *Cochrane Database Sys Rev (Online : Update Software)*. 2003;2:CD003593.

8. You are called to evaluate an 80-year-old widowed woman who was brought in to the emergency room by her son. He reports she has been increasingly reclusive, and although previously very active, over the past 6 months she has not attended her usual church groups and functions at the local senior center.

   On examination, her blood pressure is 160/72 with a pulse of 82 (lying). On standing, her blood pressure is 134/62 with a pulse of 104. The remainder of her physical examination is unremarkable. She scores 28/30 on Mini-Mental Status Examination, missing points on the day of the week and missing the calendar date by 4 days. She does acknowledge feelings of sadness, depression, and anhedonia. Screening laboratory work is within normal limits. An electrocardiogram shows first-degree atrioventricular block.

   She is being discharged from the emergency room. Arrangements are made for her to live with her son for the time being, and she is referred to a new family physician in her area. You make arrangements to see her at your office in 1 week. At this time, you wish to prescribe an antidepressant medication. Which of the following factors in this patient is the most important predictor of the development of clinically significant postural hypotension with antidepressant therapy?

   a. A history of hypertension
   b. Preexisting orthostatic hypotension
   c. A history of vertebral compression fractures
   d. An abnormal electrocardiogram
   e. None of the above

The correct answer is b.

Clinically significant orthostatic hypotension is a risk with certain antidepressant medications in older patients and is thought to be caused by antagonism of peripheral α_1-adrenergic receptors. The best predictor of postural hypotension with antidepressant therapy is preexisting orthostatic hypotension. In addition, orthostatic hypotension is more likely to develop in patients with left ventricular impairment or in patients taking other drugs like diuretics or vasodilators. Careful monitoring of orthostatic blood pressure and symptoms of hypotension is required before and during treatment with agents with this side effect. The occurrence of orthostatic hypotension may be reduced by using a low dose or divided doses and by slowly increasing the dose to reach a therapeutic effect. Paradoxically, pretreatment orthostatic hypotension has been shown to predict favorable treatment response to antidepressant therapy. Bupropion and serotonin selective reuptake inhibitors (SSRIs) do not appear to cause orthostatic hypotension. Monoamine oxidase inhibitors (MAOIs), on the other hand, may lead to orthostatic hypotension, supine hypotension, and hypertensive reactions. Tricyclic antidepressants and other agents (e.g., trazodone) can also cause significant orthostatic hypotension.

References

Glassman AH, Preud'homme XA. Review of the cardiovascular effects of heterocyclic antidepressants. *J Clin Psychiatry.* 1993;54(suppl):16–22.

Jarvik LF, Read SL, Mintz J, et al. Pretreatment orthostatic hypotension in geriatric depression: predictor of response to imipramine and doxepine. *J Clin Psychopharmacol.* 1983;3:368–372.

Scalco M, Almeida O, Hachul D, et al. Comparison of risk of orthostatic hypotension in elderly depressed hypertensive women treated with nortriptyline and thiazides versus elderly depressed normotensive women treated with nortriptyline. *Am J Cardiol.* 2000;85:1156–1158.

Tjoa HI, Kaplan NM. Treatment of hypertension in the elderly. *JAMA.* 1990; 264:1015–1018.

Chapter 12
The Neurological Evaluation in Geriatric Psychiatry

1. Parkinson's disease (PD) is associated with

   a. Bradykinesia, myoclonus, and ataxia
   b. Characteristic loss of dopaminergic neurons in the locus ceruleus
   c. Age-associated increase in prevalence, rising rapidly with each decade after 40 years of age
   d. Greater concordance between monozygotic twins than between dizygotic twins, suggesting a significant component of heritability

The correct answer is c.

Individuals with PD typically exhibit bradykinesia and shuffling gait, but not myoclonus. Dopaminergic neurons are lost in the substantia nigra. Twin studies show virtually no difference between mono- and dizygotic twin concordance—strong evidence that heritability is low, and environmental factors are critical.

Reference

Langston JW. Epidemiology versus genetics in Parkinson's disease: progress in resolving an age-old debate. *Ann Neurol.* 1998;44(suppl 1):S45–S52.

2. Dementia with Lewy bodies (DLB) can be reliably distinguished from Alzheimer's disease by which of the following:

a. Fluctuating mental status
b. Parkinsonian features
c. Hallucinations
d. All of the above
e. None of the above

The correct answer is e.

Although some patients who develop dementia exhibit more of the features a, b, and c than others, and although these patients may be somewhat more likely to exhibit cortical or brain stem Lewy bodies, the diagnostic criteria proposed for so-called dementia with Lewy bodies apparently do not reliably distinguish a specific neurodegenerative entity. Specificity of diagnostic criteria for DLB is 75%–94%, but sensitivity ranges from 34% to 79%. The heterogeneity of the clinical presentation of DLB affects interrater reliability and accuracy.

References

Knopman D, Cummings J, DeKosky S, et al. Practice parameter: diagnosis of dementia (an evidence-based review). Report of the Quality Standards Subcommittee of the American Academy of Neurology. *Neurology.* 2001; 56:1143–1153.

Lopez O, Litvan I, Catt K, et al. Accuracy of four clinical diagnostic criteria for the diagnosis of neurodegenerative dementias. *Neurology.* 1999;53: 1292–1299.

McKeith IG, Galasko D, Kosaka K, et al. Consensus guidelines for the clinical and pathological diagnosis of dementia with Lewy bodies (DLB). *Neurology.* 1996;47:1113–1124.

3. The following interventions have been shown to help in the primary prevention of stroke:

a. Carotid endarterectomy in patients with greater than 40% stenosis
b. Warfarin therapy in postmyocardial infarction patients who also have atrial fibrillation, decreased left ventricular ejection fraction, or left ventricular thrombus
c. Lowering homocysteine with B vitamin therapy
d. Answers b and c only

The correct answer is b.

Carotid endarterectomy has only been beneficial in patients with greater than 60% stenosis. Lowering homocysteine with B vitamin therapy has yet to be proven as a preventive strategy.

References

Biller J, Feinberg WM, Castaldo JE, et al. Guidelines for carotid endarterectomy: a statement for healthcare professionals from a Special Writing Group of the Stroke Council, American Heart Association. *Circulation.* 1998;97: 501–509.

Bots ML, Launer LJ, Lindemans J, et al. Homocysteine and short-term risk of myocardial infarction and stroke in the elderly: the Rotterdam Study. *Arch Intern Med.* 1999;159:38–44.

Gorelick PB, Sacco RL, Smith DB, et al. Prevention of a first stroke. A review of guidelines and a multidisciplinary consensus statement from the National Stroke Association. *JAMA.* 1999;281:1112–1120.

4. Head trauma is

a. Unlikely to produce persistent behavioral changes even when the duration of posttraumatic amnesia exceeds 1 week
b. Less likely to produce persistent symptoms in younger victims compared to older
c. An established risk factor for Alzheimer's disease
d. Often followed by depression in cases of right-side injuries

The correct answer is b.

Head trauma is more likely to produce persistent behavioral changes in cases with longer duration of loss of consciousness or of posttraumatic amnesia than if these factors do not pertain. Depression is most common after left frontal injury. Although there is evidence in favor of the hypothesis that head trauma is a risk factor for Alzheimer's disease, this has yet to be proven.

References

Launer LJ, Andersen K, Dewey ME, et al. Rates and risk factors for dementia and Alzheimer's disease: results from EURODEM pooled analyses. EURODEM Incidence Research Group and Work Groups. European Studies of Dementia. *Neurology.* 1999;52:78–84.

Mayeux R. Behavioral manifestations of movement disorders. *Neurol Clin.* 1987;2:3:527–540.

McArthur JC, Hoover DR, Bacellar H, et al. Dementia in AIDS patients: incidence and risk factors. *Neurology.* 1993;43:2245–2252.

Mortimer JA, van Duijn CM, Chandra V, et al. Head trauma as a risk factor for Alzheimer's disease: a collaborative re-analysis of case-control studies. EURODEM Risk Factors. *Int J Epidemiol.* 1991;20(suppl 2):S28–S35.

Ownsworth TL, Oei TP. Depression after traumatic brain injury: conceptualization and treatment considerations. *Brain Injury.* 1998;12:735–751.

5. Which of the following statements is true?

a. Creutzfeldt-Jakob disease and "mad cow" disease are both apparently caused by excessive transmembrane version of the prion protein called CtmPrP

b. Amyotrophic lateral sclerosis (ALS) is a trinucleotide expansion disease

c. Subacute combined degeneration can be detected by a very low serum B_{12} level

d. Human immunodeficiency virus type 1 (HIV-1)–associated dementia can be expected to occur in about 50% of patients with acquired immunodeficiency syndrome (AIDS)

The correct answer is a.

Huntington's disease is one of the trinucleotide expansion diseases. Although the familial form of ALS is associated with mutations of the gene on chromosome 21q encoding copper/zinc-binding superoxide dismutase, the cause of the sporadic form remains uncertain. A very low serum B_{12} level by no means identifies subacute combined degeneration because the vitamin level has an inconsistent relationship with the neurological findings. HIV-1-associated dementia can be expected to occur in about 15%–20% of patients with AIDS.

References

Joosten E, van den Berg A, Riezler R, et al. Metabolic evidence that deficiencies of vitamin B-12 (cobalamin), folate, and vitamin B-6 occur commonly in elderly people. *Am J Clin Nutr.* 1993;58:468–476.

Lindenbaum J, Rosenberg IH, Wilson PW, Stabler SP, Allen RH. Prevalence of cobalamin deficiency in the Framingham elderly population. *Am J Clin Nutr.* 1994;60:2–11.

McArthur JC, Sacktor N, Selnes O. Human immunodeficiency virus-associated dementia. *Sem Neurol.* 1999;19:129–150.

Nance MA. Huntington disease: clinical, genetic, and social aspects. *J Geriatr Psychiatry Neurol.* 1998;11:61–70.

6. Neurological changes commonly associated with apparently normal aging include all of the following *except*

a. Loss of ankle jerks
b. Spontaneous buccolingual dyskinesias
c. Dysmetria on finger-to-nose testing
d. Impaired lateral gaze

The correct answer is d.

Loss of ankle jerks, spontaneous buccolingual dyskinesias (especially among the edentulous), and some degree of dysmetria on finger-to-nose testing are common in apparently normal aging. It is labeled "ap-

parently" normal because the boundary between normal and pathological aging is still uncertain. Although some impairment of up- or
downgaze is common in normal aging, other impairments (e.g., lateral
gaze) are more likely to hint at intracranial pathology.

References

Gilman S, ed. *Clinical Examination of the Nervous System.* New York, NY:
McGraw Hill; 1999.

Haerer A. *Dejong's the Neurologic Examination.* New York, NY: Lippincott
Williams & Wilkins; 1992.

7. The following clinical feature helps distinguish motor system dysfunction of different etiologies:

a. Neuroleptic-induced parkinsonism is associated with more resting
tremor than is idiopathic PD
b. The psychomotor retardation of depression is usually associated
with less rigidity than is the bradykinesia of idiopathic PD
c. Neuroleptic-induced akathisia usually produces less shifting from
foot to foot than psychogenic hyperactivity
d. Progressive supranuclear palsy (PSP) frequently exhibits both rigidity and ophthalmoplegia
e. Answers b and d only

The correct answer is e.

Neuroleptic-induced parkinsonism is associated with more rigidity,
but less tremor, when compared with idiopathic PD. Depression with
psychomotor retardation is usually associated with less rigidity than is
bradykinesia in idiopathic PD. Neuroleptic-induced akathisia usually
produces more shifting from foot to foot than psychogenic hyperactivity. Classic signs of PSP include rigidity and ophthalmoplegia.

References

Gilman S, ed. *Clinical Examination of the Nervous System.* New York, NY:
McGraw Hill; 1999.

Haerer A. *Dejong's the Neurologic Examination.* New York, NY: Lippincott
Williams & Wilkins; 1992.

Keys BA, White DA. Exploring the relationship between age, executive abilities, and psychomotor speed. *J Int Neuropsychol Soc.* 2000;6:76–82.

Marsden CD, Jenner P. The pathophysiology of extrapyramidal side-effects of
neuroleptic drugs. *Psychol Med.* 1980;10:55–72.

8. Which of the following statements is correct?

a. Unilateral resting tremor is seen in idiopathic PD
b. Brain tumors usually produce papilledema in the elderly

c. Gait disorders affect less than 5% of the elderly
d. Alcoholic cerebellar degeneration produces more appendicular than truncal ataxia

The correct answer is a.

Although patients with PD may eventually exhibit bilateral tremor, it is common for them to have a primarily unilateral resting tremor in the early stages. Brain tumors usually do not produce papilledema in the elderly, making this an unreliable test to rule out increased intracranial pressure. Gait disorders affect about 13% of the elderly. Alcoholic cerebellar degeneration usually produces more truncal ataxia than appendicular cerebellar signs.

References

Gilman S, ed. *Clinical Examination of the Nervous System.* New York, NY: McGraw Hill; 1999.

Haerer A. *Dejong's the Neurologic Examination.* New York, NY: Lippincott Williams & Wilkins; 1992.

Larish DD, Martin PE, Mungiole M. Characteristic patterns of gait in the healthy old. *Ann N Y Acad Sci.* 1988;515:18–32.

Teravainen H, Calne DB. Motor system in normal aging and Parkinson's disease. In: Katzman R, Terry R, eds. *The Neurology of Aging.* Philadelphia, PA: Davis; 1983:85–109.

9. Frontal release signs

   a. Reveal frontal lobe pathology
   b. Are common in the healthy aged
   c. Include patellar hyperreflexia
   d. Do not occur with frontal lobe pathology
   e. Can distinguish basal ganglia from frontal lobe pathology

The correct answer is b.

Patients may have considerable frontal lobe damage yet have no grasp, snout, suck, rooting, hyperactive jaw jerk, or palmomental reflexes. Furthermore, the snout, glabellar, and palmomental reflexes are frequently found in the aged with no evidence of frontal pathology or in patients with basal gangliar injury.

References

Benson DF, Stuss DT, Naeser MA, et al. The long-term effects of prefrontal leukotomy. *Arch Neurol.* 1981;38:165–189.

Jacobs L, Gossman MD. Three primitive reflexes in normal adults. *Neurology.* 1980;30:184–188.

Jenkyn LR, Reeves AG, Warren T, et al. Neurologic signs in senescence. *Arch Neurol.* 1985;42:1154–1157.

Jensen JPA, Gron U, Pakkenberg H. Comparison of three primitive reflexes in neurological patients and in normal individuals. *J Neurol Neurosurg Psychiatry.* 1983;46:162–167.

Chapter 13
Neuropsychological Testing of the Older Adult

1. Following open heart surgery, a 72-year-old woman presents in her hospital room with irritability, delusions, disorientation, and memory dysfunction. During the consultation with the family, family members noted that there has been no history of memory or psychiatric dysfunction prior to the current presentation. In evaluating the cognitive functioning of the patient, it was noted that her attention was severely impaired (she could only recall two digits forward, and she was unable to perform digits backward). Given the pattern of her symptoms, the most likely diagnosis is

   a. Vascular dementia
   b. Delirium
   c. Alzheimer's disease
   d. Psychotic disorder not otherwise specified

   The correct answer is b.

   According to diagnostic criteria listed in the *Diagnostic and Statistical Manual of Mental Disorders, Fourth Edition (DSM-IV)*, a disturbance of consciousness with reduced ability to focus, sustain, or shift attention is the key cognitive symptom of an acute confusional state or delirium. Although memory, language, and executive dysfunction may be present, these deficits are often attributable to the severely impaired attention and disturbance in consciousness.

References

American Psychiatric Association. *Diagnostic and Statistical Manual of Mental Disorders*, 4th ed. Washington, DC: American Psychiatric Association; 1994.

Mesulam MM. Attentional networks, confusional states and neglect syndromes. In: Mesulam MM, ed. *Principles of Behavioral and Cognitive Neurology*. New York, NY: Oxford; 2000:174–256.

2. A 56-year-old man, currently hospitalized on the inpatient psychiatric ward for evaluation, presents with memory disturbances. On evaluation, it is noted that he also presents with several parkinsonian features, including a shuffling gait and a bilateral hand tremor. A neuropsychological evaluation was administered to determine the nature and severity of his memory dysfunction. What is a common heuristic for differentiating cortical from subcortical memory disturbances?

   a. Rapid loss of learned information versus total loss of learned information
   b. Rapid loss of learned information versus no loss of learned information
   c. Rapid loss of learned information versus impaired retrieval of learned information
   d. Intact recognition of learned information versus total loss of learned information

   The correct answer is c.

   First identified with Huntington's disease, subcortical dementia has been associated with impaired retrieval of learned information. With this, individuals with subcortical dementia benefit from recognition trials. In contrast, cortical dementia, such as Alzheimer's disease, is associated with the rapid loss of information. Although individuals with cortical dementia are often able to encode new information (such as repeating a list of words), over time there is a significant loss of learned information. In addition, individuals with a cortical dementia will not benefit from a recognition trial as the information was not encoded into long-term memory.

   References

   Kaufer DI, Cummings JL. Dementia and delirium: an overview. In: Feinberg TE, Farah MJ, eds. *Behavioral Neurology and Neuropsychology*. New York, NY: McGraw-Hill; 1997:499–520.
   Lezak MD. *Neuropsychological Assessment*, 3rd ed. New York, NY: Oxford; 1995.

3. A 71-year-old African American woman is brought into the emergency room by her son, who reported that over the past 2 weeks his mother has been leaving the stove unattended, "losing" objects around the house, and just yesterday, he was called to the local police department after his mother became lost at the mall. She is ambulatory and demonstrated no language disturbance. What is the most likely etiology of this woman's cognitive difficulties?

a. Alzheimer's disease
b. Parkinson's disease
c. Huntington's disease
d. Vascular dementia

The correct answer is d.

The best answer based on the available information suggests a rather sudden onset without any motor disturbances. With this, vascular dementia is the most likely diagnosis. Although memory problems (often demonstrated by leaving the stove on, forgetting information such as the location of the car keys and the car, or becoming disoriented and lost) can be present in all four choices, the lack of any motor signs (such as chorea, tremor, or bradykinesia) help rule out Parkinson's disease and Huntington's disease. Finally, although Alzheimer's disease remains a possibility, given the sudden onset (versus a more insidious onset), this diagnosis is unlikely.

References

Looi JC, Sachdev PS. Differentiation of vascular dementia from AD on neuropsychological tests. *Neurology*. 1999;53:670–678.

Nyenhuis DL, Gorelick PB. Vascular dementia: a contemporary review of epidemiology, diagnosis, prevention, and treatment. *J Am Geriatr Soc*. 1998; 46:1437–1448.

4. A recent neuropsychological evaluation on a 66-year-old Caucasian man reported that mild-to-moderate deficits were noted on measures of verbal fluency, drawing, and visual memory. A task of fine motor skill was noted to be slow, particularly with the left hand. The neuropsychologist concluded that there was no gross deficit in any cognitive domain, but the cognitive performance was "spotty." Which is the likely diagnosis?

a. Alzheimer's disease
b. Vascular dementia
c. Huntington's disease
d. Parkinson's disease

The correct answer is b.

"Spotty" cognitive deficits are a classic sign of vascular disease. In vascular dementia, cognitive impairments depend on the location and size of the lesion. In contrast, the cognitive deficits associated Alzheimer's disease, Huntington's disease, and Parkinson's disease are associated with specific cortical or subcortical neural degeneration, resulting in more identifiable patterns of cognitive dysfunction.

References

Looi JC, Sachdev PS. Differentiation of vascular dementia from AD on neuro-psychological tests. *Neurology.* 1999;53: 670–678.

Nyenhuis DL, Gorelick PB. Vascular dementia: a contemporary review of epidemiology, diagnosis, prevention, and treatment. *J Am Geriatr Soc.* 1998; 46:1437–1448.

5. Intellectual functioning is often thought to decline with increasing age. However, research has demonstrated that certain aspects of intellectual functioning are affected differentially. The cognitive profile associated with aging, often termed the *classic aging pattern*, is thought to present with the following:

   a. Greater decline in performance IQ in comparison to verbal IQ
   b. An equal decline in both verbal and performance IQ
   c. No decline in performance and verbal IQ
   d. A greater decline in verbal IQ in comparison to performance IQ

   The correct answer is a.

   Research has consistently demonstrated that aspects of intelligence, particularly speed of cognitive processing, are negatively related to increasing age. The more "crystallized" aspects of intelligence, such as information attained through education (i.e., vocabulary knowledge), remains relatively intact throughout the life span. With this, intelligence testing will typically note a decline in performance IQ in comparison to verbal IQ.

References

Lezak MD. *Neuropsychological Assessment*, 3rd ed. New York, NY: Oxford; 1995.

Salthouse TA. Independence of age-related influences on cognitive abilities across the life span. *Dev Psychol.* 1998;34:851–864.

6. During a yearly physical, a 65-year-old retiree expressed some concern over what she perceives is a decline in her cognitive abilities. The patient reported that several of her friends were recently diagnosed with Alzheimer's disease, and she is concerned that, since her retirement, her cognitive abilities have declined. A neuropsychological evaluation concluded that there were no gross deficits in her cognitive abilities. Cognitive changes associated with normal aging are best described as

   a. Moderate memory decline with a noticeable decline in language functions
   b. Psychomotor slowing and subtle memory changes

c. No discernible cognitive changes
d. A general decline in all cognitive domains

The correct answer is b.

Older adults are particularly sensitive to actual or perceived changes in their cognitive functioning. With their sensitivity to the potential for cognitive decline, elderly patients can misperceive changes that occur with normal aging as pathognomonic. Research has demonstrated that normal aging is associated predominantly with psychomotor slowing and only subtle memory decline. A number of cognitive skills, such as language skills, undergo little discernible decline.

References

Parkin AJ, Java RI. Deterioration of frontal lobe function in normal aging: influences of fluid intelligence versus perceptual speed. *Neuropsychology.* 1999;13:539–545.

Salthouse TA. Independence of age-related influences on cognitive abilities across the life span. *Dev Psychol.* 1998;34:851–864.

Small SA, Stern Y, Tang M, et al. Selective decline in memory function among healthy elderly. *Neurology.* 1999;52:1392–1396.

Chapter 14
Neuroimaging in Late-Life Mental Disorders

1. Positron emission tomography (PET) can be used to assess

a. Regional glucose metabolism
b. Cerebral blood flow
c. Receptor density
d. Neurotransmitter metabolism
e. All of the above

The correct answer is e.

PET is a neuroimaging technique that makes it possible to examine several biological processes. These include glucose metabolism, blood flow, receptor density, and neurotransmitter metabolism.

References

Kumar A, Schapiro M, Grady C, et al. High-resolution PET studies in Alzheimer's disease. *Neuropsychopharmacology.* 1991;4:35–46.

Phelps M, Cherry S. The changing design of positron imaging systems. *Clin Positron Imaging.* 1998;1:31–45.

2. The classical pattern of glucose hypometabolism seen early in the course of Alzheimer's disease (AD) is

   a. Cerebellar hypometabolism
   b. Frontotemporal hypometabolism
   c. Temporal-parietal hypometabolism
   d. None of the above

   The correct answer is c.

   In AD, the parietotemporal area shows early pathological changes. Hypometabolism in this region, determined by PET, is an early reflection of this pathology. As the disease progresses, other regions become involved.

   Reference

   Silverman HS, Small GW, Chang CY, et al. Positron emission tomography in evaluation of dementia. *JAMA.* 2001;286:2120–2127.

3. Parietal hypometabolism in the absence of formal diagnosis or family history of AD may be seen in patients with subjective memory complaints and

   a. High spinal fluid amyloid levels
   b. Mutations in the amyloid precursor gene *(APP)*
   c. The apolipoprotein E 4 (APOE 4) allele
   d. Hyperphosphorylated tau

   The correct answer is c.

   The APOE 4 allele predisposes to AD. Parietal hypometabolism is often detected early in the clinical process in patients with memory complaints that do not meet criteria for dementia but who have an APOE 4 allele. *APP* mutations are not usually found either in patients with the common late-life form of AD or in many forms of familial AD, although some familial forms do show the mutation.

   Reference

   Bookheimer S, Strojwas M, Cohen M, et al. Patterns of brain activation in people at risk for Alzheimer's disease. *N Engl J Med.* 2000;343:450–456.

4. Magnetic resonance spectroscopy (MRS)

   a. Is helpful as a marker of neuronal structure and function
   b. Can be used to monitor the impact of pharmacological intervention
   c. Provides information that is complementary to brain structural data

d. Uses the same principles of physics as magnetic resonance imaging (MRI)

e. All of the above

The correct answer is e.

MRS is a noninvasive neuroimaging approach that provides information on brain biochemistry that is complementary to that provided by traditional structural MRI. MRS helps us monitor several biophysical and biochemical processes in the living brain.

Reference

Moore C, Frederick B, Renshaw P. Brain biochemistry using magnetic resonance spectroscopy: relevance to psychiatric illness in the elderly. *J Geriatr Psychiatry Neurol.* 1999;12:107–117.

5. Neuroimaging findings that characterize late-life depression include

a. Small brain volumes in the prefrontal lobes, hippocampus, and caudate nucleus

b. Larger high-intensity lesion volumes

c. Smaller whole brain volume

d. Increased amyloid binding in the hippocampus

e. Both a and b

The correct answer is e.

Late-life depression is most consistently associated with smaller brain volumes (in circumscribed brain regions) and larger volumes of high-intensity lesions in the parenchyma. These are autonomous pathways to major depression in the elderly.

Reference

Kumar A, Schweizer E, Jin Z, et al. Neuroanatomical substrates of late-life minor depression. A quantitative magnetic resonance imaging study. *Arch Neurol.* 1997;54:613–617.

6. Cerebral blood flow in depression

a. Is lower than blood flow in controls in the resting, pretreatment state

b. Changes with treatment

c. Cannot be estimated in humans

d. Does not change with treatment

e. Both a and b

The correct answer is e.

Cerebral blood flow is typically lower in the resting state in patients with depression when compared with controls. Pharmacological treatment, electroconvulsive therapy, and psychotherapy alter blood flow in patients with depression.

Reference

Bonne O, Krausz Y, Shapira B, et al. Increased cerebral blood flow in depressed patients responding to electroconvulsive therapy. *J Nucl Med.* 1996;37:1075–1080.

7. Functional magnetic resonance imaging (fMRI) is

   a. Useful clinically
   b. Used in the study of genes
   c. A research tool in cognitive neuroscience
   d. Inexpensive and easy to perform

The correct answer is c.

Functional MRI helps in mapping a cerebral hemodynamic response to sensory and cognitive activation. It is a powerful research tool in cognitive neuroscience but has limited diagnostic applications.

Reference

Cohen M, Bookheimer S. Localization of brain function using magnetic resonance imaging. *Trends Neurosci.* 1994;17:268–277.

8. In vivo amyloid imaging

   a. Is readily available as a diagnostic tool
   b. Is specific for the diagnosis of vascular dementia.
   c. Is still in the development stages
   d. Can be used to effectively monitor pharmacological treatment in AD
   e. Both a and c

The correct answer is c.

In vivo amyloid imaging is an experimental approach at the present time. It helps examine and study amyloid deposits in vivo, and it has great potential in the diagnosis and treatment-monitoring aspects of AD care.

Reference

Shoghi-Jadid K, Small G, Agdeppa E, et al. Localization of neurofibrillary tangles and β-amyloid plaques in the brains of living patients with Alzheimer's disease. *Am J Geriatr Psychiatry.* 2002;10:24–35.

Chapter 15
Electroencephalography

1. The electroencephalogram (EEG) in the elderly

   a. Does not differ at all from that of young adults
   b. Defines the diagnostic gold standard in cases of dementia
   c. May be used to rule out seizures
   d. May normally show temporal slow waves
   e. Should be routinely performed in depressed patients

   The correct answer is d.

   EEG findings in the normal elderly include a slowing of the posterior dominant rhythm (alpha rhythm), as well as intermittent theta slow-wave activity over the temporal regions. EEG is an adjunct in confirming an underlying clinical picture of dementia but is not considered a gold standard. EEG cannot be used to rule out seizures. The diagnosis of epilepsy is first and foremost a clinical one, and isolated epileptiform abnormalities may not need treatment without evidence of ongoing clinical seizures. EEG may be helpful in distinguishing dementia from the cognitive decline associated with depression (pseudodementia or dementia syndrome of depression). In the latter, one would expect to see a relatively normal EEG with little or no evidence of excessive slow-wave activity, whereas the former would show more profound slow-wave activity. EEG should not, however, be considered part of the routine workup of depressed patients.

   References

   Holschneider DP, Leuchter AF. Clinical neurophysiology using electroencephalography in geriatric psychiatry: neurobiological implications and clinical utility. *J Geriatr Psychiatry Neurol.* 1999;12:150–164.
   Torres F, Faoro A, Loewenson R, Johnson E. The electroencephalogram of elderly subjects revisited. *EEG Clin. Neurophysiol.* 1983;56:391–398.

2. Common normal findings in the EEG of subjects over the age of 80 years include

   a. A posterior dominant rhythm of 8–9 Hz
   b. Isolated temporal slow waves
   c. Rare spike-and-wave foci
   d. All of the above
   e. Answers a and b only

   The correct answer is e.

EEG findings in the normal elderly include slowing of the posterior dominant rhythm (alpha rhythm) as well as intermittent theta slow-wave activity over the temporal regions. Spike-and-wave foci are not considered a normal finding.

References

Obrist WD. Problems of aging. In: Rémond A, ed. *Handbook of Electroencephalography and Clinical Neurophysiology.* Vol. 6, Part A. Amsterdam, The Netherlands: Elsevier; 1976:275–292.

Obrist WD, Henry CE, Justiss WA. Longitudinal changes in the senescent EEG: a 15-year study. In *Proceedings of the Seventh International Congress of Gerontology.* Vienna, Austria; International Association of Gerontology; 1966.

Torres F, Faoro A, Loewenson R, Johnson E. The electroencephalogram of elderly subjects revisited. *EEG Clin Neurophysiol.* 1983;56:391–398.

3. In the evaluation of cognitive impairment, an EEG should be performed

   a. Only when delirium is suspected
   b. Whenever there are focal neurological signs
   c. To document the presence of an underlying, secondary mental disorder
   d. Only to rule out possible seizures
   e. Even when the diagnosis of dementia appears to be clear

The correct answer is c.

EEG studies in the evaluation of cognitive decline are applicable not only when delirium is suspected but also in other clinical scenarios, including atypical dementia or suspected epilepsy. When there is a suspicion of an underlying secondary mental disorder (e.g., depression with underlying dementia or panic disorder with underlying temporal lobe epilepsy), EEGs should be performed to clarify the clinical diagnosis. When the diagnosis of dementia is well established and documented through clinical and other neuroimaging findings, EEG is not necessary. Focal neurological signs by themselves are not an indication for an EEG unless accompanied by clinical signs of ongoing seizures. EEG should not be used to rule out seizures. The diagnosis of seizures is first and foremost a clinical one. Isolated epileptiform abnormalities may not need treatment without evidence of ongoing clinical seizures. Furthermore, patients with epilepsy may show a normal EEG on any single EEG, particularly if this is done without activation procedures designed to accentuate epileptiform activity (e.g., sleep deprivation, hyperventilation).

References

Holschneider DP, Leuchter AF. Clinical neurophysiology using electroencephalography in geriatric psychiatry: neurobiological implications and clinical
utility. *J Geriatr Psychiatr Neurol.* 1999;12:150–164.
Group for the Advancement of Psychiatry. *The Psychiatric Treatment of Alzheimer's Disease.* New York, NY: Brunner/Mazel; 1988.

4. In an elderly patient, the presence of a normal EEG

   a. Is inconsistent with the presence of dementia
   b. Rules out the presence of an encephalopathy
   c. Is seen rarely after the age of 70 years
   d. Suggests the possibility of an underlying depression if there are co-
      existing severe cognitive deficits
   e. Usually lacks an alpha rhythm

The correct answer is d.

Normal EEGs may be seen in patients in the early stages of dementia
or mild encephalopathy. Although the posterior dominant rhythm
(alpha rhythm) may slow with normal aging, normal EEGs in the elderly do not typically lack this rhythm completely. Normal EEGs are
not uncommon in the healthy, normal elderly, even after age 70 years.
A normal EEG in the face of coexisting severe cognitive deficits suggests that the cognitive decline may be caused by an underlying depressive illness.

References

Holschneider DP, Leuchter AF. Clinical neurophysiology using electroencephalography in geriatric psychiatry: neurobiological implications and clinical
utility. *J Geriatr Psychiatry Neurol.* 1999;12:150–164.
Hubbard O, Sunde D, Goldensohn ES. The EEG in centenarians. *EEG Clin
Neurophysiol.* 1976;40:407–417.
Van Sweden V, Wauquier A, Niedermeyer E. Normal aging and transient cognitive disorders in the elderly. In: Niedermeyer E, Da Silva FL, eds. *Electroencephalography: Basic Principles, Clinical Applications, and Related
Fields.* Baltimore, MD: Williams and Wilkins; 1999:340–348.

5. The EEG in delirious patients

   a. Typically shows triphasic waves following overdoses with anticho-
      linergic agents
   b. Often shows slowing that is proportional to the level of confusion
   c. Shows many features similar to those of a demented patient
   d. All of the above
   e. Answers b and c only

The correct answer is e.

Triphasic waves are typically seen in hepatic encephalopathy, although they can also be seen in other encephalopathies, such as those of uremia. They are not typical in overdoses with anticholinergic agents. The EEG in a delirium shows many features similar to that of a demented patient and often shows slowing that is proportional to the level of confusion.

References

Holschneider DP, Leuchter AF. Clinical neurophysiology using electroencephalography in geriatric psychiatry: neurobiological implications and clinical utility. *J Geriatr Psychiatry Neurol.* 1999;12:150–164.

Jacobson SA, Leuchter AF, Walter DO, Weiner H. Serial quantitative EEG among elderly subjects with delirium. *Biol. Psychiatry.* 1993;34:135–140.

Leuchter AF, Jacobson SA. Quantitative measurement of brain electrical activity in delirium. *Int Psychogeriatr.* 1991;3:231–247.

6. Normal EEGs may be seen in

   a. Dementia
   b. Delirium
   c. Aging
   d. Seizure disorders
   e. All of the above

The correct answer is e.

Normal EEGs may be seen not only in normal aging, but also in early stages of dementia and delirium. It has been estimated in studies of late-onset epilepsy that 10% to 47% of patients with seizure disorders have normal EEGs. This may be the case particularly if studies were performed without activation procedures designed to accentuate epileptiform activity (e.g., sleep deprivation, hyperventilation).

References

Ahuja GK, Mohanta A. Late onset epilepsy. A prospective study. *Acta Neurol Scand.* 1982;66:216–226.

Cummings J, Benson D. *Dementia: A Clinical Approach.* Boston, MA: Butterworth; 1992.

Holschneider DP, Leuchter AF. Clinical neurophysiology using electroencephalography in geriatric psychiatry: neurobiological implications and clinical utility. *J Geriatr Psychiatry Neurol.* 1999;12:150–164.

Luhdorf K, Jensen LK, Plesner AM. Etiology of seizures in the elderly. *Epilepsia.* 1986;27:458–463.

Shigemoto T. (1981) Epilepsy in middle or advanced age. *Folia Psychiatr Neurol Jpn.* 1981;35:287–294.

Matching set questions

   a. Repeated loss of consciousness with generalized tonic–clonic movements
   b. Spike-and-wave complexes in the EEG
   c. Frontally predominant intermittent rhythmic delta activity
   d. Occipital spikes
   e. Focal slowing
   f. Posterior dominant rhythm of less than 10 Hz
   g. Paroxysmal lateralizing epileptiform discharges
   h. Bancaud's phenomenon

  7. Which EEG abnormality is highly suggestive of Creutzfeldt-Jakob disease in a patient with myoclonus and a rapidly progressive dementia?
  8. What is the single most reliable indicator of a seizure disorder?
  9. What finding most reliably distinguishes between the EEGs of normal older and young adults?
  10. Which is the most common EEG abnormality in vascular dementia?

7. The correct answer is g.

In Creutzfeldt-Jakob disease, the EEG reveals frontally predominant triphasic waves, paroxysmal lateralizing epileptiform discharges, or some other pseudoperiodic sharp-wave complex within 12 weeks of onset of clinical symptoms in more than 90% of cases. As the disease progresses, these sharp-wave complexes attenuate and disappear into a background of slow-wave activity. Although it is not pathognomonic of the illness, the presence of pseudoperiodic discharges in the presence of a rapidly progressive dementia is highly suggestive of the diagnosis. The absence of these periodic discharges after 10 weeks of clinical symptoms makes the diagnosis suspect.

Reference

Chiappa K, Young R. The EEG as a definitive diagnostic tool early in the course of Creutzfeldt-Jacob disease. *Electroenceph Clin Neurophysiol.* 1978;45:26.

8. The correct answer is a.

The diagnosis of seizures is first and foremost a clinical one, suggested for instance by episodes of loss of consciousness and tonic–clonic movement. Isolated epileptiform abnormalities, even isolated spike-and-wave complexes, may not need treatment without evidence of ongoing clinical seizures.

Reference

Niedermeyer E. (1999) Epileptic seizure disorders. In: Niedermeyer E, Da Silva FL, ed. *Electroencephalography: Basic Principles, Clinical Applications, and Related Fields.* Baltimore, MD: Williams and Wilkins; 1999:476–585.

9. The correct answer is f.

Slowing of the posterior dominant rhythm most reliably distinguishes between the EEGs of normal older and young adults. Findings such as spike-and-wave discharges and frontal intermittent rhythmic delta activity (FIRDA) are not considered normal findings in older adults.

References

Hubbard O, Sunde D, Goldensohn ES. The EEG in centenarians. *EEG Clin. Neurophysiol.* 1976;40:407–417.

Van Sweden V, Wauquier A, Niedermeyer E. Normal aging and transient cognitive disorders in the elderly. In: Niedermeyer E, Da Silva FL, eds. *Electroencephalography: Basic Principles, Clinical Applications, and Related Fields.* Baltimore, MD: Williams and Wilkins; 1999:340–348.

10. The correct answer is e.

Vascular dementia commonly shows focal or lateralizing abnormalities, in contrast to the diffuse and symmetric pattern of slowing seen in Alzheimer's disease (AD). However, focal abnormalities may be absent, particularly in cases of diffuse deep white matter ischemic disease (i.e., Binswanger disease) when there are no cortical infarcts or lesions "undercutting" the cortex. Here, the EEG may show a pattern indistinguishable from that of AD.

References

Erkinjuntti T, Larsen T, Sulkava R, Ketonen L, Laaksonen R, Palo J. EEG in the differential diagnosis between Alzheimer's disease and vascular dementia. *Acta Neurol Scand.* 1988;77:36–43.

Roberts MA, Mcgeorge AP, Caird FI. Electroencephalography and computerized tomography in vascular and nonvascular dementia in old age. *J Neurol Neurosurg Psychiatry.* 1978;41:903–906.

Chapter 16
Alzheimer's Disease

1. A 76-year-old woman presents to her physician with the following complaint: "My memory is not as good as it used to be." She also complains that, "I cannot remember names as well as I could 5 years ago" and "I forget where I put things." The patient reports that she retired from her job as a teacher 17 years ago and now volunteers for a special education program in a primary school. She reports no difficulty with her volunteer work. Her husband says he has not noticed any problem in his wife's mental condition, and that she still drives to her volunteer job and has continued to pay her household bills. She scores in the normal range on screening cognitive testing. The medical workup is unremarkable, and magnetic resonance imaging (MRI) shows cortical atrophy, ventricular dilatation, and white matter changes. Which of the following is the most probable diagnosis?

   a. Normal pressure hydrocephalus
   b. Mild cognitive impairment
   c. Alzheimer's disease (AD)
   d. Age-associated memory impairment

   The correct answer is d.

   Subjective cognitive complaints such as those this patient presents are very common in elderly persons. The most commonly used designation for this condition is age-associated memory impairment. This condition is relatively benign prognostically. Persons with mild cognitive impairment would generally manifest subtle changes in memory and functioning. This 76-year-old woman does not manifest changes evident to her husband or that appear to interfere with her abilities to perform her volunteer work. Patients with AD would manifest still greater impairments, for example, with managing payment of household bills, which this patient does not have. The MRI scan in this patient showed cortical atrophy and ventricular dilatation, which are typical findings in aged patients and not indicative of normal pressure hydrocephalus, in which there is disproportionate ventricular dilatation. The clinical presentation is also not indicative of normal pressure hydrocephalus in that there is no report of gait disturbance, urinary incontinence, or dementia.

References

Geerlings MI, Jonker C, Bouter LM, Ader HJ, Schmand B. Association between memory complaints and incident Alzheimer's disease in elderly people with normal baseline cognition. *Am J Psychiatry.* 1999;156:531–537.

Jorm AF, Christensen H, Korten AE, Henderson AS, Jacomb PA, Mackinnon A. Do cognitive complaints either predict future cognitive decline or reflect past cognitive decline? A longitudinal study of an elderly community sample. *Psychol Med.* 1997;27:91–98.

Petersen RC, Stevens JC, Ganguli M, Tangalos EG, Cummings JL, DeKosky ST. Practice parameter: early detection of dementia: mild cognitive impairment (an evidence-based review). Report of the Quality Standards Subcommittee of the American Academy of Neurology. *Neurology.* 2001;56:1133–1142.

2. An 89-year-old man with AD is referred by his physician to a geriatric psychiatrist for treatment. His wife reports that he can no longer pay his bills and needs considerable help in dressing and bathing himself. Cognitive assessment indicates that he knows his name and his wife's name, but he has difficulty counting backward from 10, says the president is Kennedy, and cannot recall his prior occupation. He is not receiving any medication for his dementia or other psychotropic medications. His wife says that he is manageable and asks if there is any medication that would be helpful. Which of the following medications is approved for use in persons with this degree of dementia?

a. Risperidone
b. Donepezil
c. Memantine
d. Rivastigmine

The correct answer is c.

The patient's cognitive and functional presentation is consistent with moderately severe AD. The only medication approved by the Food and Drug Administration as of 2004 for treating AD of this severity is memantine. One study indicated that donepezil might also be helpful, but neither this medication nor other cholinesterase inhibitors have been approved by regulatory agencies in the United States or the European Union for treating patients with moderately severe or severe AD. Risperidone and olanzapine can be useful in treating behavioral and psychological symptoms of dementia, such as psychosis, and aggression in Alzheimer's patients; however, the wife's description does not indicate the need for this treatment.

References

Ferris SH, Yan B. Differential diagnosis and clinical assessment of patients with severe Alzheimer disease. *Alzheimer Dis Assoc Disord.* 2003;17(suppl 3):S92–S95.

Feldman H, Gauthier S, Hecker J, et al. A 24-week, randomized, double-blind study of donepezil in moderate to severe Alzheimer's disease. *Neurology.* 2001;57:613–620.

Reisberg B, Doody R, Stoffler A, et al. Memantine in moderate-to-severe Alzheimer's disease. *N Engl J Med.* 2003;348:1333–1341.

3. Which of the following symptoms is most commonly observed in patients with AD?

   a. The belief that someone has been stealing their belongings
   b. Olfactory hallucinations, such as smelling something burning
   c. Auditory hallucinations, such as hearing the voices of dead relatives
   d. The belief that the spouse or other relatives are unfaithful
   e. The belief that people, such as the spouse, are not really who they say they are

The correct answer is a.

The most common delusion in patients with AD is that "people are stealing things." Other false beliefs such as those of infidelity and the delusion of imposters are less common. Olfactory hallucinations are rarely observed, and auditory hallucinations are uncommon.

References

Burns A, Jacoby R, Levy R. Psychiatric phenomena in Alzheimer's disease. I: Disorders of thought content. *Br J Psychiatry.* 1990a;157:72–76.

Burns A, Jacoby R, Levy R. Psychiatric phenomena in Alzheimer's disease. II: Disorders of perception. *Br J Psychiatry.* 1990b;157:76–81.

Reisberg B, Franssen EH, Sclan SG, Kluger A, Ferris SH. Stage specific incidence of potentially remediable behavioral symptoms in aging and Alzheimer's disease: a study of 120 patients using the BEHAVE-AD. *Bull Clin Neurosci.* 1989;54:95–112.

4. Hyperphosphorylated tau is most commonly found in the hippocampus in which of the following conditions?

   a. Lewy body dementia
   b. Cerebrovascular dementia
   c. Mild cognitive impairment
   d. Age-associated memory impairment
   e. AD

The correct answer is e.

Hyperphosphorylated tau is the characteristic form of tau seen in Alzheimer disease. It is a major constituent of the paired helical filaments that make up the neurofibrillary tangles of AD. A major site of this neurofibrillary pathology is the hippocampus. Lewy body dementia is accompanied by Alzheimer-type pathology, including neurofibrillary tangles, in only a minority of cases. Cerebrovascular dementia and AD appear to be on a continuum of pathology, with vascular pathology more characteristic of cerebrovascular dementia and neurofibrillary tangles with hyperphosphorylated tau more characteristic of AD. Individuals with age-associated memory impairment and mild cognitive impairment have less neurofibrillary pathology than patients with Alzheimer's disease.

References

Blessed G, Tomlinson BE, Roth M. The association between quantitative measures of dementia and senile change in the cerebral gray matter of elderly subjects. *Br J Psychiatry.* 1968;114:797–811.

McKeith IG, Perry EK, Perry RH. Report of the second Dementia with Lewy Body international workshop: diagnosis and treatment. Consortium on Dementia with Lewy Bodies. *Neurology.* 1999;902–905.

Wischik CM, Novak M, Edwards PC, Klug A, Tichelaar W, Crowther RA. Structural characterization of the core of the paired helical filament of Alzheimer disease. *Proc Natl Acad Sci U S A.* 1988;85:4884–4888.

5. You are asked to provide a one-time consultation on a 91-year-old woman who was diagnosed with AD 3 years ago and who has had high blood pressure for many years, which is under control with medication. She has been taking donepezil, sertraline, amlodipine, hydrochlorothiazide, aspirin, gingko biloba, coenzyme Q, multivitamins, and homocysteine modulators. Recently, her local physician added memantine. Her live-in caregiver states that the patient is able to bathe and dress by herself, although she needs help in selecting clothes. When she goes shopping with the caregiver, she is only able to pick items off the supermarket shelves when they are pointed to and cannot pay for them. She cannot cook but helps set the table and can feed herself. She toilets independently and is "clean" and meticulous in toileting. However, for several months she has been incontinent at night and sometimes during the day. Which of the following recommendations should be made to her referring physician?

a. Discontinue the gingko biloba
b. Discontinue the coenzyme Q
c. Suggest an alternative be found for the amlodipine
d. Suggest an alternative be found for the aspirin
e. Suggest an alternative be found for the hydrochlorothiazide

The correct answer is e.

The patient reportedly is apparently unable to shop independently or to pick out her clothes without assistance. However, she dresses independently and bathes by herself and is reported to be capable of toileting independently. The urinary incontinence is apparently occurring prematurely in the context of AD. Therefore, the urinary incontinence may be the result of an exacerbating medical condition, such as the diuretic usage. If the patient's hypertension can be controlled by medications that do not produce this side effect, the patient's quality of life would benefit markedly. Therefore, the psychiatrist should discuss alternatives to the hydrochlorothiazide with the referring physician. Gingko biloba and coenzyme Q are commonly used nonprescription substances that are generally not associated with deleterious effects. Therefore, discontinuation of these substances is unlikely to help the patient's medical condition. Similarly, there is no reason to believe the amlodipine is causing harm, and it does appear to be useful in controlling the patient's hypertension. Aspirin is commonly used for stroke prophylaxis, and the patient's history of hypertension makes the patient an excellent candidate for this prophylaxis as long as her hypertension has been controlled first to avoid increasing the risk of cerebrovascular hemorrhage. AD and cerebrovascular disease and associated risk factors are frequently related, and there appears to be a continuum between AD and vascular dementia.

References

Reisberg B. Functional assessment staging (FAST). *Psychopharmacol Bull.* 1988;24:653–659.

Skoog I, Lernfelt B, Landahl S, et al. Fifteen-year longitudinal study of blood pressure and dementia. *Lancet.* 1996;347:1141–1145.

6. Severe, end-stage AD is commonly associated with all of the following findings *except*

a. Marked slowing of electrical activity on electroencephalographic evaluation with marked delta and theta activity
b. Presence of marked rigidity in response to range-of-motion assessment of both elbows
c. Presence of an abnormal plantar reflex on neurological examination
d. Presence of marked anemia
e. Loss of ambulatory capacity

The correct answer is d.

Anemia is not a characteristic of AD. Similarly, electrolyte values and renal and hepatic function tests do not change unless additional pathology, apart from AD, is present. Progressive increments in slow-wave activity, including delta and theta wave activity, have long been recognized as concomitants of AD.

The most striking neurological concomitant of AD in the later stages is increased rigidity. Other neurological findings in severe AD include the emergence of so-called primitive, developmental, or infantile reflexes such as the grasp, sucking, rooting, and Babinski (abnormal plantar) reflex. Severe, final-stage AD is associated with loss of intelligible, volitional speech ability, and ambulatory ability.

References

Hughes JR, Shanmugham S, Wetzel LC, Bellur S, Hughes CA. The relationship between EEG changes and cognitive functions in dementia: a study in a VA population. *Clin Electroencephalogr.* 1989;202:77–85.

Reisberg, B. Functional assessment staging (FAST). *Psychopharmacol Bull.* 1988;24:653–659.

Chapter 17
Vascular Dementias

1. A 67-year-old man is brought for evaluation by his family because they think he is "getting Alzheimer's" and should make plans to wind down his business. He makes clear his feeling that their concerns are overblown but agrees to be examined to placate them. He reports he has "always been in good health," although he admits his memory "is not as good as it used to be." Which of the following historical features would provide the strongest presumption of "evidence of cerebrovascular disease . . . judged to be etiologically related to the disturbance" of cognition to support a diagnosis of vascular dementia?

   a. Elevated score (8) on the Hachinski Ischemia Scale
   b. Sudden onset of symptoms following an episode of severe arrhythmia accompanied by transient "confusion"
   c. A magnetic resonance imaging (MRI) study demonstrating "deep white matter opacities, probably ischemic"
   d. Concomitant diagnosis of diabetes mellitus with microvascular complications
   e. Identification of depressed mood and articulation of fears of "losing it"

The correct answer is b.

The presence of risk factors for cerebrovascular disease and stroke should properly alert the examiner to the possibility of cerebrovascular injury. The Hachinski scale includes several risk factors (hypertension, stroke) but omits others (diabetes mellitus, atrial fibrillation). Similarly, the findings of white matter abnormalities should increase one's level of suspicion but are not diagnostic. Precision in the diagnosis of vascular dementia remains disappointingly elusive, however. A comparison of pathological validation of four sets of clinical criteria revealed that detection and accuracy varied, and there was surprisingly little agreement among the criteria sets. A subsequent community-based study found that evidence for a clear temporal relationship between a stroke and the onset of dementia symptoms was the strongest clinical indicator of vascular dementia pathologically.

References

Gold G, Bouras C, Canuto A, et al. Clinicopathological validation study of four sets of clinical criteria for vascular dementia. *Am J Psychiatry.* 2002; 159:82–87.

Knopman DS, Parisi JE, Boeve BF, et al. Vascular dementia in a population-based autopsy study. *Arch Neurol.* 2003;60:569–575.

2. A 59-year-old man is seen in consultation in a stroke rehabilitation unit because of concern about depression and vascular dementia—without a prior history of major psychiatric disorder or cognitive impairment. He is 6 weeks post–left frontal stroke with nonfluent aphasia and right hemiparesis. He is able to comprehend and communicate and has begun to regain movement and activity in his right arm and leg. He is observed to be indifferent to the tasks of rehabilitation. He has a very poor appetite, has lost nearly 20 pounds, and sleeps up to 18 hours a day. The rehabilitation staff is frustrated by his lack of motivation and energy; he consistently "agrees" to make an effort but then begs off therapy sessions after only a few minutes and only very rarely initiates "homework."

After you waken him for the interview, you find him to be physically lethargic, but gracious; he comprehends questions and can make himself well understood despite significant and effortful difficulty expressing his thoughts. He is able, however, to convey a realistic assessment of his situation, including understanding of the importance of rehabilitation efforts. Although he appears sad, he denies overt feelings of sadness, depression, or despair but is unable to convey hope. He convincingly denies suicidal ideation. He has little emotional response, however, to this discussion and is unable to commit to modifying his behavior. Which of the following is the best diagnostic premise for initiating treatment in this case?

a. Major depressive episode
b. Apathy as a result of frontal lobe stroke injury
c. Other intercurrent medical complications

d. Vascular dementia, possibly with depression

The correct answer is a.

Although there are clearly impairments in the patient's ability to manage his affairs and process information, the only major cognitive deficit demonstrated at this time is nonfluent aphasia, and he is still in the phase of poststroke recovery. A diagnosis of vascular dementia would therefore be premature.

The issue of intercurrent medical illness is appropriately included in the differential diagnosis. The geriatric psychiatrist's consultation may prompt appropriate review of these issues for the referring physician. The major issue in this case is the proper characterization and diagnosis of mood disorder in the poststroke setting: Although the questions of apathy versus depression cannot be resolved conclusively based on the case vignette, this is a common dilemma in clinical practice. In this vignette, frankly depressed/sad mood is denied, but motivation is very poor, the patient appears sad, and there is little carry through on the patient's stated "understanding" of the goals of the therapeutic team. Such apathetic responses can be caused by depressed mood, or they can be a primary neurobehavioral deficit. From the vignette, however, one readily identifies at least five of the other seven criteria required for a diagnosis of major depressive episode without needing to include a judgment whether "diminished ability to think and concentrate" is related to depression or directly to vascular or medical conditions.

Stroke involving the left frontal lobe has most consistently been correlated with the risk of developing poststroke major depressive episode, successful treatment of which has been shown to improve overall outcome in general and efforts at rehabilitation in particular.

Reference

Robinson RG. Poststroke depression: prevalence, diagnosis, treatment, and disease progression. *Biol Psychiatry.* 2003;54:376–387.

Whyte EM, Mulsant BH. Post stroke depression: epidemiology, pathophysiology, and biological treatment. *Biol Psychiatry.* 2002;52:253–264.

3. Which of the following would be the best choice for treatment of major depression following a stroke?

   a. Tricyclic antidepressant
   b. Selective serotonin reuptake inhibitor
   c. Stimulant medication
   d. Problem-solving therapy

The correct answer is b.

Positive response of major depression caused by stroke has been demonstrated for tricyclic antidepressants, particularly nortriptyline. More recent studies, however, have also demonstrated positive response to selective serotonin reuptake inhibitor antidepressants, and because of lower side effects and better safety profile, these agents are preferred as initial therapy. Psychotherapy may also be appropriate adjunctively, especially if there are situational issues that will require adaptive responses.

References

Andersen G, Vestergaard K, Lauritzen L. Effective treatment of poststroke depression with the selective serotonin reuptake inhibitor citalopram. *Stroke.* 1994;25:1099–1104.

Robinson RG, Schultz SK, Castillo C, et al. Nortriptyline versus fluoxetine in the treatment of depression and in short-term recovery after stroke: a placebo-controlled double-blind study. *Am J Psychiatry.* 2000;157:351–359.

4. A home health care agency cares for an 82-year-old widowed woman with multiple physical problems who has "developed Alzheimer's and hallucinations" since she suffered a right hemisphere stroke several months before. Her hemiparesis persists, but her function has improved overall. Her primary care doctor added 2 mg olanzapine bid along with 2 mg benztropine mesylate bid to a regimen of 13 medications, but this has made her "worse," leading to consultation with you.

   You find a woman who is inattentive, focuses on multiple physical symptoms (diarrhea/constipation, headache, backache, loss of energy), but who clearly can recall episodes of vivid,´ usually pleasant visual images that she recognizes to be hallucinations. She is inattentive, but with cues can recall all three words you give her to remember. Your most likely initial recommendation will be

   a. Initiate 1 mg risperidone bid
   b. Obtain MRI
   c. Discontinue olanzapine and benztropine
   d. Arrange admission to a nearby experienced geriatric hospital
   e. Contact Adult Protective Services to arrange for a conservator

The correct answer is c.

The clinical problem is the emergence of hallucinations, which have *worsened* since beginning antipsychotic treatment. This is not an indication for initiating new antipsychotic medication but for reanalysis. The important clues are multiple medications, fluctuating symptoms without any sign of fixed worsening in function (therefore not suggestive of recurrent stroke), and deterioration that coincides with the administration of the anticholinergic medications olanzapine and benztropine. This anticholinergic activity was presumptively additive to her preexisting medication anticholinergic burden; older adults have been shown to have a substantial burden of anticholinergic serum activity that correlates with Mini-Mental State Examination scores. It is also to be emphasized that multiple other drugs have anticholinergic activity, and patients on multiple medications are therefore at risk for delirium from this cumulative anticholinergic activity. Therefore, readjusting her overall regimen is the preferred approach, which must include collaboration with her internist because of the potential involvement of drugs for her general medical conditions. In addition, there is no specific suggestion that she is unsafe or that her affairs are in danger, so there is no compelling need for hospitalization or conservatorship at this time, although these may be appropriate issues to address in this context. In light of the fact that the most likely explanation for these symptoms is a toxic anticholinergic reaction, MRI may be deferred until a trial of medication readjustment has been completed.

Reference

Mulsant BH, Pollock BG, Kirshner M, et al. Serum anticholinergic activity in a community-based sample of older adults: relationship with cognitive performance. *Arch Gen Psychiatry.* 2003;60:198–203.

5. A 73-year-old psychotherapist is referred for evaluation of "memory loss." She and her family are discussing whether she should retire from her sharply reduced but still professionally rewarding practice she maintains at an office in her home. She reports having suffered two strokes that she emphasizes were "small," and an MRI report describes three lacunar lesions plus a mild degree of white matter opacity. She and her family agree, however, that she has regained energy since she had a pacemaker placed 6 months previously, and that there has been no further decline. You have records from her referring physician documenting normal results on metabolic studies, and she takes no medications that would be likely to affect cognition adversely. On examination, she has mild deficits in memory testing and has difficulty copying complicated figures, scoring 26 on the Mini-Mental State Examination. However, her language functions and reasoning are fully intact, except that she complains about her ability to write since the second stroke episode. You diagnose (probable) mild and currently uncomplicated vascular dementia. You properly recommend she consider which of the following?

a. A trial of a cholinesterase inhibitor
b. A trial of a N-methyl-D-aspartate (NMDA) receptor antagonist
c. Review of her will and financial affairs, advance care directives, and arrangements
d. Further diagnostic workup, including neuropsychological testing and functional brain studies
e. Psychotherapy
f. Advice that she should stop driving and disband her practice immediately
g. Answers a and c
h. Answers a, c, d, and e
i. All of the above

The correct answer is h.

This clinical situation is a potentially important encounter and an opportunity for the geriatric psychiatrist to assist this patient and family with a major watershed in life. A first major issue is the accuracy and communication of diagnosis. Although the diagnosis of vascular dementia is compelling (patchy cognitive deficits, MRI evidence of causative cerebrovascular disease, and a history of deficits appearing in tandem with known cerebrovascular events), the possibility of coincident dementia of the Alzheimer type exists and is almost certainly a concern of patient and family. Additional information from neuropsychological testing or functional brain studies (positron emission tomography [PET], single-photon emission computed tomography [SPECT]) may be helpful in establishing a baseline for later comparative reevaluation. In terms of immediate therapy, it is appropriate to emphasize first the importance of cardiovascular disease and risk factor control— presumably managed by her internist or cardiologist. It is also appropriate to discuss the emerging evidence of the efficacy of cholinesterase inhibitors in vascular dementia. There may also be inquiries about the use of memantine, but to date evidence for use of that medication in vascular dementia is inconclusive.

Retirement and relinquishing one's professional identity and the attendant "perks" and status represent a major life transition, whether or not it is impelled by a medical or psychiatric condition. The psychiatrist is therefore advised to approach these issues generously in terms of spirit and understanding and to work with the patient and family to facilitate understanding and appreciation and to help the patient, as much as possible, retain a sense of control and motivation.

Advance directives and life planning are appropriate entries to a discussion about functional consequence of the diagnosis and appropriate life change (and patients without counsel may appreciate referral to an attorney experienced in elder law). The emphasis is on preventive steps and preserving and memorializing the patient's wishes and goals. Specific matters in this area include provisions of a trust or will and the rationale for advance health care directives, including a durable power of attorney. Supportive therapy—individual, perhaps with spouse or family involvement—can be very helpful through this transition; the need for and interest in such a recommendation can properly be assessed during the evaluation process.

The issue of professional and driving licensure is challenging. Public safety is an important responsibility for the geriatric psychiatrist in an evaluation such as described here, and the psychiatrist must consider his or her responsibilities carefully in terms of reporting a patient's disabilities. For the purposes of this vignette, however, reporting can be deferred pending the opportunity for patient initiatives and clarification of diagnosis and situation.

References

Erkinjuntti T, Kurz A, Gauthier S, Bullock R, Lilienfeld S, Damaraju CV. Efficacy of galantamine in probable vascular dementia and Alzheimer's disease combined with cerebrovascular disease: a randomised trial. *Lancet*. 2002; 359:1283–1290.

Wang CC, Kosinski CJ, Schwartzberg JG, Shanklin AV. *Physician's Guide to Assessing and Counseling Older Drivers*. Washington, DC: National Highway Traffic Safety Administration; 2003.

6. An 82-year-old retired accountant comes with his wife for evaluation out of concern he may be developing Alzheimer's disease. On questioning, you learn that the suggestion for examination came from a highway patrolman, who realized the man could not follow directions that the officer had provided at the patient's request. You elicit the specific observation that the patient has lost the ability to distinguish right from left. In other areas of mental status, you are impressed that he functions at a high level, consistent with his professional accomplishments. What features would you seek on the examination to substantiate your suspicions of the etiology of his syndrome?

a. Impaired arithmetical skills
b. Loss of the ability to spell reliably
c. History of sudden onset of symptoms following a cardiac arrest
d. Inability to identify his different fingers
e. All of the above

The correct answer is e.

This man has acquired elements of the Gerstmann syndrome: right–left disorientation, finger agnosia, acalculia, and agraphia (manifest by loss of spelling). Although the validity of the syndrome has been disputed, this constellation of symptoms localizes a defect to the dominant left parietal lobe, particularly the angular gyrus, as has been demonstrated by functional brain imaging (PET scanning). Alzheimer's disease is unlikely in this man because of the preservation of memory and other cognitive functions. In general, knowledge of focal neurological symptoms and a careful history reduce the inaccurate diagnoses of degenerative disorders.

References

Benson DF, Cummings JL, Tsai SY. Angular gyrus syndrome simulating Alzheimer disease. *Arch Neurol.* 1982;39:616–620.

Fisher CM. Lacunar strokes and infarcts: a review. *Neurology.* 1982;32:871–876.

Roux FE, Boetto S, Sacko O, et al. Writing, calculating, and finger recognition in the region of the angular gyrus: a cortical stimulation study of Gerstmann syndrome. *J Neurosurg.* 2003;99:716–727.

Chapter 18
Delirium

1. A 75-year-old man with Parkinson's disease treated with carbidopa/levodopa has minimal cognitive impairment. He has a long history of bipolar disorder treated with lithium carbonate despite mild chronic renal failure. He is hospitalized for a transurethral resection of the prostate, and an indwelling catheter is placed postoperatively. He is eating and drinking poorly. The next day, he is somnolent and grossly confused with an ataxic gait. The most likely cause of his confusion is

   a. Urinary tract infection
   b. Dehydration
   c. Worsening renal failure
   d. Lithium toxicity
   e. Worsening Parkinson's disease

The correct answer is d.

A urinary tract infection is certainly a possibility in a patient with an indwelling catheter, but it is unlikely it would cause confusion by the first postoperative day. Dehydration can also cause confusion, but it is also unlikely to develop over 1 day. Worsening renal failure is a possibility, but there is no evidence to suggest this. Worsening Parkin-

son's disease could cause the ataxic gait but is unlikely to cause somno-
lence. Lithium toxicity is the most likely cause in an elderly man who
already has impaired renal function and is drinking poorly.

References

Brauer C, Morrison RS, Silberzwerg SB, et al. The cause of delirium in patients
    with hip fracture. *Arch Intern Med.* 2000;160:1856–1860.
Francis J, Martin D, Kapoor WN. A prospective study of delirium in hospital-
    ized elderly. *JAMA.* 1990; 263: 1097–1101.

2. An 80-year-old man presents to the emergency room with a cough and
   fever. His wife reports that he has been showing progressive memory
   problems for several years. In addition, for many years he has had two
   to three cocktails with dinner every night. Chest x-ray shows pneumonia, and he is admitted and given intravenous antibiotics. On his third
   day in the hospital, he is disoriented and inattentive and complains of
   seeing bugs on the wall; he becomes agitated, sweaty, and tachycardic.
   The most likely diagnosis is

   a. Delirium caused by pneumonia
   b. Delirium caused by alcohol withdrawal
   c. Delirium caused by an allergy to antibiotics
   d. New onset of late-life schizophrenia
   e. Worsening dementia

   The correct answer is b.

   Pneumonia can cause delirium, but that diagnosis would be more
   likely if he presented delirious to the emergency room. Delirium is
   unlikely to be caused by a drug allergy. Late-life schizophrenia does
   not present with disorientation and inattention. Dementia is usually
   slowly progressive and not associated with tachycardia. Alcohol withdrawal is the most likely cause given the time course, the tachycardia,
   and the visual hallucinations.

   References

   American Psychiatric Association. Practice guideline for the treatment of pa-
       tients with delirium. *Am J Psychiatry.* 1999;156(5 suppl):1–20.
   Lipowski ZJ. *Delirium: Acute Confusional States.* New York, NY: Oxford
       University Press; 1990.

3. For a delirious 80-year-old man who is in the intensive care unit and
   showing signs of alcohol withdrawal, what would be the most appropriate specific treatment for his delirium?

   a. Intravenous haloperidol
   b. Intravenous lorazepam

c. Reassurance
d. Intravenous carbamazepine
e. Intravenous hydration

The correct answer is b.

Reassurance is always appropriate and helpful in the management of delirium but is nonspecific. Intravenous hydration is also nonspecific. Intravenous haloperidol is often used for treating delirium but is not specific to delirium caused by alcohol withdrawal. Currently, intravenous lorazepam is the treatment of choice, with carbamazepine used if the patient is having seizures.

Reference

Mayo-Smith MF. Pharmacological management of alcohol withdrawal: a meta-analysis and evidence-based practice guideline. *JAMA*. 1997;278:144–151.

4. An 89-year-old woman presents to an emergency room after slipping on the ice outside her apartment. X-rays show swelling but no fracture. She has difficulty walking, is weak and hypotensive, and is admitted to the hospital. She is given acetaminophen with codeine for her pain. Electrocardiogram shows new atrial fibrillation, and she is started on digoxin. She complains that she cannot fall asleep and is given 5 mg zolpidem. The next morning, her nephew comes in to see her and finds her somnolent and quite confused. He tells the doctor that for the last year he has been paying her bills because she was forgetting to do so, and her electricity was almost shut off. The most important predisposing factor in the development of her delirium is

a. Preexisting cognitive impairment
b. Vision impairment
c. Severe illness
d. Age

The correct answer is a.

This patient clearly has preexisting cognitive impairment that predisposes her to develop delirium. Age alone is not an independent risk factor for delirium. She has no severe illness, and there is no mention of vision impairment.

Reference

Inouye SK, Viscoli CM, Horwitz RI, et al. A predictive model for delirium in hospitalized elderly medical patients based on admission characteristics. *Ann Intern Med*. 1993;119:474–481.

5. Considering the vignette in question 4 and putting aside the importance of preexisting cognitive impairment as a predisposing factor, the
most important *precipitating* factor associated with the development
of her delirium is

    a. Atrial fibrillation
    b. Soft-tissue injury
    c. Sleep deprivation
    d. Addition of three new medications

The correct answer is d.

Whenever multiple new medications are added to a patient's regimen
and the patient develops delirium, it is likely that the medications are
the cause. If possible, the medications should be stopped to see if the
delirium clears. New onset atrial fibrillation on it own is unlikely to
induce delirium. Chronic sleep disturbance may worsen preexisting
cognitive impairment but does not produce this degree of cognitive
interference. Significant physical injury such as a major fracture may
precipitate delirium but bruising and soft-tissue swelling is unlikely to
do so.

Reference

Inouye SK, Charpentier PA. Precipitating factors for delirium in hospitalized
    elderly persons: predictive model and interrelationship with baseline vul-
    nerability. *JAMA.* 1996;275:852–857.

Chapter 19
Other Dementias and Mental Disorders
Due to General Medical Conditions

1. A 64-year-old married lawyer was assessed at a psychiatric outpatient
clinic. He was referred by his family doctor because of a "personality
change." He had always been perfectionistic, hardworking, and highly
professional, but over the previous 12 months, he had become less
motivated and less interested in his practice. He had become overly
familiar with his clients and was noted to make inappropriate comments, often with a sexual connotation. He was much less careful with
his appearance and was somewhat disheveled. He voiced no concerns.
He had become unreliable and had begun to drink excessive amounts
of alcohol. He had experienced one episode of depression a year and
a half earlier, which had lasted for a period of about 2 months. He
scored 27/30 on the Mini-Mental State Examination, losing 2 points
for attention and 1 point for recall. He was able to recall the forgotten

word with cuing. Neurological examination was normal except for the presence of palmomental and snout reflexes. Laboratory tests were unremarkable, and a computerized tomographic (CT) scan showed mild nonspecific cerebral atrophy. A single-photon emission computed tomographic scan of the brain showed decreased perfusion in frontal regions. The most likely diagnosis in the case is

a. Major depressive episode
b. Vascular dementia
c. Mixed dementia
d. Frontotemporal dementia (FTD)
e. Dementia with Lewy bodies (DLB)

The correct answer is d.

Mr. A demonstrates elements of all of the core diagnostic features of FTD, which include (a) insidious onset and gradual progression; (b) early decline in social interpersonal conduct; (c) early impairment in regulation of personal conduct; (d) early emotional blunting; and (e) early loss of insight (Neary et al., 1998). His clinical presentation would suggest features of the "disinhibited form" of FTD, which may be associated with pathological changes in the orbital-medial-frontal and anterior-temporal regions. The presence of primitive reflexes is also characteristic of FTD. Major depressive episode is a consideration but is unlikely to present with sexual disinhibition and primitive reflexes. Vascular dementia can coexist with other forms of dementia, but there are no risk factors noted, such as hypertension, cardiovascular impairment, or history of transient ischemic attack. The features of DLB are not noted, such as parkinsonism and psychosis with hallucinations.

References

Galasko D, Katzman R, Salmon D, et al. Clinical and neuropathological findings in Lewy body dementias. *Brain Cogn.*1996;31:166–175.
McKhann GM, Albert MS, Grossman M, et al. Clinical and pathological diagnosis of frontotemporal dementia: report of the Work Group on Frontotemporal Dementia and Pick's Disease. *Arch Neurol.* 2001;58:1803–1809.
Neary D, Snowden JS, Gustafson L, et al. Frontotemporal lobar degeneration: a consensus on clinical diagnostic criteria. *Neurology.* 1998;51:1546–1554.

2. A patient who has a frontotemporal dementia has recently begun to display more behavioral problems. He had become increasingly disinhibited and intrusive. He was very inappropriate, asking strangers for money and was highly agitated on occasion, swearing and making hos-

tile gestures. There is conclusive evidence that the best medication for first-line treatment is

a. An atypical antipsychotic
b. A serotonergic antidepressant
c. A benzodiazepine
d. A cholinesterase inhibitor
e. None of the above

The correct answer is e.

Medication treatment for this disorder remains an area in which few controlled trials have been done. Some data but not all suggest that serotonergic antidepressants may offer symptomatic benefits. Also, a randomized, controlled trial with trazodone in dosages up to 300 mg qd found a significant decrease in the Neuropsychiatric Inventory total score. Clinical reports suggest some utility for cholinesterase inhibitors, but this is unconfirmed in controlled studies, and there are few data on other drugs.

References

Deakin JB, Rahman S, Nestor PJ, Hodges JR, Sahakian BJ. Paroxetine does not improve symptoms and impairs cognition in frontotemporal dementia: a double-blind randomized controlled trial. *Psychopharmacology (Berl)*. 2004;172:400–408.

Lebert F, Stekke W, Hasenbroekx C, Pasquier F. Frontotemporal dementia: a randomised, controlled trial with trazodone. *Dement Geriatr Cogn Disord*. 2004;17:355–359.

Moretti R, Torre P, Antonello R, et al. Frontotemporal dementia: paroxetine as a possible treatment of behavior symptoms. *Eur Neurol*. 2003;49: 13–19.

Swartz JR, Miller BL, Lesser IM, Darby AL. Frontotemporal dementia: treatment response to serotonin selective reuptake inhibitors. *J Clin Psychiatry*. 1997;58:212–216.

3. A 72-year-old married retired seamstress was referred to a memory clinic because of increasing forgetfulness with significant symptoms of anxiety and distress. She complained that she saw "mites" flying around her apartment. She noted that these mites would sometimes talk to her, and she believed that they were "dead souls" who had come back to life. She also described seeing children running around her sofa. Her family reported that at times she seemed reasonably alert and oriented, but at other times she appeared to be totally confused. On examination, there was evidence of a mild pill-rolling tremor and some bradykinesia, which had been present for about 6 months. She was anxious but denied significant depression. She scored 24/30 on

the Mini-Mental State Examination, losing points for attention, short-term memory, and visuospatial function. She had great difficulty drawing the face of a clock, in particular having difficulty spacing the numbers. Her family doctor had started her on low-dose loxapine because of the hallucinations. Shortly thereafter, she had developed an acute dystonic reaction, especially a very stiff neck. The most likely diagnosis in this case is

a. Alzheimer's disease
b. Mixed dementia
c. Frontotemporal dementia
d. Late-onset schizophrenia
e. Dementia with Lewy bodies

The correct answer is e.

This lady presents with at least two of the three core features essential for a diagnosis of probable DLB. She has recurrent visual hallucinations, which are well formed and detailed and has spontaneous motor features of parkinsonism. She also has possible evidence of fluctuating cognition, with pronounced variations in attention and alertness, as described by her family. Other features, which can be supportive of DLB, include repeated falls, syncope, transient loss of consciousness, neuroleptic sensitivity, systematized delusions, and hallucinations in other modalities (McKeith et al., 1996). Alzheimer's disease is not likely to present with early symptoms of psychosis with florid visual hallucinations and marked parkinsonism. Frontotemporal dementia is more likely to present with personality changes rather than psychosis. The psychosis of late-onset schizophrenia is more likely to be characterized by paranoid delusions and auditory hallucinations than florid visual hallucinations and is not usually associated with parkinsonism or exquisite sensitivity to neuroleptic medication.

Reference

McKeith IG, Galasko D, Kosaka K, et al. Consensus guidelines for the clinical and pathologic diagnosis of dementia with Lewy bodies (DLB): report of the Consortium on DLB International Workshop. *Neurology.* 1996;47: 1113–1124.

4. You are asked for a treatment recommendation for a patient with DLB who is experiencing vivid visual hallucinations accompanied by significant distress and agitation. Her family doctor had started her on low-dose haloperidol because of the hallucinations. Shortly thereafter, she developed marked parkinsonism. Which of the following class of medication would you initially recommend to her family physician?

a. An atypical antipsychotic
b. A serotonergic antidepressant
c. A mood stabilizer
d. A benzodiazepine
e. A cholinesterase inhibitor

The correct answer is e.

There is evidence of significant cholinergic deficit in DLB. One large, randomized, controlled trial of the cholinesterase inhibitor rivastigmine demonstrated significant effectiveness compared to placebo in reducing the core neuropsychiatric symptoms of DLB (McKeith et al., 2000). The subjects were less apathetic, had less anxiety, and had fewer delusions and hallucinations while receiving treatment. Although more data are necessary, based on current data the treatment of choice would be a cholinesterase inhibitor. There may be an occasional role for atypical antipsychotic medications in patients with severe psychotic symptoms that are causing extreme distress or dysfunction. Because patients with DLB frequently have extreme sensitivity to the extrapyramidal side effects of neuroleptics, clinicians are advised to explore other treatments and generally avoid antipsychotic medications. Even atypical antipsychotics are used with caution. Many clinicians consider quetiapine to be the antipsychotic medication of choice in DLB because of its very low propensity to cause extrapyramidal symptoms.

References

Fernandez HH, Wu CK, Ott BR. Pharmacotherapy of dementia with Lewy bodies. *Expert Opin Pharmacother*. 2003;4:2027–2037.

Masterman D. Cholinesterase inhibitors in the treatment of Alzheimer's disease and related dementias. *Clin Geriatr Med*. 2004;20:59–68.

McKeith I, Del Ser T, Spano P, et al. Efficacy of rivastigmine in dementia with Lewy bodies: a randomised, double-blind, placebo-controlled international study. *Lancet*. 2000;356:2031–2036.

McKeith JG, Galasko D, Kosaka K, et al. Consensus guidelines for the clinical and pathologic diagnosis of dementia with Lewy bodies (DLB): Report of the Consortium on DLB International Workshop. *Neurology*. 1996;47: 1113–1124.

Wild R, Pettit T, Burns A. Cholinesterase inhibitors for dementia with Lewy bodies. *Cochrane Database Syst Rev*. 2003;3:CD003672.

5. A 54-year-old engineer was referred to a psychiatric outpatient clinic because of apathy and irritability. He also complained of some mild memory loss. In recent months, he had developed some unusual movements of his arms and legs, which were nonrepetitive, jerky, and abrupt. He admitted to feelings of depression. On examination, he had

mild word-finding difficulty, and there was evidence of mild memory loss with delayed responses to questions. He also demonstrated difficulty with frontal systems tasks, including visual pattern completion tests, tests of alternating motor patterns, and the go/no go test. There was a family history of mood disorders, suicide, and presenile dementia. His father developed dementia in his late 40s and died in a nursing home at age 60. The most likely diagnosis is

a. Parkinson disease
b. Frontotemporal dementia
c. Amyotrophic lateral sclerosis
d. Huntington disease
e. Toxic encephalopathy

The correct answer is d.

The abnormal movements and family history strongly suggest a diagnosis of Huntington's disease, which is an idiopathic degenerative disease characterized by dementia and chorea. It is inherited as an autosomal dominant trait, with approximately 50% of the children affected. The first mental status changes are usually irritability, untidiness, loss of interest, and other personality changes. The pattern of dementia is primarily subcortical. Language problems include mild word-finding difficulty, impaired verbal fluency, and dysarthria. Subjects tend to perform poorly on frontal systems tasks. In this case, a CT scan demonstrated atrophy of the caudate nuclei, which is a common finding. Affective illness occurs in more than 50% of patients, and many also develop psychotic features. In the early stages of the disorder, the patient may be misdiagnosed. In a recent case report, diagnoses of depression, Ganser syndrome, and schizophrenia were made before the development of chorea.

References

Caine ED, Shoulson I. Psychiatric syndromes in Huntington's disease. *Am J Psychiatry*. 1983;140:728–733.

MacDonald ME, Gines S, Gusella JF, Wheeler VC. Huntington's disease. *Neuromolecular Med*. 2003;4:7–20.

Pflanz S, Besson JA, Ebmeier KP, Simpson S. The clinical manifestation of mental disorder in Huntington's disease: a retrospective case record study of disease progression. *Acta Psychiatr Scand*. 1991;83:53–60.

Tost H, Wendt CS, Schmitt A, Heinz A, Braus DF. Huntington's disease: phenomenological diversity of a neuropsychiatric condition that challenges traditional concepts in neurology and psychiatry. *Am J Psychiatry*. 2004;161:2834.

Chapter 20
Grief and Bereavement

1. The duration of "normal" grief is

    a. 4–8 weeks
    b. 2–12 months
    c. 12–24 months
    d. >2 years

    The correct answer is d.

    Although the intensity of mourning lessens with time, for many individuals grief is lifelong; pangs of grief continue to be triggered by reminders of the deceased person or by anniversaries. Many bereaved individuals maintain continuing "contact" with the deceased in various symbolic and psychological ways. Studies lasting for 2 years postbereavement have found manifestation of grief lasting at least that long for a number of bereaved individuals.

    References

    Goin MK, Burgoyne RW, Goin JM. Timeless attachment to a dead relative. *Am J Psychiatry.* 1979;136:988–989.
    Harlow SD, Goldberg EL, Comstock GW. A longitudinal study of the prevalence of depressive symptomatology in elderly widowed and married women. *Arch Gen Psychiatry.* 1991;48:1065–1068.
    Klass D, Goss R. Spiritual bonds to the dead in cross-cultural and historical perspective: comparative religion and modern grief. *Death Stud.* 1999;23: 6:547–567.
    Zisook S, Shuchter SR. Major depression associated with widowhood. *Am J Geriatr Psychiatry.* 1993;1:316–326.

2. The percentage of bereaved individuals meeting symptomatic criteria for major depression 2 months after the death of their spouse is

    a. 5%–10%
    b. 10%–30%
    c. 30%–50%
    d. >50%

    The correct answer is b.

    Although almost all widows and widowers consider themselves to be grieving 2 months after their loss, only 30% experience "dysphoria" most of the time, on most days, for 2 or more weeks. Only two thirds of these, or 20% of the total widowed population, meet full criteria for major depression at 2 months.

References

Futterman A, Gallagher D, Thompson LW, et al. Retrospective assessment of marital adjustment and depression during the first two years of spousal bereavement. *Psychol Aging.* 1990;5:277–283.

Gilewski MJ, Farberow NL, Gallagher DE, et al. Interaction of depression and bereavement on mental health in the elderly. *Psychol Aging.* 1991;6:67–75.

Zisook S, Shuchter SR. Depression through the first year after the death of a spouse. *Am J Psychiatry.* 1991;148:1346–1352.

3. The best clue for differentiating normal bereavement from major depression are

   a. Time since death
   b. Feelings of worthlessness, psychomotor retardation, and suicidal ideation
   c. A positive dexamethone suppression test
   d. The nature of the relationship with the deceased

The correct answer is b.

The *Diagnostic and Statistical Manual of Mental Disorders, Fourth Edition* (DSM-IV; 1994) says that if a major depressive syndrome begins after the death of a spouse and ends within 2 months, it may be compatible with a V-Code of bereavement rather than major depression. Even within that time frame, however, severity of depression, marked impairment, and the symptoms of morbid worthlessness or guilt, psychomotor retardation, or suicidal ideation should prompt the consideration of a major depressive episode.

References

American Psychiatric Association. *Diagnostic and Statistical Manual of Mental Disorders.* 4th ed. Washington, DC: American Psychiatric Association; 1994.

Breckenridge JN, Gallagher D, Thompson LW, et al. Characteristic depressive symptoms of bereaved elders. *J Gerontol.* 1986;41:163–168.

Bruce M, Kim K, Leaf P, et al. Depressive episodes and dysphoria resulting from conjugal bereavement in a prospective community sample. *Am J Psychiatry.* 1990;147:608–611.

Gallagher-Thompson DE, Breckenridge JN, Thompson LW. Similarities and differences between normal grief and depression in older adults. *Essence.* 1982;5:127–140.

4. Which of the following is most likely to be associated with grief complications?

   a. Looking for the deceased in crowds more than 2 months after the death
   b. Visual images of the deceased
   c. Dreams of the deceased
   d. A past history of recurrent major depression

The correct answer is d.

There are many ways bereaved individuals continue to maintain relationships with their deceased loved ones. These include thoughts that the deceased is looking out for them, searching for the deceased in crowds (for months, if not years, in some cases), and dreams of the deceased (which actually increase in frequency over the first year or two). These have no pathological significance and may be adaptive. On the other hand, a past history of major depression is a significant risk for depression precipitated by loss.

References

Field NP, Nichols C, Holen A, et al. The relation of continuing attachment to adjustment in conjugal bereavement. *J Consult Clin Psychol.* 1999;67: 212–218.

Klass D, Goss R. Spiritual bonds to the dead in cross-cultural and historical perspective: comparative religion and modern grief. *Death Stud.* 1999;23: 547–567.

Shuchter SR. *Dimensions of Grief: Adjusting to the Death of a Spouse.* San Francisco, CA: Jossey-Bass; 1986.

Zisook S, Shuchter SR. Major depression associated with widowhood. *Am J Geriatr Psychiatry,* 1993;1:316–326.

5. For bereaved persons who develop a bereavement-related depression,

   a. Pharmacological treatment alone is ineffective
   b. Psychotherapy interferes with the grief work
   c. Antidepressant medication plus psychotherapy is a preferred treatment
   d. Treatment may prolong grief reaction

The correct answer is c.

Although bereavement-related depressions are rarely treated, sometimes because of the outdated notion that treatment interferes with grief, several open and one controlled study consistently showed efficacy of treatment. In all cases, improvement in grief intensity occurred simultaneously with treatment for the depression. The only controlled study found a combination of interpersonal psychotherapy and/or antidepressant medication to be the most effective approach.

References

Jacobs SC, Nelson JC, Zisook S. Treating depression of bereavement with antidepressants: a pilot study. *Psychiatr Clin North Am.* 1987;10:501–510.

Pasternak RE, Reynolds CF III, Schlernitzauer M, et al. Acute open-trial nortriptyline therapy of bereavement-related depression in late life. *J Clin Psychiatry.* 1991;52:307–310.

Reynolds CF III, Miller MD, Pasternak RE, et al. Treatment of bereavement-related major depressive episodes in later life: a controlled study of acute and continuation treatment with nortriptyline and interpersonal psychotherapy. *Am J Psychiatry.* 1999;156:202–208.

Zygmont M, Prigerson HG, Houck PR, et al. A post hoc comparison of paroxetine and nortriptyline for symptoms of traumatic grief. *J Clin Psychiatry.* 1998;59:241–245.

6. Posttraumatic stress disorder (PTSD) following bereavement

   a. By definition does not exist; bereavement does not fulfill the A (stressor) criterion
   b. Occurs only after an unnatural death (e.g., suicide, homicide, or accident)
   c. Is the most frequently seen form of PTSD in Detroit, Michigan
   d. Is benign

The correct answer is c.

A change in *DSM-IV* (American Psychiatric Association, 1994) from previous diagnostic manuals is that it allows for bereavement to be considered a stress criterion. Using the new criteria in a community-dwelling Detroit sample, Breslau et al. (1998) found that PTSD after the sudden/unexpected loss of a loved one was the most common form of PTSD. Two other investigators found that PTSD occurs in the wake of bereavement, even when the death was caused by a chronic illness.

References

American Psychiatric Association. *Diagnostic and Statistical Manual of Mental Disorders.* 4th ed. Washington, DC: American Psychiatric Association; 1994.

Breslau N, Kessler RC, Chilcoat HD, et al. Trauma and posttraumatic stress disorder in the community: the 1996 Detroit Area Survey of Trauma. *Arch Gen Psychiatry.* 1998; 55:626–632.

Schut HAW, de Keijser J, van den Bout J. Incidence and prevalence of post traumatic stress symptomatology in the conjugally bereaved. Paper pre-

sented at: Third International Conference on Grief and Bereavement in
Contemporary Society; June/July 1991; Sydney, Australia.

Zisook S, Chentsova-Dutton Y, Shuchter SR. PTSD following bereavement.
Ann Clin Psychiatry. 1998;10:157–163.

7. After the death of a spouse

   a. Many (>20%) men develop a new intimate relationship or remarry
      within 2 years
   b. Most (>50%) women develop a new intimate relationship or re-
      marry within 2 years
   c. Widows should be discouraged from getting involved in new rela-
      tionships for at least 1 year after the death of a spouse
   d. Widowers who remarry have higher rates of depression than wid-
      owers who do not

The correct answer is a.

After the death of a spouse, many widows and widowers develop new
intimate relationships or remarry. Widowers are more likely than widows to find a mate, especially men with good education and income.
Older widows are less likely than younger widows to find new intimate partners or remarry. For both widows and widowers, remarriage
has been associated with positive outcomes.

Reference

Schneider DS, Sledge PA, Shuchter SR, et al. Dating and remarriage over the
first 2 years of widowhood. *Ann Clin Psychiatry.* 1996;8:51–57.

8. The strongest predictors of making a good adjustment to bereavement
   include

   a. Gender and age
   b. Positive self-esteem and personal competencies
   c. An ambivalent relationship with the deceased
   d. Intense early grief reactions

The correct answer is b.

Personal resources, such as resiliency, self-esteem, and competence in
managing the tasks of daily life have been the strongest predictors of
good adjustment to bereavement. The data on gender and age are
equivocal. Some had found overly ambivalent or dependent relationships predicted poor outcome. Often, individuals who grieve intensely
early on continue to grieve intensely at follow-up; on the other hand,

the long-term effects of a relatively attenuated grief reaction likely are benign.

References

Clayton PJ. Bereavement and depression. *J Clin Psychiatry*. 1990;51:34–40.

Cleirin MPHD. *Adaption After Bereavement*. Leiden, The Netherlands: DSWO Press; 1991.

Lund DA, Caserta MS, Dimond MF. The course of spousal bereavement in later life. In: Stroebe MS, Stroebe W, Hansson RO, eds. *Handbook of Bereavement: Theory, Research and Intervention*. Cambridge, UK: Cambridge University Press; 1993:240–254.

Norris FH, Murrell SA. Social support, life events, and stress as modifiers of adjustment to bereavement by older adults. *Psychol Aging*. 1990;5:429–436.

Wortman CB, Silver RC. The myths of coping with loss. *J Consult Clin Psychol*. 1989;57:349–357.

Zisook S, Shuchter SR. Depression through the first year after the death of a spouse. *Am J Psychiatry*. 1991;148:1346–1352.

9. Among women aged 65 years or older, what percentage have been widowed one or more times?

   a. 10%
   b. 20%
   c. 30%
   d. 40%
   e. 50%

The correct answer is e.

According to US Census Bureau(1997) statistics, 50% of women and 10% of men 65 years and older have been widowed at least once. There are over 900,000 new widows and widowers every year in the United States.

Reference

US Bureau of the Census. *Statistical Abstract of the United States*. 117th ed. Washington, DC: US Government Printing Office; 1997.

10. All of the following are risk factors for bereavement-related depression *except*

    a. Early intense reactions soon after the loss
    b. Female gender
    c. Family history of depression
    d. Increased alcohol use soon after the loss
    e. Poor physical health

The correct answer is b.

The risk factors listed above, as well as the presence of a major depressive syndrome soon after the loss, classified over 90% of widows and widowers in terms of major depression 2 years after the loss. Data on the association of gender with risk for bereavement-related depression are conflicting.

References

Bruce M, Kim K, Leaf P, et al. Depressive episodes and dysphoria resulting from conjugal bereavement in a prospective community sample. *Am J Psychiatry*. 1990;147:608–611.

Clayton PJ. Bereavement and depression. *J Clin Psychiatry*. 1990;51:34–40.

Gallagher-Thompson DE, Breckenridge J, Thompson LW, et al. Effects of bereavement on indicators of mental health in elderly widows and widowers. *J Gerontol*. 1983;38:565–571.

Zisook S, Shuchter SR. Depression through the first year after the death of a spouse. *Am J Psychiatry*. 1991;148:1346–1352.

Zisook S, Shuchter SR. Major depression associated with widowhood. *Am J Geriatr Psychiatry*. 1993;1:316–326.

Chapter 21
Late-Life Mood Disorders

1. Which of the following statements about pseudodementia in geriatric patients is correct?

   a. It is common in depressed elderly patients with histrionic personality disorder
   b. It represents a catastrophic reaction
   c. It has a benign long-term outcome
   d. After the initial cognitive improvement, a considerable number of patients progress to dementia over a period of a few years
   e. It occurs principally in patients with recurrent depression

The correct answer is d.

Unlike pseudodementia of younger adults, which occurs in the context of a variety of psychiatric diagnoses, geriatric pseudodementia develops during severe major depression. Most elders with depressive pseudodementia have their first depressive episode in late life. Many depressed elderly patients remain with some cognitive impairment even after improvement of depression, although they may not meet criteria for dementia. Even patients with significant cognitive recovery have high rates of irreversible dementia (about 40% within 3 years) on follow-up. Most of these patients do not meet criteria for dementia for 1–2 years after the initial episode of depression with reversible dementia. Therefore, identification of a reversible dementia syndrome in elderly depressives constitutes an indication for thorough diagnostic workup aimed at the identification of treatable dementing disorders and for frequent follow-up.

Reference

Alexopoulos GS, Meyers BS, Young RC, Mattis S, Kakuma T. The course of geriatric depression with "reversible dementia": A controlled study. *Am J Psychiatry.* 1993;150:1693–1699.

2. Which of the following statements about the medical burden of depression in elderly patients is correct?

   a. Geriatric depression occurs in the context of multiple medical illnesses
   b. Depression increases mortality
   c. Depression increases medical morbidity
   d. Depression worsens the outcomes of medical disorders
   e. All of the above

The correct answer is e.

The prevalence of geriatric depression is much higher in medical settings than in the community. In medically hospitalized patients, major depression occurs in 11%, and less severe, yet clinically significant, depressive symptomatology is identified in 25% of the population. Elders who reside in long-term care settings suffer higher rates of depression than those living in the community, and half of those relocated to nursing homes are at increased risk for depression. Depression estimates in nursing home residents range from 12% to 22.4% for major depression and an additional 17%–30% for minor depression. Primary care patients with any medical diagnosis were twice as likely to have depression as patients without a medical diagnosis. The total mean number of medical diagnoses in depressed patients was 7.9 compared to 3.0 medical diagnoses in nondepressed patients. These differences persisted when the elderly group was examined separately.

Depression is associated with increased mortality. Increased mortality has been documented in hospitalized patients even when the severity of medical illnesses and disability is controlled. It has been reported that presence of major depression on admission to a nursing home increases the likelihood of death 1 year later by 59%. The effect of depression on mortality was independent of other medical health parameters.

Depressive symptoms, especially chronic symptoms, are associated with more medical morbidity than other psychiatric disorders of late life. In older community residents, long-term depressive symptoms had an adverse impact on health. In contrast, medical burden contributed only to short-lived depressive symptoms. In elderly medical inpatients, those with six depressive symptoms had greater comorbid illness, cognitive impairment, and functional impairment.

Depression adversely affects the prognosis of comorbid disease, as suggested by evidence of prolonged recovery from illness, long hospital stays, increased medical complications, and earlier mortality in depressed patients. Increased mortality risk has been reported in depressed compared to nondepressed medical and psychiatric patients. Depression after surgery has been associated with poorer recovery in both functional and psychosocial status.

References

Burrows AB, Satlin A, Salzman C, Nobel K, Lipsitz L. Depression in a long-term care facility: clinical features and discordance between nursing assessment and patient interviews. *J Am Geriatr Soc.* 1995;43:1118–1122.

Cooper PL, Crum RM, Ford DE. Characteristics of patients with major depression who received care in general medical and specialty mental health settings. *Med Care.* 1994;32:15–24.

Covinsky KE, Kahana E, Chin MH, Palmer RM, Fortinsky RH, Landefeld CS. Depressive symptoms and 3-year mortality in older hospitalized medical patients. *Ann Intern Med.* 1999;130:563–569.

Covinsky KE, Palmer RM, Kresevic DM, et al. Improving functional outcomes in older patients: lessons from an acute care for elders unit. *J Qual Improve.* 1998;24:63–76.

Jorm AF, Henderson AJ, Kaye DW, Jacomb PA. Mortality in relation to dementia, depression and social interaction in an elderly community sample. *Int J Geriatr Psychiatry.* 1991;6:5–11.

Katz IR, Parmelee PA, Streim JE. Depression in older patients in residential care: significance of dysphoria and dimensional assessment. *Am J Geriatr Psychiatry.* 1995;3:161–169.

Lacro JP, Jeste DV. Physical comorbidity and polypharmacy in older psychiatric patients. *Biol Psychiatry.* 1994;36:146–152.

Luber MP, Hollenberg JP, Williams-Russo P, et al. Diagnosis, treatment, comorbidity, and resource utilization in patients in a general medical practice. *Int J Psychiatry Med.* 2000;30:1–13.

Meeks S, Murrell SA, Mehl RC. Longitudinal relationships between depressive symptoms and health in normal older and middle-aged adults. *Psychol Aging.* 2000;15:100–109.

Mossey JM, Mutran E, Knott K, Craik R. Determinants of recovery 12 months after hip fracture: the importance of psychosocial factors. *Am J Public Health.* 1989;79:279–286.

Murphy E, Smith R, Lindesay J, Slattery J. Increased mortality rates in late-life depression. *Br J Psychiatry.* 1988;152:347–353.

Parmelee PA, Katz IR, Lawton MP. Depression among institutionalized aged: assessment and prevalence estimation. *J Gerontol.* 1989;44:M22–M29.

Rovner BW. Depression and increased risk of mortality in the nursing home patient. *Am J Med.* 1993;94:19–22.

Shamash K, O'Connell K, Lowy MM, Katona CLE. Psychiatric morbidity and outcome in elderly patients undergoing emergency hip surgery: a 1 year follow-up study. *Int J Geriatr Psychiatry.* 1992;7:505–509.

3. Which of the following statements about disability is correct?

   a. Depression is the ninth leading cause of disability in the United States
   b. Deficits in initiation and perseveration seem to have a stronger relationship to instrumental activities of daily living (IADL) impairment than other cognitive impairments in depressed elderly patients
   c. Although disability compromises quality of life, it does not increase the risk for specific medical disorders
   d. Once disability develops, improvement of depressive symptoms rarely leads to a substantial reduction of disability
   e. In most depressed elders, disability can be fully explained by the severity of depression, medical burden, and cognitive impairment

The correct answer is b.

Depression is the second leading cause of disability in the United States. Disability has various negative outcomes, including increased morbidity for specific medical conditions (e.g., gastrointestinal bleeding). Severity of depression, cognitive impairment, and medical burden appear to predict approximately 40% of the variance in IADL. Therefore, although disability has a reciprocal relationship with psychiatric and medical disorders, it constitutes a distinct dimension of health status. Nonetheless, the course of disability parallels the course of depression. Reduction in the levels of depression was shown to result in approximately 50% reduction in days burdened by disability 1 year later. In depressed patients with chronic obstructive pulmonary disease, nortriptyline was superior to placebo in improving both depression and day-to-day function, although it did not influence the physiological measures of pulmonary insufficiency. Executive dysfunction (initiation–perseveration) was found to have a stronger relationship to IADL impairment than other cognitive impairments in depressed elderly patients. A similar association between executive dysfunction and disability was reported in nondepressed patients with mild-to-moderate Alzheimer's disease.

References

Alexopoulos GS, Vrontou C, Kakuma T, et al. Disability in geriatric depression. *Am J Psychiatry*. 1996d;153:877–885.

Borson S, McDonald GJ, Gayle T, Deffenbach M, Lakshminarayan S, Van Tuinen C. Improvement in mood, physical symptoms, and function with nortriptyline for depression in patients with chronic obstructive pulmonary disease. *Psychosomatics*. 1992;33:190–201.

Chen ST, Sultzer DL, Hinkin CH, Mahler ME, Cummings JL. Executive dysfunction in Alzheimer's disease: association with neuropsychiatric symptoms and functional impairment. *J Neuropsychiatr Clin Neurosci*. 1998; 10:426–432.

Guralnik JM, LaCroix AZ, Branch LG, Kasl SV, Wallace RB. Morbidity and disability in older persons in the years prior to death. *Am J Public Health*. 1991;81:443–447.

Kiosses DN, Alexopoulos GS, Murphy C. Symptoms of striatofrontal dysfunction contribute to disability in geriatric depression. *Int J Geriatr Psychiatry*. 2000;15:992–999.

Murray CGL, Lopez AD. Alternative projections of mortality and disability by cause 1990–2020: global burden of disease study. *Lancet*. 1997;349: 1498–1504.

Ormel J, Von Koroff M, Van Den Brink W, Katon W, Brilman E, Oldehinkel T. Depression, anxiety and social disability show synchrony of change in primary care patients. *Am J Public Health*. 1993;83:385–390.

Pahor M, Guralnik JM, Salive ME, Chrischilles EA, Manto A, Wallace RB. Disability and severe gastrointestinal hemorrhage. A prospective study of community-dwelling older persons. *J Am Geriatr Soc*. 1994;42:816–825.

Von Korff M, Omel J, Katon W, Lin EHB. Disability and depression among high utilizers of health care: a longitudinal analysis. *Arch Gen Psychiatry*. 1992;49:91–100.

4. Which of the following statements about suicide and suicidal ideation in the elderly is correct?

   a. Female suicide rates continue to increase slightly during late life
   b. The rate of suicide for elderly individuals steadily decreased from the 1930s until today
   c. Suicide attempts and suicidal ideation decrease with aging
   d. Depression is the most common psychiatric diagnosis of suicide victims across the life span
   e. None of the above

The correct answer is c.

Suicide rates consistently increase in males and reach their highest level in the oldest age group. In contrast, female suicide rates increase slightly with age, peak in middle adulthood, and decline in late life. Although suicide is more frequent in elderly patients than in younger patients, the rate of suicide for elderly individuals steadily decreased from the 1930s to 1980. However, the suicide rate began to rise again in the 1980s. Despite the high frequency of suicide in late life, suicidal attempts and suicidal ideation decrease with aging. Older adults commit more carefully planned and lethal self-destructive acts and give fewer indications of suicidal intent. Therefore, although suicide attempts are more rare in old than young age, their lethality is increased. Depression is the most common psychiatric diagnosis in elderly suicide victims, unlike younger adults, for whom substance abuse alone or with comorbid mood disorders is the most frequent diagnosis.

References

Allen A, Blazer DG. Mood disorders. In: Sadavoy J, Lazarus LW, Jarvik LF, eds. *Comprehensive Review of Geriatric Psychiatry*. Washington, DC: American Psychiatric Press; 1991:337–351.

Carney SS, Rich CL, Burke PA, Fowler RC. Suicide over 60: The San Diego Study. *J Am Geriatr Soc*. 1994;42:174–180.

Conwell Y, Brent D. Suicide and aging I: patterns of psychiatric diagnoses. *Int Psychogeriatr*. 1995;7:149–164.

Conwell Y, Duberstein PR, Herrmann J, Forbes N, Caine ED. Age differences in behaviors leading to completed suicide. *Am J Geriatr Psychiatry*. 1998; 6:122–126.

Dennis MS, Lindesay J. Suicide in the elderly: the United Kingdom perspective. *Int Psychogeriatr*. 1995;7:263–274.

Henriksson MM, Marttunen MJ, Isometsä ET, et al. Mental disorders in elderly suicide. *Int Psychogeriatr*. 1995;7:275–286.

Meyers BS. Late-life delusional depression: acute and long-term treatment. *Int Psychogeriatr*. 1995;7(suppl):113–124.

Moscicki EK. Epidemiologic surveys as tools for studying behavior: a review. *Suic Life Threat Behav*. 1989;19:131–146.

National Center for Health Statistics. Advance report of final mortality statistics, 1989. *NCHS Monthly Vital Stat Rep*. 1992;40(8, suppl 2).

Wallace J, Pfohl B. Age-related differences in the symptomatic expression of major depression. *J Nerv Ment Dis*. 1995;183:99–102.

5. Which of the following statements about geriatric bipolar disorder is correct?

   a. Unlike early-onset mania, late-onset mania is associated with medical disorders or drug treatment
   b. Bipolar disorder is extremely uncommon in geriatric populations because of selective mortality

c. Late-onset bipolar patients have an equal rate of mood disorders among relatives as those with early-onset mania
d. Bipolar disorder increases mortality but not to the level of unipolar depressive disorder
e. None of the above

The correct answer is a.

No manic cases were identified in a sample of elderly persons participating in the Epidemiologic Catchment Area Study. Nonetheless, mania or hypomania constitutes 5%–10% of the diagnoses of elderly patients. It has been suggested that mania associated with medical disorders or drug treatment as a rule has onset after 40 years of age. Mania with onset during senescence is associated with coarse brain disease. Cerebrovascular disease, especially right-sided lesions, has been implicated in late-onset mania. Late-onset bipolar disorder patients have a lower rate of affective disorders among relatives compared with early-onset mania patients. The mortality rate for elderly bipolar disorder patients seems to be greater than the community base rate for this age group and appears to exceed that of geriatric patients with depression.

References

Dhingra U, Rabins PV. Mania in the elderly: a 5–7 year follow-up. *J Am Geriatr Soc.* 1991;39:581–583.

Kramer M, German PS, Anthony JC, Von Korff M, Skinner EA. Patterns of mental disorders among the elderly residents of eastern Baltimore. *J Am Geriatr Soc.* 1985;33:236–245.

Krauthammer C, Klerman GL. Secondary mania: manic syndromes associated with antecedent physical illness or drugs. *Arch Gen Psychiatry.* 1978;35: 1333–1339.

Shulman KI, Tohen M, Satlin A, Mallya G, Kalunian D. Mania compared with unipolar depression in old age. *Am J Psychiatry.* 1992;149:341–345.

Starkstein SE, Boston JD, Robinson RG. Mechanisms of mania after brain injury. Twelve case reports and review of the literature. *J Nerv Ment Dis.* 1988;176:87–100.

Young RC, Klerman GL. Mania in late life: focus on age at onset. *Am J Psychiatry.* 1992;149:867–876.

Chapter 22
Psychoses

1. Compared to patients with early-onset schizophrenia, those with late-onset schizophrenia

   a. Are more refractory to treatment with antipsychotic medications
   b. Are more likely to be diagnosed with the disorganized subtype of schizophrenia
   c. Are less likely to have held a job and have children
   d. Show less-severe negative symptoms
   e. Have a higher risk of suicide

   The correct answer is d.

   Compared to patients with early-onset schizophrenia, patients with late-onset schizophrenia (onset after age 40 or 45 years) show less-severe negative symptoms, tend to require lower doses of antipsychotic medications, and are more likely to have held a job and have children. Patients with late-onset schizophrenia are more likely to have paranoid schizophrenia and less likely to be diagnosed with the disorganized subtype of schizophrenia. Patients with late-onset schizophrenia do not have a higher risk of suicide compared to patients with early-onset schizophrenia; the increased rate of mortality in both groups is approximately equal.

   References

   Howard R, Rabins PV, Seeman MV, Jeste DV, and the International Late-Onset Schizophrenia Group. Late-onset schizophrenia and very-late-onset schizophrenia-like psychosis: an international consensus. *Am J Psychiatry.* 2000;157:172–178.

   Jeste DV, Caligiuri MP, Paulsen JS, et al. Risk of tardive dyskinesia in older patients: a prospective longitudinal study of 266 patients. *Arch Gen Psychiatry.* 1995;52:756–765.

   Jeste DV, Harris MJ, Pearlson GD, et al. Late-onset schizophrenia: studying clinical validity. *Psychiatr Clin North Am.* 1988;11:1–14.

2. Late-onset schizophrenia is characterized by all of the following statements *except*

   a. Higher incidence in women than men
   b. Association with premorbid antisocial personality
   c. Response to low doses of antipsychotic medications
   d. Stable cognitive deficits in most patients
   e. None of the above

The correct answer is b.

Abnormal premorbid personality traits of a paranoid or schizoid nature have been found in a sizable proportion of patients with late-onset schizophrenia. Premorbid antisocial personality traits have not been associated with late-onset schizophrenia.

References

Herbert ME, Jacobson S. Late paraphrenia. *Br J Psychiatry.* 1967;113:461–469.

Kay DWK, Roth M. Environmental and hereditary factors in the schizophrenias of old age ("late paraphrenia") and their bearing on the general problem of causation in schizophrenia. *J Ment Sci.* 1961;107:649–686.

3. Patients with very-late-onset schizophrenia-like psychosis (onset after age 60 years)

    a. Are more likely than patients with younger onset schizophrenia to have an underlying medical or neurological illness
    b. Usually have a history of poor premorbid social functioning
    c. Are difficult to treat with conventional or atypical antipsychotic medications
    d. Tend to have a family history of schizophrenia
    e. Show prominent negative symptoms

The correct answer is a.

Patients with very-late-onset schizophrenia-like psychosis (onset after age 60 years) are thought to represent a heterogeneous group whose illnesses represent underlying medical or neurological conditions predisposing these patients to psychotic symptoms. These patients are not more likely to have a history of poor premorbid social functioning and do not have higher rates of family history of schizophrenia. They respond to treatment with antipsychotic medications.

References

Howard R, Rabins PV, Seeman MV, Jeste DV, and the International Late-Onset Schizophrenia Group. Late-onset schizophrenia and very-late-onset schizophrenia-like psychosis: an international consensus. *Am J Psychiatry.* 2000;157:172–178.

Murray RM, O'Callaghan E, Castle DJ, Lewis SW. A neurodevelopmental approach to the classification of schizophrenia. *Schizophr Bull.* 1992;18:319–332.

4. Psychosocial therapies for schizophrenia

a. Include cognitive behavioral therapy but not family interventions
b. Should only be utilized in patients with good insight
c. Are less effective in combination with antipsychotic drug therapy
d. May help reduce relapse and improve coping skills
e. None of the above

The correct answer is d.

Family interventions, cognitive behavioral therapy, and social skills training are the most widely studied psychosocial therapies for schizophrenia. These interventions have been shown to reduce relapse and improve coping skills. There is no evidence that psychosocial interventions are less effective in patients with poor insight or in those on antipsychotic medications.

References

Dickerson FB. Cognitive behavioral psychotherapy for schizophrenia: a review of recent empirical studies. *Schizophr Res.* 2000;43:71–90.

Lauriello J, Bustillo J, Keith SJ. A critical review of research on psychosocial treatment of schizophrenia. *Biol Psychiatry.* 1999;46:1409–1417.

5. Psychosis of Alzheimer's disease (AD) is a distinct syndrome characterized most commonly by

a. Reduced risk of aggressive behaviors
b. Greater severity in the late stages of AD
c. Olfactory hallucinations
d. Delusions or visual or auditory hallucinations
e. Signs of delirium

The correct answer is d.

Psychosis of AD is most commonly characterized by delusions or hallucinations, which may be auditory or visual. This syndrome has important consequences, including increased caregiver distress, higher rates of institutionalization, and an increased risk of agitation, wandering, and other disruptive behaviors. A delirium should be ruled out in patients with dementia who develop psychotic symptoms, but psychosis of AD is a syndrome distinct from delirium. The severity of psychotic symptoms tends to decrease in the later stages of AD, a phenomenon that has been termed *pseudoremission* because it is thought that patients in the later stages may lack the cognitive or verbal abilities to express their delusions or hallucinations.

References

Cummings JL, Miller B, Hill MA, Neshkes R. Neuropsychiatric aspects of multi-infarct dementia and dementia of the Alzheimer type. *Arch Neurol.* 1987;44:389–393.

Jeste DV, Finkel SI. Psychosis of Alzheimer's disease and related dementias: diagnostic criteria for a distinct syndrome. *Am J Geriatr Psychiatry.* 2000; 8:29–34.

6. Delusional disorder

    a. Usually begins in patients' teens to early 20s
    b. Is often associated with prominent auditory hallucinations
    c. Is characterized by the presence of nonbizarre delusions
    d. Has a somewhat earlier age of onset in women than in men
    e. Occurs in about 5%–8% of the elderly population

The correct answer is c.

Delusional disorder is characterized by the presence of nonbizarre delusions (e.g., delusions of infidelity). The presence of auditory hallucinations should suggest other diagnoses, including schizophrenia. The *Diagnostic and Statistical Manual of Mental Disorders, Fourth Edition* (*DSM-IV*; American Psychiatric Association, 1994) estimated the population prevalence of delusional disorder at 0.03%, with a lifetime risk of 0.05% to 0.1%. Delusional disorder can occur in young adults but usually presents first in mid-to-late adulthood. The average age of onset is somewhat earlier for men (40–49 years) than for women (60–69 years).

Reference

American Psychiatric Association. *Diagnostic Criteria from* DSM-IV. Washington, DC: American Psychiatric Association; 1994.

7. For the older patient with schizophrenia or other psychotic disorders, atypical antipsychotic medications

    a. Are as likely as conventional neuroleptics to cause acute extrapyramidal symptoms (EPS)
    b. Should be considered second-line agents after high-potency antipsychotic agents such as haloperidol
    c. Should be prescribed in doses equivalent to those prescribed for younger patients with schizophrenia
    d. Are unlikely to cause sedation and orthostasis
    e. Are less likely to carry a risk of causing tardive dyskinesia

The correct answer is e.

In older patients with schizophrenia, the atypical antipsychotic agents have become first-line treatments, largely because of their more favorable side-effect profile compared to the conventional antipsychotics. The atypicals are less likely to cause acute EPS and tardive dyskinesia in both younger and older patients with schizophrenia. Side effects that are most commonly experienced by patients taking atypical antipsychotics include sedation and orthostasis. Dosing recommendations for older patients follow the "start low, go slow" principle of geriatric medicine: Initial and target doses are generally one quarter to one half those recommended for younger patients.

References

Jeste DV, Eastham JH, Lacro JP, Gierz M, Field MG, Harris MJ. Management of late-life psychosis. *J Clin Psychiatry.* 1996;57(suppl 3):39–45.

Jeste DV, Finkel SI. Psychosis of Alzheimer's Disease and related dementias: diagnostic criteria for a distinct syndrome. *Am J Geriatr Psychiatry.* 2000; 8:29–34.

8. Prominent visual hallucinations and non-drug-induced EPS are most commonly associated with which of the following late-life disorders?

   a. Delusional disorder
   b. Dementia with Lewy bodies (DLB)
   c. Brief psychotic reaction
   d. Late-onset schizophrenia
   e. Bipolar disorder

The correct answer is b.

DLB is most commonly associated with the combination of visual hallucinations, parkinsonian features that precede use of antipsychotic agents, and fluctuating cognition. Early in the course of the illness, patients with DLB are more likely to experience visual hallucinations compared to patients with AD.

Reference

Samuel W, Caligiuri M, Galasko D, et al. Better cognitive and psychopathologic response to donepezil in patients prospectively diagnosed as dementia with Lewy bodies: a preliminary study. *Int J Geriatr Psychiatry.* 2000;15: 794–802.

9. A patient with AD develops the delusion that his caregiver daughter is stealing from him. He has become increasingly difficult to manage at home, destroying papers around the home. He once wandered from the house and was found several blocks away, disoriented to his loca-

tion. There is no evidence from the physical examination and laboratory workup of an underlying medical illness such as an infection. Which of the following interventions would be most useful initially?

a. Use of a low-potency antipsychotic agent such as chlorpromazine
b. Supportive psychotherapy for the patient
c. Prescribing 100 mg trazodone tid
d. A low dose of an atypical antipsychotic agent
e. Reassurance to the daughter that the symptoms are transient

The correct answer is d.

Although data are still somewhat limited, the atypical antipsychotics are now considered first-line agents for the pharmacological treatment of psychosis and severe agitation in dementia patients. Although the atypical agents are generally well tolerated by older individuals, recommended dose ranges are considerably lower than for younger patients. Low-potency conventional antipsychotics such as chlorpromazine carry a significant risk of sedation, and orthostasis that may be particularly troublesome in dementia patients. Trazodone has been used in the treatment of agitation accompanying dementia; however, the dose range should be considerably lower. Family support and psychoeducation should be provided, but the symptoms listed cannot be considered transient.

References

Jeste DV, Rockwell E, Harris MJ, Lohr JB, Lacro J. Conventional versus newer antipsychotics in elderly patients. *Am J Geriatr Psychiatry.* 1999;7: 70–76.

Katz IR, Jeste DV, Mintzer JE, Clyde C, Napolitano J, Brecher M. Comparison of risperidone and placebo for psychosis and behavioral disturbances associated with dementia: a randomized, double-blind trail. *J Clin Psychiatry.* 1999;60:107–115.

Street JS, Clark WS, Gannon KS, et al. Olanzapine treatment of psychotic and behavioral symptoms in patients with Alzheimer disease in nursing care facilities: a double-blind randomized, placebo-controlled trial. *Arch Gen Psychiatry.* 2000;10:968–976.

10. As patients with early-onset schizophrenia age, the most common pattern is one of

a. Stability or even improvement in symptoms
b. Increased severity of positive symptoms
c. Complete "burnout" of symptoms
d. Appearance of visual hallucinations
e. Development of new types of delusions

The correct answer is a.

Studies of the long-term course of schizophrenia have demonstrated that only approximately 20% of patients appear to experience the functional decline described by Kraepelin; another 20%–30% show substantial improvement and even remission. Outcome heterogeneity is a consistent finding. Furthermore, in the majority of patients, initial deterioration usually occurs shortly after the onset of the disorder and is frequently limited to the first 5 or 10 years after illness, whereas aging is accompanied by stability or even improvement in symptoms. In a study of institutionalized patients, Davidson and colleagues (1995) reported that, although positive symptoms abated somewhat with age, they were still present, calling into question the concept of complete "burnout" of symptoms, at least in institutionalized patients.

References

Belitsky R, McGlashan TH. The manifestations of schizophrenia in late life: a dearth of data. *Schizophr Bull.* 1993;19:683–685.

Bleuler M. *The Schizophrenic Disorders: Long-Term Patient and Family Studies* (Clemens SM, trans). New Haven, CT: Yale University Press; 1978. Originally published 1972.

Ciompi L. Catamnestic long-term study on the course of life and aging of schizophrenics. *Schizophr Bull.* 1980;6:606–618.

Davidson M, Harvey PD, Powchik P, et al. Severity of symptoms in chronically institutionalized geriatric schizophrenic patients. *Am J Psychiatry.* 1995;152:197–207.

McGlashan TH. A selective review of recent North American long-term follow-up studies of schizophrenia. *Schizophr Bull.* 1988;14:515–542.

Chapter 23
Anxiety Disorders

1. A 75-year-old woman in generally good health reports that she fell on the sidewalk 6 months ago. She was not injured, but since then she has feared having another fall and has restricted her level of activity. Because of her fear of falling, she no longer goes for walks by herself and will only leave her house when absolutely necessary. As a result, she has less social contact than previously. What is the most likely diagnosis?

   a. Posttraumatic stress disorder
   b. Panic disorder with agoraphobia
   c. Agoraphobia without history of panic disorder
   d. Social phobia
   e. Major depressive disorder

The correct answer is c.

Older people with agoraphobia rarely report a current or past history of panic attacks. Current data suggest that most people with late-onset agoraphobia attribute the start of their disorder to an abrupt onset of physical illness or a traumatic event, such as a fall or being mugged. Although this woman was traumatized by the fall, she does not report symptoms of posttraumatic stress disorder such as distressing recollections, flashbacks, numbing of general responsiveness, or symptoms of hyperarousal. Her reduced level of social activity is secondary to her reluctance to leave home and is not because she fears humiliation or embarrassment in a social situation. Therefore, a diagnosis of social phobia does not apply. Finally, major depression is important to consider in the differential diagnosis of an elderly person who becomes housebound. However, in this case, her reduced level of activity is caused by phobic avoidance not depression-related anhedonia, anergia, or apathy.

References

Burvill PW, Johnson GA, Jamrozik KD, Anderson CS, Stewart-Wynne EG, Chakera TM. Anxiety disorders after stroke: results from the Perth Community Stroke Study. *Br J Psychiatry.* 1995;166:328–332.

Lindesay J. Phobic disorders in the elderly. *Br J Psychiatry.* 1991;159:531–541.

Lindesay J, Banerjee S. Phobic disorders in the elderly: a comparison of three diagnostic systems. *Int J Geriatr Psychiatry.* 1993;8:387–393.

Livingston G, Watkin V, Milne B, Manela MV, Katona C. The natural history of depression and the anxiety disorders in older people: the Islington community study. *J Affect Disord.* 1997;46:255–262.

2. For the person described in question 1, what is the most appropriate treatment?

   a. Lorazepam
   b. Sertraline
   c. Relaxation therapy
   d. Exposure therapy

The correct answer is d.

Exposure therapy is the treatment of choice for agoraphobia without a history of panic disorder. Exposure therapy encourages the patient to face the feared situation. Exposure usually occurs in a graded fashion over a period of several weeks. Best results are obtained when the exposure is prolonged rather than brief, takes place in real life rather than fantasy, and is regularly practiced by the patient with self-exposure homework.

By itself, relaxation therapy is not effective in treating agoraphobic avoidance. Controlled studies in younger adults have found that lorazepam and sertraline are efficacious treatments for panic disorder with agoraphobia. However, there is no current evidence that these medications are an effective treatment for agoraphobia when there is no history of panic disorder.

References

Antony MM, Swinson RP. *Anxiety Disorders and Their Treatment: A Critical Review of the Evidence-Based Literature.* Ottawa: Health Canada; 1996
Lindesay J, Banerjee S. Generalized anxiety and phobic disorders. In: Chiu E, Ames D, eds. *Functional Psychiatric Disorders of the Elderly.* Cambridge, UK: Cambridge University Press; 1994:78–92.

3. A 72-year-old man suffers a left hemispheric stroke. Several months after the stroke, he starts to feel anxious, worried, keyed up, and on edge. In addition, he becomes preoccupied with physical sensations in his body and reports light-headedness, hot flashes, pressure in his head, and nausea. He is referred to a psychiatrist, who establishes that the patient also has depressed mood, anhedonia, initial and middle insomnia, anergia, anorexia, and feelings of hopelessness. The most likely diagnosis is

a. Major depressive disorder with associated generalized anxiety
b. Panic disorder
c. Hypochondriasis
d. Somatization disorder
e. Adjustment disorder

The correct answer is a.

Generalized anxiety disorder has been identified in approximately 25% of patients within the first year following a stroke. However, most of these patients also have a diagnosis of major depression. Longitudinal studies in older patients with or without stroke suggest that when generalized anxiety and depression coexist, the anxiety is usually symptomatic of the depressive illness. Key symptoms of generalized anxiety are excessive worry accompanied by motor tension and hypervigilance. However, symptoms of autonomic hyperarousal can also be a feature of generalized anxiety and may account for this patient's complaints of light-headedness, hot flashes, and nausea.

Anxious mood and somatic symptoms also can be features of panic disorder, hypochondriasis, and somatization disorder. In panic disorder, the symptoms occur as discrete episodes that develop abruptly, have a crescendo and decrescendo of severity, and usually reach a peak within 10 minutes. In this man's case, his symptoms are ongoing and pervasive and do not occur as discrete episodes. In hypochondriasis, the individual misinterprets his or her physical symptoms as evidence of a serious disease, which this man does not. Somatization disorder usually starts before the age of 30 years. It is characterized by multiple physical complaints in multiple organ systems, and symptoms persist for several years. Clearly, this diagnosis does not apply in this case. Finally, a diagnosis of adjustment disorder with depressed and anxious mood is excluded on the basis that the symptoms meet criteria for an episode of major depression.

References

Aström M. Generalized anxiety disorder in stroke patients. A 3-year longitudinal study. *Stroke.* 1996;27:270–275.

Blazer D, George LK, Hughes D. Generalised anxiety disorder. In: Robins LN, Regier DA, eds. *Psychiatric Disorders in America: The Epidemiological Catchment Area Study.* New York, NY: Free Press; 1991;180–203.

Castillo CS, Schultz SK, Robinson RG. Clinical correlates of early-onset and late-onset poststroke generalized anxiety. *Am J Psychiatry.* 1995;152: 1174–1179.

Parmelee PA, Katz IR, Lawton MP. Anxiety and its association with depression among institutionalized elderly. *Am J Geriatr Psychiatry.* 1993;1: 46–58.

4. A 67-year-old man has a 45-year history of obsessive-compulsive disorder (OCD), which is treated with clomipramine. He is referred to a urologist for evaluation and management of symptoms of prostatic hypertrophy. The urologist prescribes tamsulosin hydrochloride and questions whether the patient's OCD could be treated with a medication that is less likely to aggravate symptoms of prostatic hypertrophy. Given the circumstances, what medication would be the most appropriate alternative treatment of this patient's OCD?

a. Sertraline
b. Paroxetine
c. Venlafaxine
d. Buspirone
e. Lorazepam

The correct answer is a.

Controlled studies undertaken in mixed-aged patients have found that selective serotonin reuptake inhibitors (SSRIs) are an effective alternative to clomipramine in the treatment of OCD. Because of its potent anticholinergic effects, clomipramine has the potential to exacerbate symptoms of prostatic hypertrophy. As a group, SSRIs have less anticholinergic activity than tricyclic antidepressants. Nevertheless, there may be differences between SSRIs in this regard, and in vitro data suggest that paroxetine has more anticholinergic activity than sertraline. Thus, sertraline is a reasonable choice in this case. To date, there have been no controlled trials of venlafaxine as a treatment for OCD. By itself, buspirone is not an effective treatment for OCD, but it is sometimes used as an adjuvant to SSRIs in treatment-refractory cases. Benzodiazepines such as lorazepam are not effective for OCD.

References

Jenike MA. Geriatric obsessive-compulsive disorder. *J Geriatr Psychiatry Neurol.* 1991;4:34–39.

Kohn R, Westlake RJ, Rasmussen SA, Marsland RT, Norman WH. Clinical features of obsessive-compulsive disorder in elderly patients. *Am J Geriatr Psychiatry.* 1997;5:211–215.

Piccinelli M, Pini S, Bellantuono C, Wilkinson G. Efficacy of drug treatment in obsessive-compulsive disorder. A meta-analytic review. *Br J Psychiatry.* 1995;166:424–443.

Skoog G, Skoog I. A 40-year follow-up of patients with obsessive-compulsive disorder. *Arch Gen Psychiatry.* 1999;56:121–127.

5. Which of the following anxiety disorders is most prevalent in people aged 65 years or older?

a. Panic disorder
b. Social phobia
c. Agoraphobia
d. Obsessive-compulsive disorder

The correct answer is c.

Some community-based epidemiological studies have found that phobic disorders are the most prevalent anxiety disorder in older people, whereas others have found that phobic disorders are less common than generalized anxiety disorder. The median period prevalence of phobic disorders in the general elderly population is approximately 3.0%. Agoraphobia is more common than specific phobia or social phobia. Many elderly people with agoraphobia develop their disorder late in life, and they often have moderate or severe social impairment as a result of the phobia.

Most epidemiological studies have found that the period prevalence of panic disorder in people aged 65 years or older is less than 0.5%, and very few cases of this disorder start after the sixth decade of life.

Obsessive-compulsive disorder is also uncommon in later life; studies have reported period prevalence rates of between 0% and 0.8%.

References

Flint AJ. Epidemiology and comorbidity of anxiety disorders in the elderly. *Am J Psychiatry*. 1994;151:640–649.

Flint AJ, Cook JM, Rabins PV. Why is panic disorder less frequent in late-life? *Am J Geriatr Psychiatry*. 1996;4:96–109.

6. An 82-year-old woman, living independently at home, is admitted to the hospital after she falls and fractures her hip. The day after surgical repair of her hip, she suddenly becomes anxious, fearful, and agitated. She reports that during the night she heard the nurses laughing about her, and she believes they are planning to harm her. On examination, she is inattentive and distractible and is temporally disoriented. What is the most likely cause of this woman's anxiety?

   a. Dementia
   b. Delirium
   c. Major depressive disorder
   d. Delusional disorder
   e. Adjustment disorder

The correct answer is b.

The abrupt onset of anxiety, fear, and agitation in response to persecutory ideation in an elderly person who has just undergone emergency surgery is highly suggestive of delirium. The diagnosis is further supported by the presence of temporal disorientation and signs suggesting an altered level of consciousness. The acute nature of these symptoms and signs is not consistent with dementia, major depression, or delusional disorder. Psychotic symptoms are not a feature of adjustment disorder.

Reference

Jacobson S. Delirium in the elderly. *Psychiatr Clin North Am*. 1997;20:91–110.

7. A 65-year-old man presents with mixed symptoms of major depression and generalized anxiety. His physician prescribes nefazodone, starting with a dose of 50 mg bid. Because of the patient's high level of anxiety and disturbing insomnia, the physician also initiates treatment with a benzodiazepine, to be given on a short-term basis until the antidepressant becomes effective. Which of the following benzodiazepines is most suitable?

a. Alprazolam
b. Clonazepam
c. Diazepam
d. Lorazepam

The correct answer is d.

Two factors that guide the selection of a benzodiazepine are its duration of action and hepatic metabolic pathway. Benzodiazepines are metabolized in the liver by either oxidation or conjugation. Oxidation is slowed by aging, with the result that compounds metabolized by this route can accumulate in elderly people, with the potential for toxicity. On the other hand, conjugation is unaffected by aging. For older adults, recommended benzodiazepines are those with elimination half-lives of intermediate duration and those that are metabolized by conjugation. Lorazepam is such a drug, as are oxazepam and temazepam. Diazepam and clonazepam have long half-lives and are metabolized by oxidation and are not recommended for this man. Alprazolam has an intermediate duration of action (12–15 hours), but it is metabolized by oxidation and thus has the potential to accumulate in an older person. Furthermore, alprazolam is metabolized by the hepatic isoenzyme P450 3A4, which is inhibited by nefazodone. Thus, if alprazolam was given to this man, it is possible that its metabolism would be further impaired as a result of an interaction with the antidepressant.

References

Burke WJ, Folks DG, McNeilly DP. Effective use of anxiolytics in older adults. *Clin Geriatr Med.* 1998;14:47–65.

Flint AJ, Rifat SL. Anxious depression in elderly patients: response to antidepressant treatment. *Am J Geriatr Psychiatry.* 1997;5:107–115.

Nutt D. Management of patients with depression associated with anxiety symptoms. *J Clin Psychiatry.* 1997;58(suppl 8):11–16.

Shorr RI, Robin DW. Rational use of benzodiazepines in the elderly. *Drugs Aging.* 1994;4:9–20.

8. A 70-year-old widow with a long-standing history of generalized anxiety disorder is brought by her daughter to a new primary care physician. The patient recently relocated after the death of her husband 6 months earlier. The woman asks the physician for a prescription for 10 mg qd diazepam, a medication that she has taken for the past 30 years. The physician is concerned about her taking diazepam because it can contribute to cognitive impairment, falls, and hip fractures in older people. What is the physician's most appropriate course of action at this point?

a. Stop the diazepam
b. Continue the diazepam
c. Substitute buspirone for the diazepam
d. Substitute paroxetine for the diazepam

The correct answer is b.

Given that this is the woman's first contact with the physician, she is adjusting to a move that has taken place after the death of her husband, and there is no imminent risk from continuing with the diazepam, it would be prudent to maintain the diazepam. However, it also would be appropriate to arrange a follow-up visit with her to discuss the possibility of withdrawing the diazepam in the future. It would be important to establish whether she still experiences symptoms of generalized anxiety disorder, whether she currently has symptoms of depression, and whether she has a recent history of falls or cognitive impairment. It also would be important to determine whether she has previously tried withdrawing the diazepam, and if so, whether this was associated with an exacerbation or recurrence of anxiety.

If she is relatively asymptomatic and has not recently tried discontinuing the diazepam, then a slow withdrawal over several weeks (or even months) would be appropriate. If the history or withdrawal attempt suggest that she needs ongoing treatment for generalized anxiety, options that are available to the patient include (a) continue with the diazepam, cognizant of the potential risks as she grows older; (b) attempt substitution of buspirone if she does not have significant depressive symptoms; (c) attempt substitution of paroxetine, escitalopram, or venlafaxine (which are effective treatments for generalized anxiety disorder), especially if she has comorbid depressive symptoms. Buspirone and antidepressants have a delayed onset of action and do not suppress the withdrawal symptoms of benzodiazepines. Thus, if these medications are substituted for a benzodiazepine, they need to be given at a therapeutic dose for 2–4 weeks before the benzodiazepine is gradually withdrawn. However, despite this approach, some patients are less satisfied with the anxiolytic effects of buspirone compared with a benzodiazepine.

References

Davidson JRT, DuPont RL, Hedges D, Haskins JT. Efficacy, safety, and tolerability of venlafaxine extended release and buspirone in outpatients with generalized anxiety disorder. *J Clin Psychiatry*. 1999;60:528–535.

DeMartinis N, Rynn M, Rickels K, Mandos L. Prior benzodiazepine use and buspirone response in the treatment of generalized anxiety disorder. *J Clin Psychiatry*. 2000;61:91–94.

Schweizer E, Rickels K. The long-term management of generalized anxiety disorder: issues and dilemmas. *J Clin Psychiatry.* 1996;57(suppl 7):9–12.

Steinberg JR. Anxiety in elderly patients. A comparison of azapirones and benzodiazepines. *Drugs Aging.* 1994;5:335–345.

Chapter 24
Personality Disorders

1. Which of the following personality disorders has been the most prevalent in patients over the age of 50 years?
   a. Avoidant
   b. Obsessive-compulsive
   c. Schizoid
   d. Paranoid
   e. Dependent

The correct answer is d.

The epidemiology of personality disorder in late life has not been well defined. In elders with major depressive disorder or dysthymia, dependent and avoidant personality disorder has been the most frequent, but Abrams and Horowitz's meta-analytic study (1999) showed paranoid personality was the most common form of personality disorder in those over age 50 years.

Reference

Abrams R, Horowitz S. Personality disorders after age 50: a meta-analytic review of the literature. In: Rosowsky E, Abrams R, Zweig R, Eds. *Personality Disorders in Older Adults: Emerging Issues in Diagnosis and Treatment.* Mahwah, NJ: Erlbaum; 1999.

2. An 81-year-old man with no prior history of depression or clinically significant personality dysfunction suffered a cerebrovascular accident, resulting in an infarct in the right frontotemporal region. He subsequently experienced a major depressive episode, for which he was successfully treated with venlafaxine and psychotherapy. However, he then developed occasional irritability (unusual for him) and louder than normal speech and began to tell jokes with inappropriate sexual content to his school-aged grandchildren. Sleep and appetite remained normal. Score on the Mini-Mental State Examination was 30/30. The disinhibited behavior continued after lowering the venlafaxine dose and adding a mood stabilizer but was somewhat moderated after 4 months by the use of 1 mg risperidone qd. The clinical picture would best be characterized as

a. Late-onset bipolar disorder (mania)
b. Residual depressive symptomatology
c. Posttraumatic stress disorder
d. Narcissistic personality disorder
e. Personality change caused by a general medical condition

The correct answer is e.

A pharmacologically induced mania or other change of polarity might be possible, but disinhibition rather than frank mania is described, and there was no response to mood-stabilizing medication. Similarly, the symptoms are not distinctly depressive, and there is no evidence of typical posttraumatic anxiety features. The picture cannot be described as a personality disorder, narcissistic or other, because it is unrelated to the patient's long-term functioning and therefore fails to meet a general criterion for diagnosis of personality disorder. Therefore, the rubric that best applies is personality change caused by a general medical condition.

Reference

American Psychiatric Association. *Diagnostic and Statistical Manual of Mental Disorders*, 4th ed. Washington, DC: American Psychiatric Association; 1994.

3. Individuals with late-onset schizophrenia or delusional disorder are likely to have had which of the following personality disorders premorbidly?

a. Borderline with "minipsychotic" episodes
b. Narcissistic
c. Histrionic
d. Antisocial
e. Paranoid or schizotypal

The correct answer is e.

Although patients with severe symptoms of borderline personality disorder may experience transient episodes of psychosis, patients with paranoid or schizotypal personality disorders are the most likely patients with personality disorder to develop frank psychoses in late life.

References

Tyrer P. *Personality Disorders: Diagnoses, Management and Course.* London: Wright; 1988.

Yassa R, Suranyi-Cadotte B. Clinical characteristics of late-onset schizophrenia and delusional disorder. *Schizophr Bull.* 1993;19:701–707.

4. Which of the following statements about personality traits in normal aging is *incorrect*?

   a. A quiet, inner-directed attitude can be found in many individuals
   b. In cross-sectional studies, older persons score lower on scales assessing impulsivity and hostility
   c. In cross-sectional studies, criminality and sociopathy decline with age
   d. With respect to personality traits, individuals develop more exaggerated manifestations of their adult personalities
   e. In longitudinal studies of personality traits, individuals tend to show overall stability as they age

The correct answer is d.

All other statements are factually accurate. Cross-sectional data from the Minnesota Multiphasic Personality Inventory and other assessment instruments show that older individuals are quieter and less likely to have high levels of impulsiveness or sociopathy than groups of younger adults. On the other hand, individuals studied longitudinally tend to be stable with respect to basic personality traits over long periods of time.

References

Costa P, McCrae R. Set like plaster? Evidence for the stability of adult personality. In: Heatherton T, Weinberger J, eds. *Can Personality Change?* Washington, DC: American Psychological Association; 1994:21–40

Neugarten B. Personality and aging. In: Birren JE, Schaie KW, eds. *Handbook of the Psychology of Aging.* New York, NY: Van Nostrand Reinhold; 1977.

Swenson WM, Pearson JS, Osborne D. *An MMPI Source Book: Basic-Item, Scale and Pattern Data on 50,000 Medical Patients.* Minneapolis, MN: University of Minnesota Press; 1973.

Woodruff J, Guze SE, Clayton PJ. The medical and psychiatric implications of antisocial personality. *Dis Nerv Syst.* 1971;32:712–714.

5. Based on clinical data and theoretical constructs, which of the following statements best characterizes the relationship between geriatric personality disorders and depressive disorders?

   a. Personality and depressive disorders may coexist but otherwise are clinically independent of one another
   b. Personality and depressive disorders are synergistic
   c. Personality disorders represent a *form fruste* of depressive disorders
   d. There is a scarring relationship; that is, repeated depressive episodes alter or scar the personality
   e. All of the above

The correct answer is e.

Each of the above relationships can be demonstrated in individual cases and are believed to be equally possible theoretically.

References

Black DW, Bell S, Hulbert J, Nasrallah A. The importance of axis II in patients with major depression: a controlled study. *J Affect Disord*. 1988;14:115–122.

Sadavoy, J. The effect of personality disorder on axis I disorders in the elderly. In: Duffy M, ed. *Handbook of Counselling and Psychotherapy With Older Adults*. New York, NY: Wiley; 1999:397–413.

6. A 69-year-old man developed rapid onset of decreased interest, poor concentration, impaired appetite, and mild weight loss. His sleep and energy are undisturbed, and he denied suicidal ideation and substance abuse. However, he strongly endorsed feelings of tension, shortness of breath, stomach tightness, nausea, and leg weakness. Cognitive abilities and activities of daily living were unimpaired, and there were no other symptoms of anxiety or psychosis. There was a prior history of similar feelings when he was left by his wife many years before. Medical history was unremarkable. There was no family history of depression. Preoccupations focused on concerns that, because of business problems, he would not be able to maintain his income, and that this would cause him to lose his girlfriend, who he thought was most interested in his money and business. In the initial exploratory sessions in treatment, he would rock back and forth in his chair, moaning like a child, and focus on abdominal complaints. Past history revealed a cold, distant, and unavailable mother and few emotional supports. He had strong feelings of betrayal and abandonment throughout his life. Formal assessment of personality revealed strong dependency characteristics as well as some dramatic cluster B characteristics. The therapist diagnosed major depression with personality disorder not otherwise specified. Antidepressant medication produced some remission of the major affective symptoms but left significant residual anxiety. Regarding this case, which of the following statements is most true?

   a. Despite the poor emotional support, life stress, and frequent separations in this patient's history, there is no specific evidence to link these factors with personality disorder in someone of his age
   b. This patient demonstrates depression comorbid with a personality disorder, but it is an atypical presentation because this association is less typical in elderly patients compared to younger adult patients
   c. Compared to younger adults, this patient's depressive symptoms are likely to be chronic despite adequate antidepressant therapy and concurrent psychotherapy

d. The presence of residual symptoms following antidepressant therapy is unusual in patients with this type of clinical profile.

The correct answer is c.

Devanand et al. (1994) showed increased chronicity of affective symptoms in elderly patients with associated personality disorder, and Thompson et al. (1988) showed poor short-term outcome in psychotherapy associated with personality disorder.

Answer a is false. One study by Schneider et al. (1992) showed that the factors underlying disturbed personality traits in elders are similar to those in younger patients, and that lack of emotional support, frequent life stress, and the presence of frequent separations are found in recovered depressed elders as they are in younger individuals. Answer b is false. Based on a meta-analytic study, the rates of personality disorder appear to be highest among depressed elderly. Abrams and Horowitz (1999) found that the prevalence of personality disorder comorbid with depression in elderly patients was approximately 33%. Answer d is false. Abrams et al. (1998) showed that the presence of a personality disorder in elderly patients is a key component in predisposition to residual symptoms following treatment of depression.

References

Abrams RC, Horowitz SV. Personality disorders after age 50: a meta-analytic review of the literature. In: Rosowsky E, Abrams RC, Zweig RA, eds. *Personality Disorders in Older Adults: Emergency Issues in Diagnosis and Treatment.* Mahwah, NJ: Erlbaum: 1999.

Abrams RC, Spielman LA, Alexopoulos GS, Klausner E. Personality disorder symptoms and functioning in elderly depressed patients. *Am J Geriatr Psychiatry.* 1998;6:24–30.

Devanand DP, Nobler MS, Singer T, et al. Is dysthymia a different disorder in the elderly? *Am J Psychiatry.* 1994;151:1592–1599.

Schneider LS, Zemansky MF, Bender M, Sloane RB. Personality in recovered depressed elderly. *Int Psychogeriatr.* 1992;4:177–185.

Thompson LW, Gallagher D, Czirr R. Personality disorder and outcome in the treatment of late life depression. *J Geriatr Psychiatry.* 1988;21:133–146.

Chapter 25
Substance Abuse

1. A 68-year-old man is referred because of persistently troubling bereavement 6 months after his spouse's death. He does not meet criteria for a depressive disorder and experiences relief after several psychotherapy sessions focusing on the marriage relationship and his loss. In the initial workup, he indicated that for years he has regularly con-

sumed a 750-cc bottle of table wine in the evening, five or six evenings per week (about 25 to 30 standard drinks a week) but never more than this per occasion. He suffers no hangovers or other perceived ill effects. He exercises and is in good physical health according to his referring primary physician, has never had any obvious alcohol-related problems, and is CAGE negative. He seems surprised and interested when you inform him that his level of drinking is much higher than recommended safe levels and could eventually result in health problems. What step in management is indicated next regarding this patient's use of alcohol?

a. Refer back to primary physician
b. Advise reduction in alcohol use
c. Prescribe naltrexone
d. Refer for alcoholism assessment

The correct answer is b.

This patient demonstrates a pattern of risky drinking, rather than problem drinking or an alcohol use disorder. The proper management of risky drinking is brief intervention, a technique consisting of several steps. Step 1 is education, discussing with the patient how his or her alcohol consumption pattern differs from norms and safe drinking guidelines and the possible adverse health consequences that might occur if this drinking pattern continues. The second step is to advise the patient to reduce alcohol intake. Most research on brief intervention has focused on primary care physicians, but many primary physicians are reluctant to undertake brief intervention because of the extra time it takes, discomfort about advising patients to change their behavior, specific aversion to managing alcohol-related matters, or reimbursement limits for prevention efforts. There is no reason why a general or geriatric psychiatrist should not undertake this intervention when an obvious opportunity occurs.

Referral back to the primary physician for brief intervention (answer a) would only be justified if you, as the consulting psychiatrist, were sure that the primary physician has experience and comfort in this role. Naltrexone (answer c) is an adjunct to treatment for patients with an alcohol use disorder who are also involved in other elements of an alcoholism treatment or rehabilitation program. There is already enough information available that further assessment by an alcoholism expert is not necessary (answer d). Such a referral could also be counterproductive, unnecessarily and inaccurately "pathologizing" the patient's drinking.

References

Center for Substance Abuse Treatment. *Brief Interventions and Brief Therapies for Substance Abuse: Treatment Improvement Protocol 34.* Rockville,

MD: US Dept of Health and Human Services, Public Health Service, Substance Abuse and Mental Health Services Administration; 1999. DHHS Publication (SMA) 99–3353.

Fleming MF, Barry KL, Adams WL, Stauffacher EA. Brief physician advice for alcohol problems in older adults: a randomized community-based trial. *Am J Fam Pract.* 1999;48:378–384.

2. A 72-year-old man is referred because of depression for the past several months. Evaluation shows that he clearly meets criteria for current major depression, with moderately severe symptoms but no evidence of suicidal intent, agitation, or psychotic features. This appears to be the first episode. In the past 2 years, there have been no adverse life events. Further history reveals that he was treated for alcohol dependence 20 years earlier, remained abstinent for 10 years, but resumed drinking after retirement. For the past 2 years, he has consumed about a pint of vodka on drinking days (about 10 standard drinks), but the number of drinking days per week has increased from three or four to nearly daily, up to and including the evening before this evaluation. He says that his father and a paternal uncle were "alcoholic" and also suffered from depression, although neither was ever treated for these conditions. What is the most likely diagnosis of this patient's mood disorder?

a. Alcohol-induced depression
b. Major depression
c. Major depression complicated by alcohol effects
d. Diagnosis cannot yet be determined

The correct answer is d.

This patient could be suffering from alcohol-induced or major depression alone or in combination (answers a, b, and c, respectively). One cannot be certain which of these diagnoses is correct because heavy alcohol use has continued up to the present. Only time will permit resolution of the differential diagnosis. Alcohol-induced depression can be serious enough to fulfill criteria for major depression. Even then, alcohol-induced depression resolves without specific antidepressant treatment after 3 to 4 weeks of sobriety, and often a trend toward improvement is evident after just several days of sobriety. On the other hand, true comorbid major depression is much more likely to persist with little change beyond 3 weeks. Some patients may partially improve over the first few weeks without antidepressant treatment but reach a plateau of significant residual depression that persists. This would be the expected course for a patient with true comorbid depression further aggravated by alcohol effects.

Patients who suffer severely painful depressive symptoms or suicidal impulses that persist unchanged after the first 2 to 3 days should be treated vigorously with antidepressant medications even though the differential diagnosis may not be resolved, as should all patients who continue to be depressed after 3 to 4 weeks of sobriety. Effective treatment of depression also tends to improve drinking outcomes in alcoholics and heavy drinkers. When initial depressive symptoms are mild to moderate and there is no evidence of suicidal intent or psychotic features, it is appropriate to withhold antidepressants until sufficient time has passed to permit an accurate diagnosis. This may not only avoid misdiagnosis but also protect the patient from a costly and potentially hazardous lengthy course of antidepressant drug therapy.

References

Atkinson RM. Depression, alcoholism and ageing: a brief review. *Int J Geriatric Psychiatry.* 1999;14:905–910.

Brown SA, Inaba RK, Gillin JC, Schuckit MA, Stewart MA, Irwin MR. Alcoholism and affective disorder: clinical course of depressive symptoms. *Am J Psychiatry.* 1995;152:45–52.

Dupree LW, Schonfeld L. Cognitive-behavioral and self-management treatment of older problem drinkers. *J Mental Health Aging.* 1998;4:215–232.

3. A 69-year-old woman is referred because of memory loss for the past 2 years. Mental examination shows that she suffers from dementia, with significant deficits in memory, object recognition, and executive functioning; there is no evidence of anomia. Neurological examination reveals coarse horizontal nystagmus, gait ataxia, and peripheral neuropathy with a stocking distribution in the lower extremities. Computerized tomographic scan of the brain shows generalized moderate cortical atrophy. What new information will be most useful as an aid to diagnosis?

a. Family history of neurological disorder
b. Personal history of alcohol use
c. Neuropsychological evaluation
d. Imaging study of the cerebellum

The correct answer is b.

Evidence of cerebellar dysfunction and bilateral peripheral neuropathy, rare in Alzheimer's dementia (AD) and unusual in vascular dementias, strongly raises the possibility of alcohol-induced dementia. Further evidence for this possibility is the sparing of naming (lack of anomia or dysnomia), a deficit that tends to be both early and prominent in AD but absent or mild in alcohol-induced dementia. Memory loss and other clinical criteria for dementia, as well as cortical atrophy on imaging studies, may be similar in both conditions, especially in early AD. The alcohol amnestic disorder (Wernicke-Korsakoff syndrome) may also present with memory loss, cerebellar dysfunction, and peripheral polyneuropathy, but memory loss tends to be much more dense and is more often covered by confabulation, and other deficits in higher mental functioning required for the diagnosis of dementia are absent or very mild.

Answers a (family history of neurological disorders) and c (neuropsychological evaluation) of course are indicated as part of a complete workup, but neither is as critical a next step as learning the history of the patient's exposure to alcohol. Prolonged heavy drinking, over many years, is the factor most likely to be associated with this pattern of clinical findings; of course, direct or indirect proof of heavy alcohol exposure is required for the diagnosis of alcohol-induced dementia. Establishing an accurate history of alcohol use may require interviewing relatives or friends who are familiar with the patient's drinking history. An imaging study of the cerebellum (answer d) would be costly and would not contribute to either management or prognosis. On the other hand, if alcohol has been ruled out as a cause of the findings, such a study may be indicated.

References

Atkinson RM. Substance abuse. In: Coffey CE, Cummings JL, eds. *Textbook of Geriatric Neuropsychiatry.* 2nd ed. Washington, DC: American Psychiatric Press; 2000:367–400.

Oslin D, Atkinson RM, Smith DM, Hendrie H: Alcohol related dementia: proposed clinical criteria. *Int J Geriatr Psychiatry.* 1998;13:203–212.

4. Several studies have demonstrated that moderate alcohol consumption is associated with reduced overall mortality compared to both heavy drinking and abstention. What is the most important explanation of this finding?

   a. Abstainers include persons who are ill
   b. Abstainers include former alcoholics
   c. Moderate drinking benefits cognitive status
   d. Moderate drinking reduces coronary heart disease
   e. Heavy drinkers have more accidents

The correct answer is d.

When plotted on a graph, there is a U- or J-shaped relationship between current alcohol consumption and mortality. People who drink nothing or who drink heavily have higher mortality rates than people who drink moderately (one or two standard drinks per day). There are several reasons for this finding; in fact, all five answers given here are technically correct. But, reduction in mortality from coronary heart disease (answer d) accounts for most of the overall effect of moderate drinking on mortality. There is increasing evidence for a variety of mechanisms to help explain how alcohol protects against coronary heart disease. The other options refer to valid findings but ones that have less influence in explaining the relationship between drinking level and overall mortality.

References

Mertens JR, Moos RH, Brennan PL. Alcohol consumption, life context, and coping predict mortality among late-middle-aged drinkers and former drinkers. *Alcoholism (New York)*. 1996;20:313–319.

Thun MJ, Peto R, Lopez AD, et al. Alcohol consumption and mortality among middle-aged and elderly US adults. *N Engl J Med*. 1997;337:1705–1714.

5. Several pharmacological variables increase the risk of benzodiazepine dependence, including long duration of treatment, higher daily dose level, shorter elimination half-life, and higher milligram potency. Several patient variables also increase this risk, including prior history of substance abuse, personality disorder, and major presenting symptoms that require treatment. Which chronic disorder is most highly associated with risk of dependence when a benzodiazepine is prescribed?

   a. Social anxiety disorder
   b. Generalized anxiety disorder
   c. Sleep disorder
   d. Panic disorder

The correct answer is c.

Although not necessarily the drugs of choice, especially in elderly patients, benzodiazepines are quite effective in the treatment of anxiety and panic symptoms, and little tolerance develops over time to these antianxiety and antipanic effects with continuing use. In contrast, the sleep-enhancing effects of benzodiazepines tend to wane after several weeks, indicating the development of significant tolerance to the hypnotic effect of these drugs. Thus, dose escalation over time is more likely in clinical situations in which these drugs are prescribed for chronic insomnia. Patients treated for insomnia, compared to those with an anxiety disorders, are also more likely to receive benzodiazepines that are short acting, that is, that have a short elimination half-life and high milligram potency. High dose, short elimination half-life, and high milligram potency all increase risk of dependence.

Reference

American Psychiatric Association. *Benzodiazepine Dependence, Toxicity, and Abuse.* Washington, DC: American Psychiatric Press; 1990.

6. Compared to typical clinical presentations of benzodiazepine withdrawal in younger adults, which one of the following is probably more likely to occur in an older patient?

   a. Delirium
   b. Psychosis
   c. Depression
   d. Anxiety

The correct answer is a.

There is some evidence that when benzodiazepines are tapered gradually, aging patients may experience discontinuance symptoms with similar or even less intensity compared to younger adults, but abrupt cessation of these agents tends to produce distressing symptoms in a majority of patients of all ages. True withdrawal symptoms occur in 20% to 50% of users. The clinical presentation of benzodiazepine discontinuance varies from one patient to the next.

Delirium, psychosis, depression, and anxiety can all occur as features of benzodiazepine discontinuance. Depression and anxiety are not true withdrawal symptoms; delirium and psychosis are. Of these four, only delirium (answer a) appears to be a more common manifestation of benzodiazepine discontinuance in elderly patients. This is not surprising. Marginal cognitive reserve in the aging brain makes delirium a more common sign of many acute systemic disorders that can compromise brain function (e.g., infectious diseases or thyroid dysfunction) in geriatric patients compared to younger adults.

References

American Psychiatric Association. *Benzodiazepine Dependence, Toxicity, and Abuse.* Washington, DC: American Psychiatric Press; 1990.

Foy A, Drinkwater V, March S, Mearrick P. Confusion after admission to hospital in elderly patients using benzodiazepines. *Br Med J (Clin Res Ed).* 1986;293:1072.

Foy A, O'Connell D, Henry D, Kelly J, Cocking S, Halliday J. Benzodiazepine use as a cause of cognitive impairment in elderly hospital inpatients. *J Gerontol.* 1995;50A:M99–M106.

7. A 75-year-old woman has taken 5 mg diazepam tid for 8 years for generalized anxiety symptoms that occur in conjunction with her chronic obstructive pulmonary disease. The medication effectively controls her anxiety and aids her sleep. You are asked to consult about whether to

continue this regimen by her primary physician, who you know provides close medical supervision to his patients. What is the most important issue requiring assessment?

a. Prior alcohol or substance dependence
b. Prior response to alternative treatments
c. Current evidence of diazepam toxicity
d. Patient's reliability and adherence

The correct answer is c.

Although older patients vary in their central nervous system (CNS) sensitivity to benzodiazepines, in general persisting or cumulative drug toxicity is much more likely with increasing age, even at conventional therapeutic dose levels. The major manifestations of CNS toxicity are daytime sedation, impaired memory and other cognitive dysfunction, and disturbed gait. General functional decline is not unusual. Depression can also occur, and occasionally in severe cases, a frank dementia may be engendered by benzodiazepine toxicity. The presence or absence of benzodiazepine toxicity is a critical factor in determining whether to continue, reduce, or discontinue drugs of this class.

History of prior alcohol or sedative-hypnotic dependence (answer a), previous responses to alternative treatments for anxiety (answer b), the patient's record of reliability in using the drug and general capacity for informed adherence to medical recommendations (answer d), the efficacy of the current treatment in relieving symptoms, and the availability of close medical supervision are all additional factors that must be weighed when deciding to initiate or sustain a long-term course of benzodiazepine treatment.

The information provided in the case vignette already addresses most of these issues. The fact that this patient has faithfully complied with the same diazepam dosing regimen for 8 years effectively addresses issues of drug dependence and reliability. Information about her prior response to alternative treatments (answer b) is not provided and should be ascertained. However, the possible presence and extent of current benzodiazepine toxicity is a far more important immediate focus for assessment. If she demonstrates signs of drug toxicity, the regimen must be changed, at least by trying a reduced dosage of her diazepam. It would have been preferable to initiate treatment with a selective serotonin reuptake inhibitor (SSRI), and it is this class of drugs that merits first consideration should her anxiety symptoms reoccur as diazepam is phased out.

References

American Psychiatric Association. *Benzodiazepine Dependence, Toxicity, and Abuse.* Washington, DC: American Psychiatric Press; 1990.

Ancill RJ, Carlyle WW. Benzodiazepine use and dependency in the elderly: striking a balance. In: Hallstrom C, ed. *Benzodiazepine Dependence*. Oxford, UK: Oxford University Press; 1993:238–251.

Higgitt AC, Lader MH, Fonagy P. Clinical management of benzodiazepine dependence. *Br Med J*. 1985;291:688–690.

8. Beliefs about smoking influence readiness to quit. Older adult smokers share in common with younger adult smokers certain attitudes and beliefs about smoking and quitting, but in other important respects, smokers differ in beliefs by age. For example, older smokers are *more* likely than younger smokers to perceive smoking as a positive habit to enhance coping, reduce stress, and control weight. What other important belief is *less* characteristic of older smokers when compared to younger smokers?

   a. Smoking influences children
   b. Smoking impairs health
   c. Smoking reduces irritability
   d. Smoking improves concentration

The correct answer is b.

Many surviving smokers have quit spontaneously by their 60s. Among the residual smoking group, many have attempted to quit or are interested in quitting, but a serious barrier is the well-validated finding that older smokers as a group are distinctly less inclined to view smoking as hazardous to health compared to younger adult smokers. Many older smokers believe that it is more hazardous to be 20 pounds overweight (their experience during past attempts to quit) than to smoke. It is true that improvements in health after quitting may be both too subtle and slow to emerge to affect motivation to quit. Younger and older smokers are equally likely to believe that quitting would set a positive example for young children or grandchildren. Troubles with irritability and concentration are frequently cited as reasons for relapse among smokers of all ages who have tried to quit.

References

Orleans CT, Jepson C, Resch N, Rimer BK. Quitting motives and barriers among older smokers. *Cancer*. 1994;74:2055–2061.

Schoenbaum M. Do smokers understand the mortality effects of smoking? Evidence from the Health and Retirement Survey. *Am J Public Health*. 1997;87:755–759.

9. In 1981, it was first proposed that smoking (nicotine dependence) might protect against AD. Since then, more than 30 studies have examined the relationship between smoking and dementia. How can the findings to date best be summarized?

a. Population-based prospective studies and most case–control studies demonstrate no protective effect of smoking against AD
b. At least two recent case–control studies affirmed a protective effect of smoking against AD
c. In prospective studies, the risk of AD is lower in smokers who possess the E [APOE]-ε4 allele than in those who lack this allele
d. Senile plaque formation is less prominent in the brains of patients with AD who were smokers than in those who were nonsmokers

The correct answer is a.

In fact, each of the four options is correct, but only answer a meets the requirement of best explaining the overall findings in the literature on the relationship between smoking and dementia. The fact that a few more recently published case–control studies suggest a protective effect (answer b) adds little to our knowledge because there are uncontrollable variables in such studies that confound the interpretation of findings. The moderating effect of the E [APOE]-ε4 allele on the relationship of smoking to AD risk (answer c) is interesting, but this finding speaks to a much narrower question than the overall findings of research on the relationship between smoking and AD risk. A postmortem study has found reduced senile plaque formation (but increased neurofibrillary tangles) in smokers with AD when compared to nonsmokers with AD (answer d), but this finding has not been replicated and, like answer c, this finding also speaks to a narrower question than the overall findings of research on the relationship between smoking and AD risk.

References

Broe GA, Creasey H, Jorm AF, et al. Health habits and risk of cognitive impairment and dementia in old age: a prospective study on the effects of exercise. *Aust N Z J Public Health*. 1998;22:621–623.

Doll R, Peto R, Boreham J, Sutherland I. Smoking and dementia in male British doctors: a prospective study. *BMJ*. 2000;320:1097–1102.

Wang HX, Fratiglioni L, Frisoni GB, Viitanen M, Winblad B. Smoking and the occurrence of Alzheimer's disease: cross-sectional and longitudinal data in a population-based study. *Am J Epidemiol*. 1999;149:640–644.

Chapter 26
Sleep Disorders in Geriatric Psychiatry

1. All of the following statements are true *except*

   a. Some of the change in sleep patterns of older people is caused by alteration in the circadian rhythm
   b. Older people may live in settings that are not conducive to uninterrupted sleep
   c. Caregiving roles may require older people to be up all night
   d. One of the best predictors of future depression in older people who are not currently depressed is current sleep disturbance
   e. In older people, there is usually only one significant cause of insomnia

The correct answer is e.

One of the best predictors of future depression in older people who are not currently depressed is current sleep disturbance. Some older people develop poor sleep habits, and up to one half of elderly persons use some kind of sleeping medicine. Elderly people are prone to develop sleep phase disorder and may sleep during the day and stay awake at night. Some of the change in sleep patterns is caused by alteration in the circadian rhythm. However, many factors are involved, including the fact that many older people no longer have structured activities during retirement. Older people may live in settings that are not conducive to uninterrupted sleep. Poor sleep is highly correlated with poor health status, and poor health is more common in the elderly. Finally, many elderly people are caregivers for spouses and other relatives. These caregiving roles may require them to be up all night.

References

Dijk DJ, Duffy JF. Circadian regulation of human sleep and age-related changes in its timing, consolidation and EEG characteristics. *Ann Med.* 1999;31: 130–140.

Dijk DJ, Duffy JF. Sleep and sleep disorders in older adults. *J Clin Neurophysiol.* 1995;12:139–146.

Morgan K, Clarke D. Longitudinal trends in late-life insomnia: implications for prescribing. *Age Ageing.* 1997;26:179–184.

Schnelle JF, Alessi CA, Al-Samarrai NR, Fricker RD Jr, Ouslander JG. The nursing home at night: effects of an intervention on noise, light, and sleep. *J Am Geriatr Soc.* 1999;47:430–438.

Use the following list to answer questions 2 through 4.

  a. Decreased amounts of stage 3 and 4 sleep
  b. Significant medical morbidity if untreated
  c. Daytime sleepiness usually present and may be present early in the
     course of the illness
  d. Associated with sundowning
  e. Decreased rapid eye movement (REM) latency
  f. Paradoxical daytime alertness

2. Which of the features are most often associated with dementia?

  a. Answers a and e
  b. Answers a, b, and c
  c. Answers a and d
  d. Answers a, b, c, d
  e. Answer f
  f. None
  g. All are true

The correct answer is c.

3. Which of the features are most often associated with depression?

  a. Answers a and e
  b. Answers a, b, and c
  c. Answers a and d
  d. Answers a, b, c, d
  e. Answer f
  f. None
  g. All are true

The correct answer is b.

4. Which of the features are most often associated with sleep apnea?

  a. Answers a and e
  b. Answers a, b, and c
  c. Answers a and d
  d. Answers a, b, c, d
  e. Answer f
  f. None
  g. All are true

The correct answer is b.

Depression and dementia, particularly dementia of the Alzheimer's
type, demonstrate decreased amounts of stage 3 and 4 sleep. This is

the restorative phase of sleep; therefore, both depressed and mildly demented people are likely to complain of fatigue. When demented and nondemented elderly persons are compared, demented patients are found to have more sleep disruption and arousals, lower sleep efficiency, a higher percentage of stage 1 sleep, and decreases in stage 3 and 4 sleep. These findings worsen as the dementia progresses. Later in the course of the dementia, patients also have increased daytime sleepiness. The result is complete fragmentation of sleep/wakefulness during the night and day.

A high level of sleep-disordered breathing is an extremely significant risk factor for mortality during sleep phase in these patients. In addition, untreated sleep apnea causes loss of daytime cognitive abilities. Sleepiness may lead to mistakes in judgment, motor vehicle accidents, falls, and other misfortunes and deleteriously affect social and marital life.

References

Dew MA, Reynolds CF 3rd, Buysse DJ, et al. Electroencephalographic sleep profiles during depression. Effects of episode duration and other clinical and psychosocial factors in older adults. *Arch Gen Psychiatry.* 1996;53: 148–156.

Ohayon MM, Caulet M, Philip P, Guilleminault C, Priest RG. How sleep and mental disorders are related to complaints of daytime sleepiness. *Arch Intern Med.* 1997;157:2645–2652.

Peker Y, Hedner J, Kraiczi H, Loth S. Respiratory disturbance index: an independent predictor of mortality in coronary artery disease. *Am J Respir Crit Care Med.* 2000;162:81–86.

Reynolds CF, Kupfer DJ, Tasksa LS. EEG sleep in healthy elderly, depressed, and demented subjects. *Biol Psychiatry.* 1988;20:431–442.

Reynolds CF 3rd, Kupfer DJ, Taska LS, Hoch CC, Sewitch DE, Spiker DG. Sleep of healthy seniors: a revisit. *Sleep.* 1985;8:20–29.

5. All of the following statements are false *except*

   a. Caregivers rarely report that nocturnal difficulties played an important role in their decision to institutionalize their elderly relative
   b. In most patients who are placed in a nursing home, the first sign of sleep disorder occurs after placement
   c. The nursing home environment is usually conducive to good sleep
   d. Nursing practices related to incontinence are particularly helpful
   e. On average, nursing home residents only get 40 minutes of sleep for every hour spent in bed

The correct answer is e.

Not only are nursing home residents likely to have a sleep disorder before placement, but also sleep disturbance becomes more common as patients become more impaired in the institution. People in nursing homes regularly use sedatives for sleep. Nonetheless, they have abnormal sleep-wake patterns and increased amounts of time spent in bed. Unfortunately, the nursing home environment may be partially responsible for some of these problems. Nighttime arousals of residents are often associated with noise and light disturbances. The major source of these disturbances is often the nursing staff. More than half of nursing home residents wake up as often as two to three times per hour during the night. Nursing practices related to incontinence are particularly disruptive. On average, nursing home residents only get 40 minutes of sleep for every hour spent in bed.

References

Monane M, Glynn RJ, Avorn J. The impact of sedative-hypnotic use on sleep symptoms in elderly nursing home residents. *Clin Pharmacol Ther*. 1996; 59:83–92.

Pat-Horenczyk R, Klauber MR, Shochat T, Ancoli-Israel S. Hourly profiles of sleep and wakefulness in severely versus mild-moderately demented nursing home patients. *Aging (Milano)*. 1998;10:308–315.

Schnelle JF, Alessi CA, Al-Samarrai NR, Fricker RD Jr, Ouslander JG. The nursing home at night: effects of an intervention on noise, light, and sleep. *J Am Geriatr Soc*. 1999;47:430–438.

6. All of the following are true *except*

   a. Transient, situational insomnia may respond to sedatives
   b. An elderly person who has trouble with maintaining sleep should try a small amount of alcohol before bed
   c. Sedative/hypnotics cause falls both at night and during the day
   d. Sedative/hypnotic use in elderly patients may cause cognitive problems, performance problems, and irritability
   e. A trial of improved sleep hygiene is often the best initial approach

The correct answer is b.

Transient, situational insomnia may respond to sedatives. Treatment of elderly people with sedatives is fraught with danger. In fact, the use of medication to promote sleep is associated with increased mortality. Older patients with chronic sleep complaints should not be started on a sedative-hypnotic agent without a careful clinical assessment to identify the cause of the sleep disturbance. Sedative-hypnotics cause falls both at night and during the day. Daytime symptoms of sedative-hypnotic use in elderly patients include cognitive problems, performance problems, and irritability. Tolerance often develops to longer-acting agents. In the patient with chronic insomnia, it is imperative that the clinician excludes primary sleep disorders and reviews medications and other medical conditions that may be contributory. If the initial history and physical examination do not suggest a serious underlying cause for the sleep problem, a trial of improved sleep hygiene is the best initial approach.

References

Holbrook AM, Crowther R, Lotter A, Cheng C, King D. Meta-analysis of benzodiazepine use in the treatment of insomnia. *CMAJ.* 2000;162:225–233.

Morgan K, Clarke D: Longitudinal trends in late-life insomnia: implications for prescribing. *Age Ageing.* 1997;26:179–184.

Seppala M, Hyyppa MT, Impivaara O, Knuts LR, Sourander L. Subjective quality of sleep and use of hypnotics in an elderly urban population. *Aging (Milano).* 1997;9:327–334.

Chapter 27
Sexuality and Aging

1. Mr. S is a 76-year-old man with a history of coronary artery disease and hypertension, for which he is currently taking atenolol, isosorbide dinitrate, and verapamil. He visits his doctor seeking treatment for erectile dysfunction. He reports no previous history of sexual dysfunction prior to the last 6 months. He denies that he is experiencing any marital discord. What would be the most appropriate treatment for his sexual dysfunction?

   a. Sildenafil
   b. Sex therapy
   c. Penile prosthesis
   d. Penile injection therapy

The correct answer is d.

The most likely cause of Mr. S's erectile dysfunction is either an underlying organic impairment in erectile function or perhaps the use of the β-blocker atenolol. As a result, sex therapy would not be the most appropriate first line of treatment, especially with an otherwise intact and harmonious relationship with a partner. Because Mr. S is taking isosorbide dinitrate, the use of sildenafil (Viagra) would be contraindicated. The most appropriate treatment would be penile injection therapy. The placement of a penile prosthesis would be the last resort treatment if other, less-invasive, treatments fail.

References

Althof SE, Seftel AD. The evaluation and management of erectile dysfunction. *Psychiatr Clin North Am.* 1995;18:171–192.

Boolell M, Gepi-Attee S, Gingell JC, Allen MJ. Sildenafil, a novel effective oral therapy for male erectile dysfunction. *Br J Urol.* 1996;78:257–261.

Evans C. The use of penile prostheses in the treatment of impotence. *Br J Urol.* 1998;81:591–598.

Mobley DF, Baum N. Sildenafil in elderly men: advice and caveats. *Clin Geriatr.* 1999;7:34–41.

Segraves RT. New treatment for erectile dysfunction. *Curr Psychiatry Rep.* 2000;2:206–210.

2. Mr. R is a 70-year-old man complaining of delayed orgasm and erectile dysfunction. Which of the following medications is a likely cause?

    a. Sildenafil
    b. Papaverine
    c. Imipramine
    d. Bupropion
    e. Buspirone

The correct answer is c.

Sildenafil is an oral agent, and papaverine is an injectable agent; they are used to treat erectile dysfunction. Buproprion is an antidepressant that is not associated with sexual dysfunction; buspirone is an antianxiety medication that is also not associated with significant sexual dysfunction. Imipramine, however, is a tricyclic antidepressant associated with various forms of sexual dysfunction in both men and women.

References

Crenshaw TL, Goldberg JP. *Sexual Pharmacology: Drugs That Affect Sexual Function.* New York, NY: Norton; 1996.

Gitlin MJ. Psychotropic medications and their effects on sexual function: diagnosis, biology, and treatment approaches. *J Clin Psychiatry.* 1994;55:406–413.

Margolese HC, Assalian P. Sexual side effects of antidepressants: a review. *J Sex Marital Ther.* 1996; 22(3): 209–224.

3. A 90-year-old man who is a resident at a nursing home was described by nurses as "sexually aggressive" because he grabbed at a nurse's chest and appeared to have a lewd facial expression. What would be the most appropriate initial step to address the situation?

    a. Treat with estrogen to decrease sexual aggression
    b. Treat with 0.5 mg risperidone qd to reduce agitated, aggressive behaviors
    c. Interview staff to determine whether behavior actually represented sexual aggression

d. Develop a behavioral plan to prevent further episodes of sexual aggression

e. Treat with 10 mg fluoxetine to reduce libido

The correct answer is c.

All of these responses are potential treatments for sexual aggression. However, the first step is always to confirm that the behavior was indeed an episode of sexual aggression and not merely an attempt to get staff attention or a misdirected motor movement. It would not be appropriate to treat the individual with medication until the context of the behavior was better understood.

References

Hashmi FH, Krady AI, Qayum F, Grossberg GT. Sexually disinhibited behavior in the cognitively impaired elderly. *Clin Geriatr.* 2000;8:61–68.

Kumar A, Koss E, Metzler D, et al. Behavioral symptomatology in dementia of the Alzheimer type. *Alzheimer's Dis Assoc Disord.* 1988;2:363–365.

Redinbaugh EM, Zeiss AM, Davies HD, Tinklenberg JR. Sexual behavior in men with dementing illnesses. *Clin Geriatr.* 1997;5:45–50.

4. Mr. and Mrs. P live together in a nursing home. Mr. P suffers from Parkinson disease and mild cognitive impairment; Mrs. P suffers from Alzheimer's disease and has a history of depression. A nursing aide walked in on the couple engaged in sexual activity. She was upset by seeing this and reported it to the charge nurse, who then brought up the issue with the couple's physician. How should staff respond to the situation?

a. Contact the children of the couple to discuss the situation

b. Move the couple into separate rooms

c. Nothing; leave them alone

d. Maintain privacy for the couple and consider having the social worker or physician initiate a discussion with them regarding their sexual needs

e. Discipline the nursing aid for invading their privacy

The correct answer is d.

Sexual activity is a fundamental right of nursing home residents, and the facility has a responsibility to provide privacy for consenting couples when appropriate. Staff more often than residents have inappropriate reactions to sexual behaviors in the facility. It is never appropriate to breach privacy or confidentiality with respect to a consenting couple's sexual activity. It is also inappropriate to punish such individuals. Staff should be educated regarding residents' rights and institutional responsibilities rather than disciplined for a lack of understanding. When a couple is engaged in a sexual relationship, staff not only must always maintain privacy, but also be vigilant to a situation in which one or both partners suffer from cognitive impairment that may limit their ability to consent to the relationship. A staff member such as a social worker or physician who has a relationship with such individuals might consider having a discussion with both partners to make sure that they understand the nature of the relationship, have the ability to decline any unwanted aspects of a relationship, and are being provided with appropriate privacy and confidentiality.

References

Kaas MJ. Sexual expression of the elderly in nursing homes. *Gerontologist.* 1978;18:372–378.

Lichtenberg PA, Strzepek DM. Assessments of institutionalized dementia patient's competencies to participate in intimate relationships. *Gerontologist.* 1990;30:117–120.

Reingold DA. Rights of nursing home residents to sexual expression. *Clin Geriatr.* 1997;5:52–63.

5. Normal age-associated changes in male sexual functioning include

   a. Erectile dysfunction and anorgasmia
   b. Decreased libido and decreased refractory period
   c. Decreased erectile durability and increased refractory period
   d. Increased libido and increased duration of plateau stage
   e. Decline in sexual pleasure associated with reduced penile sensitivity

The correct answer is c.

The most consistently described normal changes in male sexual function associated with aging include a decline in erectile frequency, durability, and reliability; increased stimulation needed for orgasm; declines in ejaculatory force and emission; and prolonged refractory period in which further erection and ejaculation is inhibited. Levels of sexual libido or desire do not change appreciably. Despite some loss of penile sensitivity and need for increased stimulation to achieve erection, sexual pleasure does not appear to decline.

References

Butler RN, Lewis MI. *Love and Sex After 40: A Guide for Men and Women for Their Mid- and Later Years.* New York, NY: Harper and Row; 1986.

Masters WH. Sex and aging: expectations and reality. *Hosp Pract.* 1986;15:175–198.

Metz ME, Miner MH. Male menopause, aging, and sexual function: a review. *Sexuality Disabil. 1995;13:287–307.*

6. Which of the following statements best characterizes sexuality in late life?

   a. Predictors of sexual activity include physical health and partner availability
   b. The rates of sexual intercourse decrease equally for married and single individuals
   c. Sex therapy is usually unsuccessful in late life
   d. A major problem is the lack of available partners for men

The correct answer is a.

Married couples tend to be more sexually active than single individuals according to most surveys. The best predictors of sexual activity include health of the individual and the partner, previous level of sexual activity, and the availability of a partner. This becomes a problem for women in late life, who outnumber men by 2:1 by the age of 85.

References

Comfort A, Dial LK. Sexuality and aging: an overview. *Clin Geriatr Med.* 1991;7:1–7.

Jacoby S. Great sex. What's age got to do with it? *Modern Maturity* [serial online]. September/October 1999. Available at: http://www.aarp.org/press/1998/nr100198.html. Accessed November 1, 2000.

Marsiglio W, Donnelly D. Sexual relations in later life: a national study of married persons. *J Gerontol.* 1991;46:S338–S344.

7. Surveys of sexual activity in late life have indicated that

   a. Rates of sexual activity increase from ages 65 to 75 years, but taper off thereafter
   b. In general, men are more sexually active than women in late life
   c. Despite high levels of sexual activity, most individuals are not fully satisfied with their sexual performance
   d. Compared to younger individuals, older cohorts are equally approving of sex between unmarried partners

The correct answer is b.

In the last decade, there have been several major surveys of sexual activity in late life. All have indicated that over half of respondents in late life continue to be sexually active, although men are somewhat more sexually active. However, rates of sexual activity decline for both sexes after age 65 years. Respondents continue to describe sexuality as a satisfying aspect of their lives and indicate a high degree of satisfaction with their partners. Generational differences are seen in attitudes toward oral sex, masturbation, and sex between unmarried partners, with older cohorts being less likely to approve of such behaviors.

References

Jacoby S. Great sex. What's age got to do with it? *Modern Maturity* [serial online]. September/October 1999. Available at: http://www.aarp.org/press/1998/nr100198.html. Accessed November 1, 2000.

Marsiglio W, Donnelly D. Sexual relations in later life: a national study of married persons. *J Gerontol.* 1991;46:S338–S344.

Michael RT, Gagnon JH, Laumann EO, Kolata G. *Sex in America: A Definitive Survey.* Boston, MA: Little, Brown; 1994.

National Council on the Aging. *Healthy Sexuality and Vital Aging. Executive Summary.* Washington, DC: National Council on the Aging; 1998.

8. Mr. F is a 78-year-old man with a history of chronic obstructive pulmonary disease, coronary artery disease, diabetes mellitus, and morbid obesity. He wants to continue a sexual relationship with his wife but describes sex as physically difficult and exhausting. What would be the most appropriate suggestions to improve his situation?

   a. Attempt sexual foreplay only and cease sexual intercourse
   b. Focus on foreplay and choose a more comfortable sexual position
   c. Start taking sildenafil to increase erectile strength and endurance
   d. Start a rigorous exercise program to build up endurance and strength

The correct answer is b.

Sexual activity can often be physically challenging in individuals with certain medical problems or disabilities. Still, sex can be enjoyed by focusing on sexual strengths, such as the ability to engage in relaxing and less-strenuous sexual foreplay (e.g., erotic massage, cuddling, kissing, etc.). A couple does not need to give up sexual intercourse but should adapt their position to be less strenuous or uncomfortable (such as side by side or having one partner leaning on a pillow in front of the other). The use of oral erectogenic agents will treat erectile dysfunction but will not help to increase physical endurance during sex. Although exercise can help increase strength and endurance, the initiation of a rigorous exercise regimen solely for the purpose of sexual activity can potentially lead to injury or exacerbation of underlying physical disability.

References

Butler RN, Lewis MI. *Love and Sex After 40: A Guide for Men and Women for Their Mid- and Later Years.* New York, NY: Harper and Row; 1986.

Goodwin AJ, Agronin ME. *A Women's Guide to Overcoming Sexual Fear and Pain.* Oakland, CA: New Harbinger Press; 1997.

Schover LR, Jensen SB. *Sexuality and Chronic Illness.* New York, NY: Guilford Press; 1988.

IV Treatment

Chapter 28
The Practice of Evidence-Based Geriatric Psychiatry

1. A primary characteristic that distinguishes evidence-based medicine from traditional medical paradigms is the use of

   a. Local opinion on preferred practice
   b. A hierarchy of evidence to aid decision making
   c. Internal clinical skills, judgment, and experience
   d. Clinical wisdom and opinion of experts

   The correct answer is b.

   Evidence-based medicine utilizes a hierarchy of evidence to guide clinical decision making and to classify the level of evidence that supports an intervention. Evidence-based medicine draws heavily on the use of external evidence to support, but not replace, internal clinical skills, judgment, and experience. Moreover, evidence-based medicine applies rigor to health care evaluation that supercedes that provided in a traditional medical paradigm representing local opinions for preferred practices, expert opinion, and personal beliefs and preferences.

   References

   Friedland DJ, Go AS, Davoren JB, et al. *Evidence-Based Medicine: A Framework for Clinical Practice.* Stamford, CT: Appleton and Lange; 1998.
   Guyatt G, Rennie D. *Users' Guides to the Medical Literature : A Manual for Evidence-Based Clinical Practice/The Evidence-Based Medicine Working Group.* Chicago, IL: AMA Press; 2002.
   Sackett DL, Rosenberg WM, Gray JA, Haynes RB, Richardson WS. Evidence based medicine: what it is and what it isn't. *BM J.* 1996;312:71–72.

2. The use of evidence-based practices specific to older adults is important because

   a. Cognitive changes of aging can affect response to psychotherapy
   b. There is substantial variation in competence and practice
   c. Changes associated with aging can alter pharmacological response
   d. Older adults are generally more susceptible to medication side effects
   e. All of the above

The correct answer is e.

The identification of mental health interventions tailored for older adults is important because aging is associated with a variety of changes in physiological, cognitive, and social functioning that may affect response to treatment. Cognitive impairment affects responses to psychotherapeutic interventions, and pharmacological response and sensitivity to medication side effects change as individuals age. Finally, older adults receive mental health services in a variety of health care settings (primary care, aging network services, long-term care, home care, specialty mental health care, family caregiver, hospitals, criminal justice system), and there are significant differences between providers in these settings. Identification and use of evidence-based treatments in these settings can help improve the care that older adults receive.

References

Banerjee S, Dickinson E. Evidence based health care in old age psychiatry. *Int J Psychiatry Med.* 1997;27:283–292.

Burns BJ, Taube CA. Mental health services in general medical care and nursing homes. In: Fogel B, Furino A, Gottlieb G, eds. *Mental Health Policy for Older Americans: Protecting Minds at Risk.* Washington, DC: American Psychiatric Press; 1990:63–84.

Gatz M, Smyer MA. The mental health system and older adults in the 1990s. *Am Psychol.* 1992;47:741–751.

3. Meta-analyses find support for the effectiveness of the following treatment(s) of cognitive impairment in dementia of the Alzheimer type

   a. Atypical antipsychotics
   b. Cholinesterase inhibitors
   c. Cognitive remediation therapy
   d. Estrogen

The correct answer is b.

Meta-analyses and evidence-based reviews suggest that cholinesterase inhibitors have a significant, but modest, effect in diminishing the rate of cognitive decline among individuals with mild-to-moderate Alzheimer's dementia when compared to placebo over a period of 6 to 12 months. In contrast, a 2002 Cochrane Review concluded that the use of estrogen replacement is not indicated for cognitive improvement or maintenance in women with Alzheimer's disease. Moreover, although cognitive retraining programs can temporarily slow decline in functional skills for a limited subset of individuals, they do not result in sustained effects.

References

Doody RS, Stevens JC, Beck C, et al. Practice parameter: management of dementia (an evidence-based review): report of the Quality Standards Subcommittee of the American Academy of Neurology. *Neurology.* 2001;56: 1154–1166.

Hogervorst E, Yaffe K, Richards M, Huppert F. Hormone replacement therapy to maintain cognitive function in women with dementia. (Cochrane Review.) In: *The Cochrane Library.* Oxford, UK: Update Software; 2002, Issue 4.

National Institute for Clinical Excellence. *Technology Appraisal Guidance No. 19: Guidance on the Use of Donepezil, Rivastigmine and Galantamine for the Treatment of Alzheimer's Disease.* London: National Institute for Clinical Excellence; 2001.

Spector A, Orrell M, Davies S, Woods B. Reality orientation for dementia. (Cochrane Review.) In: *The Cochrane Library.* Oxford, UK: Update Software; 2001, Issue 2.

4. Based on meta-analyses and evidence-based reviews of the literature, the following show comparable efficacy and tolerability in the treatment of older adults with major depression *except*

 a. Tricyclic antidepressants (TCAs)
 b. Non-selective serotonin reuptake inhibitor norepinephrine reuptake inhibitors (NSSRIs)
 c. Benzodiazepines
 d. Selective serotonin reuptake inhibitors (SSRIs)

The correct answer is c.

Among studies comparing different types of antidepressants in the treatment of geriatric depression, comparable efficacy and tolerability have been reported among TCAs, SSRIs, and NSSRIs. Moreover, meta-analyses comparing SSRIs and TCAs showed no significant differences between agents with respect to efficacy or discontinuation because of side effects. However, clinically significant differences in side-effect profiles between TCAs and SSRIs exist. In contrast, although benzodiazepines are a commonly prescribed treatment for older adults with anxiety disorders, caution is warranted because of their association with falls, memory impairment, and paradoxical agitation.

References

Alexopoulos GS, Katz IR, Reynolds CF III, Carpenter D, Docherty JP. The expert consensus guideline series: pharmacotherapy of depressive disorders in older patients. *Postgrad Med.* October 2001:1–86.

Anderson IM. Selective serotonin reuptake inhibitors versus tricyclic antidepressants: a meta-analysis of efficacy and tolerability. *J Affect Disord.* 2000;58:19–36.

McCusker J, Cole M, Keller E, Bellavance F, Berard A. Effectiveness of treatments of depression in older ambulatory patients. *Arch Intern Med.* 1998; 158:705–712.

Mittmann N, Herrmann N, Einarson TR, et al. The efficacy, safety and tolerability of antidepressants in late life depression: a meta-analysis. *J Affect Disord.* 1997;46:191–217.

5. Based on meta-analyses and evidence-based reviews the use of cognitive-behavioral therapy (CBT) has empirical support for individuals with all of the following *except*

   a. Depression
   b. Alcohol abuse
   c. Anxiety
   d. Schizophrenia

The correct answer is d.

CBT has established efficacy in the treatment of geriatric depression, alcohol abuse, and anxiety. The effectiveness of CBT has been examined among older adults with schizophrenia; however, empirical support is limited to a controlled pilot study that suggested potential benefits of a combination of CBT and skills training.

References

Gatz M, Fiske A, Fox LS, et al. Empirically validated psychological treatments for older adults. *J Ment Health Aging.* 1998;4:9–46.

Granholm E, McQuaid JR, McClure FS, Pedrelli P, Jeste DV. A randomized controlled pilot study of cognitive behavioral social skills training for older patients with schizophrenia. *Schizophr Res.* 2002;53:167–169.

Stanley MA, Novy DM. Cognitive-behavior therapy for generalized anxiety in late life: an evaluative overview. *J Anxiety Disord.* 2000;14:191–207.

6. Which of the following has empirical support from multiple studies as an effective geriatric mental health service?

   a. Geropsychiatric inpatient units
   b. Community-based, multidisciplinary, geriatric mental health treatment teams
   c. Geriatric psychiatry consultation services to nursing homes
   d. Hospital-based geriatric psychiatry consultation-liaison services

The correct answer is b.

Hospital-based geriatric psychiatry consultation-liaison services appear to be effective, although further research is necessary to evaluate such programs comprehensively. The effectiveness of geropsychiatric inpatient units or day hospital programs has not been adequately examined through rigorous studies. Although one randomized controlled trial (RCT) has examined the effectiveness of geriatric psychiatry consultation services to nursing homes, it failed to find clinically different outcomes compared to usual care. An evidence-based review of multiple published studies found support for the effectiveness of community-based, multidisciplinary, geriatric mental health treatment teams. In addition, a more recent systematic review of community-based mental health outreach services found five RCTs, one quasi-experimental study, and six uncontrolled cohort studies. This review confirmed the positive effect of home- and community-based treatment of psychiatric symptoms in improving or maintaining psychiatric status (including depressive symptoms and overall psychiatric symptoms).

References

Bartels SJ, Moak GS, Dums AR. Mental health services in nursing homes: models of mental health services in nursing homes: a review of the literature. *Psychiatr Serv.* 2002;53:1390–1396.

Draper B. The effectiveness of old age psychiatry services. *Int J Geriatr Psychiatry.* 2000;15:687–703.

Van Citters AD, Bartels SJ. Effectiveness of community-based mental health outreach services for older adults: a systematic review. *Psychiatr Serv.* 2004;55(11):1237–1249.

7. Meta-analytic procedures can be negatively affected by

   a. Differences in the duration of studies
   b. Ignoring important differences between studies
   c. Lack of interchangeable instruments
   d. Excluding informative studies
   e. All of the above

The correct answer is e.

Meta-analytic procedures are affected by all of the above and need to be evaluated for methodological rigor and clinical significance. Aggregate analyses are prone to excluding informative studies and may cluster studies without sufficient attention to important differences. Meta-analyses can be affected by small sample sizes, lack of interchangeable instruments and extractable data, and duration of studies. Despite these problems, a rigorous meta-analysis has the ability to provide an estimate of the effect of an intervention.

References

Friedland DJ, Go AS, Davoren JB, et al. *Evidence-Based Medicine: A Framework for Clinical Practice.* Stamford, CT: Appleton and Lange; 1998.

Guyatt G, Rennie D. *Users' Guides to the Medical Literature : A Manual for Evidence-Based Clinical Practice/The Evidence-Based Medicine Working Group*. Chicago, IL: AMA Press; 2002.

8. For the busy, practicing geriatric clinician, which source provides the most objective summarized information on empirically tested, effective interventions?

   a. Clinical guidelines from professional societies
   b. Treatment algorithms from expert consensus panels
   c. Prefiltered databases (e.g., Cochrane Data Base, Best Evidence, Evidence-Based Mental Health)
   d. MEDLINE or PubMed

The correct answer is c.

The Cochrane Data Base of Systematic Reviews, Best Evidence, and Evidence-Based Mental Health are examples of prefiltered databases of systematic reviews that provide the most objective summarized information on empirically evaluated, effective interventions. However, these reviews exist for only a limited number of interventions. As such, it is often necessary to evaluate additional sources of information. Although clinical guidelines developed by professional societies or treatment algorithms prepared by expert consensus panels provide an overview of the effectiveness of interventions in a specific topic area, they are subject to a variety of biases. Medical literature databases such as MEDLINE can assist in finding information when prefiltered resources do not provide satisfactory information. Because of the relatively comprehensive nature of MEDLINE, the clinician must conduct an efficient search of the literature, select the best of the relevant studies, apply rules of evidence to determine their validity, and extract the clinical message. Guyatt and Rennie (2002) provided a step-by-step manual with detailed instruction on using and appraising the evidence base, including conducting Web-based searches, reviewing resources that synthesize research, and evaluating individual research studies.

Reference

Guyatt G, Rennie D. *Users' Guides to the Medical Literature: A Manual for Evidence-Based Clinical Practice/The Evidence-Based Medicine Working Group*. Chicago, IL: AMA Press; 2002.

9. In the hierarchy of evidence, the highest level of evidence is

   a. Case reports
   b. A single well-designed RCT
   c. A meta-analysis or evidence-based systematic review

d. Quasi-experimental designed studies

e. Pre–post or matched case–control studies

The correct answer is c.

According to a hierarchical classification of evidence proposed by Gray (1997), meta-analyses or systematic review of well-designed RCTs are most highly supported, followed by a single properly designed RCT, studies without randomization (such as a single group pre–post, cohort, time series, or matched case–control studies), other quasi-experimental studies from more than one center or research group, and expert reports and authorities' recommendations based on descriptive studies or clinical evidence.

Reference

Gray JAM. *Evidence-based Healthcare: How to Make Health Policy and Management Decisions.* New York, NY: Churchill Livingston; 1997.

10. In general, treatment guidelines

a. Are unlikely to be biased when produced by professional societies

b. Have been shown to be effective in changing clinical practice

c. Are an objective and reliable summary of the evidence base

d. Should be critically evaluated for sources of supporting evidence

The correct answer is d.

Guidelines are subject to biases that include potential poor quality of development and under- or overestimation of treatment effects or side effects. Guidelines produced by professional societies are not immune to these potential biases. To avoid these limitations, clinicians are advised to examine the developmental procedures associated with the guideline of interest, with attention to the presence of a supporting systematic review of evidence linking treatment options to outcomes; discussion of relevant patient groups and preferences or values associated with treatment recommendations; and an indication of the strength of the authors' recommendations. Of note, providing practice guidelines to clinicians in the absence of additional educational efforts is unlikely to change treatment practices

References

Grilli R, Margrini N, Penna A, Mura G, Liberati A. Practice guidelines developed by specialty societies: the need for a critical appraisal. *Lancet.* 2000; 355:103–106.

Grimshaw JM, Russell IT. Effect of clinical guidelines on medical practice: a systematic review of rigorous evaluations. *Lancet.* 1993;342:1317–1322.

Oxman TE. Effective educational techniques for primary care providers: application to the management of psychiatric disorders. *Int J Psychiatry Med.* 1998;28:3–9.

Shaneyfelt TM, Mayo-Smith MF, Rothwangl J. Are guidelines following guidelines? The methodological quality of clinical practice guidelines in the peer-reviewed medical literature. *JAMA.* 1999;281:1900–1905.

11. All of the following have been associated with interactions between physicians and representatives from the pharmaceutical industry *except*

    a. Requests to add medications to formularies
    b. Decreased prescribing of generic drugs
    c. Higher prescribing costs
    d. Underpublication of unfavorable research findings
    e. Greater use of an evidence-based approach to clinical decision making

The correct answer is e.

Industry provides at least 70% of the financial resources for clinical drug trials conducted in the United States. Interactions with pharmaceutical representatives have been associated with (a) requests for additions to formularies (some of which have little to no advantage over existing formulary drugs); (b) increased awareness, preference, and prescribing of new drugs (combined with decreased prescribing of generic drugs); (c) higher prescribing costs; (d) attitudes that support interactions with pharmaceutical representatives; (e) favorable publications and research findings; and (f) underpublication of unfavorable findings.

References

Bodenheimer T. Uneasy alliance—clinical investigators and the pharmaceutical industry. *N Engl J Med.* 2000;342:1539–1544.

Choudhry NK, Stelfox HT, Detsky AS. Relationships between authors of clinical practice guidelines and the pharmaceutical industry. *JAMA.* 2002;287:612–617.

Wazana A. Physicians and the pharmaceutical industry: is a gift ever just a gift? *JAMA.* 2000;283:373–380.

12. Which of the following are accurate statements with respect to potential conflicts of interest associated with published clinical guidelines?

    a. Most of the time, authors of guidelines report existing or potential conflicts of interest
    b. More than 4/5 authors of clinical guidelines have a financial relationship with at least one pharmaceutical manufacturer

c. Published guidelines frequently list potential conflicts of interest with pharmaceutical manufacturers by the authors or participating experts

d. Users of published guidelines can generally assume that major conflicts of interest are uniformly disclosed

The correct answer is b.

Among 100 authors of clinical guidelines published between 1991 and 1999 for common medical diseases, 87% had a relationship with at least one pharmaceutical manufacturer. Of the 44 published guidelines with authors surveyed, only 1 reported a financial conflict of interest with the pharmaceutical industry, 1 reported no conflicts of interest, and the remaining 42 did not indicate the existence of potential conflicts of interest. As such, readers cannot assume that conflicts of interest are uniformly disclosed. Conflicts of interest can lead to biased reporting of research on effectiveness of interventions. Clinicians should take care in reviewing published reports to identify and weigh potential investigator conflicts of interest.

References

Choudhry NK, Stelfox HT, Detsky AS. Relationships between authors of clinical practice guidelines and the pharmaceutical industry. *JAMA.* 2002;287: 612–617.

McCrary SV, Anderson CB, Jakovljevic J, et al. A national survey of policies on disclosure of conflicts of interest in biomedical research. *N Engl J Med.* 2000;343:1621–1626.

Chapter 29
Electroconvulsive Therapy

1. A 68-year-old man with a history of recurrent psychotic depression is referred for electroconvulsive therapy (ECT) after failing four adequate medication trials, including a tricyclic antidepressant and antipsychotic combination. Which of the following statements is true regarding his likelihood of response to ECT?

   a. His age makes him less likely to respond than a younger patient

   b. The presence of psychosis indicates a severe illness that is less likely to respond

   c. Medication resistance may decrease the likelihood of ECT response

   d. Multiple prior depressive episodes increase the likelihood of ECT response

   e. He has greater than a 90% chance of complete response to ECT regardless of prior treatment history

The correct answer is c.

Although relative medication resistance is a common reason for ECT referral, patients who have failed one or more adequate medication trials have a diminished (although still substantial) rate of ECT response.

References

Prudic J, Haskett RF, Mulsant B, et al. Resistance to antidepressant medications and short-term clinical response to ECT. *Am J Psychiatry.* 1996;153: 985–992.

Prudic J, Sackeim HA, Devanand DP. Medication resistance and clinical response to electroconvulsive therapy. *Psychiatry Res.* 1990;31:287–296.

2. A 68-year-old man with a history of recurrent psychotic depression is referred for ECT after failing four adequate medication trials, including a tricyclic antidepressant and antipsychotic combination. Which of the following factors is associated with a lower risk of relapse following ECT?

   a. Bilateral electrode placement
   b. Final Hamilton Depression Rating Scale (HAM-D) scores less than 7
   c. Lack of postictal confusion
   d. Lowered seizure threshold over the course of treatment
   e. Seizure durations of at least 60 seconds

The correct answer is b.

Residual depressive symptoms can have a negative impact on the quality of life and may lead to chronic depression or increased likelihood of relapse. Although not proven, it is likely that full remission of depression is more common with ECT than with pharmacotherapy, and an ECT series should generally be continued until there is either complete remission of depression or a plateau in improvement is reached. Electrode placement, seizure duration, and postictal confusion are not related to relapse, and seizure threshold generally increases over a course of ECT.

References

American Psychiatric Association. *The Practice of Electroconvulsive Therapy: Recommendations for Treatment, Training and Privileging.* 2nd ed. Washington, DC: American Psychiatric Association; 2000.

Devanand DP, Nobler MS, Singer T, et al. Subjective side effects during electroconvulsive therapy. *Convulsive Ther.* 1995;11:232–240.

Hamilton M. The effect of treatment on the melancholic depressions. *Br J Psychiatry.* 1982;140:223–230.

Prien R, Kupfer D. Continuation drug therapy for major depressive episodes: how long should it be maintained? *Am J Psychiatry.* 1986;143:18–23.

3. A 70-year-old man with a history of recurrent depression shows a rapid response to ECT, with complete remission of depressive symptoms following his sixth treatment. The best next step would be

   a. Immediately initiate continuation/maintenance treatment (pharmacotherapy and/or ECT)
   b. Stop ECT because such a rapid improvement indicates a likely placebo response
   c. Stop ECT only if he has reached his lifetime maximum of 100 treatments
   d. Continue the ECT series for a total of at least eight treatments because this is the average number of treatments needed for full response
   e. Continue ECT until he shows evidence of cognitive impairment

The correct answer is a.

The risk of relapse following ECT is high, especially in the first few months, and the need for aggressive continuation therapy is compelling. An ECT series should generally be continued until there is maximal improvement, without any predetermined minimum or maximum number. There is no "lifetime maximum" of ECT treatments.

References

American Psychiatric Association. *The Practice of Electroconvulsive Therapy: Recommendations for Treatment, Training and Privileging.* 2nd ed. Washington, DC: American Psychiatric Association; 2000.

Sackeim HA, Prudic J, Devanand DP, et al. The impact of medication resistance and continuation pharmacotherapy on relapse following response to electroconvulsive therapy in major depression. *J Clin Psychopharmacol.* 1990;10:96–104.

4. A 67-year-old man with depression is taking propranolol for hypertension and ischemic heart disease. Stimulus dosage titration is performed at the first ECT treatment to estimate initial seizure threshold. The first stimulus results in a missed seizure, and within seconds the patient develops sinus bradycardia with a heart rate of 20 beats per minute. Which of the following is the most likely explanation for this arrhythmia?

   a. Relative increased activity of the sympathetic and parasympathetic nervous systems
   b. Relative increased activity of the sympathetic nervous system
   c. Relative increased activity of the parasympathetic nervous system
   d. Relative increased activity of the sympathetic nervous system and decreased activity of the parasympathetic nervous system

e. Relative decreased activity of the sympathetic and parasympathetic nervous systems

The correct answer is c.

There is a vagally mediated increase in parasympathetic tone immediately following administration of the electrical stimulus. This may be more pronounced in patients taking β-blockers and when there is no subsequent ictally induced increase in sympathetic tone as in the case of a subconvulsive stimulation.

References

American Psychiatric Association. *The Practice of Electroconvulsive Therapy: Recommendations for Treatment, Training and Privileging.* 2nd ed. Washington, DC: American Psychiatric Association; 2000.

Applegate RJ. Diagnosis and management of ischemic heart disease in the patient scheduled to undergo electroconvulsive therapy. *Convulsive Ther.* 1997;13:128–144.

5. With increasing patient age, ECT seizure threshold can be expected to

   a. Decrease, with associated longer seizure duration
   b. Decrease, with associated shorter seizure duration
   c. Increase, with associated longer seizure duration
   d. Increase, with associated shorter seizure duration
   e. Show no change

The correct answer is d.

Seizure threshold generally increases with age, and there is an inverse correlation between seizure threshold and seizure duration.

References

American Psychiatric Association. *The Practice of Electroconvulsive Therapy: Recommendations for Treatment, Training and Privileging.* 2nd ed. Washington, DC: American Psychiatric Association; 2000.

Boylan LS, Haskett RF, Mulsant BF, et al. Determinants of seizure threshold in ECT: benzodiazepine use, anesthetic dosage, and other factors. *J ECT.* 2000;16:3–18.

Sackeim HA, Decina P, Kanzler M, et al. Effects of electrode placement on the efficacy of titrated, low-dose ECT. *Am J Psychiatry.* 1987;144:1449–1455.

6. An 80-year-old man, 2 months after coronary artery bypass surgery with significantly impaired left ventricular function and severe major depression with psychotic features, is referred for ECT. On further

cardiac testing, ejection fraction is 15%. To decrease cardiac risk, which of the following anesthetic medications might be considered?

a. Droperiodol
b. Fentanyl
c. Lidocaine
d. Etomidate
e. Nitrous oxide

The correct answer is d.

Etomidate generally causes fewer hemodynamic consequences than other anesthetic agents and should be considered in some patients with severely impaired cardiac output.

Reference

American Psychiatric Association. *The Practice of Electroconvulsive Therapy: Recommendations for Treatment, Training and Privileging.* 2nd ed. Washington, DC: American Psychiatric Association; 2000.

7. In combining maintenance lithium therapy with outpatient maintenance ECT

a. Lasix should be given as pretreatment to clear the lithium
b. Patients should receive an additional 300 to 600 mg of lithium on the day of ECT to prevent drug washout
c. Lithium must be tapered off (to a level of 0 Meq) before each ECT
d. Lithium should be held for at least 24 hours before each ECT
e. Intravenous fluids should be minimized to prevent causing a subtherapeutic lithium level

The correct answer is d.

Patients receiving lithium during ECT may be at higher risk for prolonged seizures or postictal delirium. However, many patients have received lithium during ECT without incident, and risk rapidly diminishes with dose reduction. At moderate lithium levels, holding lithium for at least 24 hours prior to ECT is generally sufficient to minimize risk of complications.

References

American Psychiatric Association. *The Practice of Electroconvulsive Therapy: Recommendations for Treatment, Training and Privileging.* 2nd ed. Washington, DC: American Psychiatric Association; 2000.

Kellner CH, Nixon DW, Bernstein HJ. ECT–drug interactions: a review. *Psychopharmacol Bull.* 1991;27:595–609.

Mukherjee S, Sackeim HA, Schnur DB. Electroconvulsive therapy of acute manic episodes: a review of 50 years experience. *Am J Psychiatry.* 1994; 151:169–176.

Weiner RD, Whanger AD, Erwin CW, et al. Prolonged confusional state and EEG seizure activity following concurrent ECT and lithium use. *Am J Psychiatry.* 1980;137:1452–1453.

8. Which of the following statements generally characterizes right unilateral ECT compared to bilateral ECT?

   a. Decreased efficacy in all patients
   b. Increased seizure threshold
   c. Decreased cognitive impairment
   d. Increased prolactin release
   e. Increased ECT course length in all patients

The correct answer is c.

There is abundant evidence that right unilateral ECT is associated with less cognitive impairment than bilateral ECT. Its efficacy may match that of bilateral ECT at stimulus intensities that are sufficiently above seizure threshold. Compared with bilateral ECT, right unilateral placement is associated with a lower seizure threshold and less prolactin release. Speed of response is related to dosing relative to seizure threshold with unilateral and bilateral electrode placement.

References

American Psychiatric Association. *The Practice of Electroconvulsive Therapy: Recommendations for Treatment, Training and Privileging.* 2nd ed. Washington, DC: American Psychiatric Association; 2000.

McCall WV, Reboussin DM, Weiner RD, et al. Titrated, moderately suprathreshold versus fixed, high dose RUL ECT: acute antidepressant and cognitive effects. *Arch Gen Psychiatry.* 2000;57:438–444.

Sackeim HA, Prudic J, Devanand DP, et al. Effects of stimulus intensity and electrode placement on the efficacy and cognitive effects of electroconvulsive therapy. *N Engl J Med.* 1993;328:839–846.

Sackeim HA, Prudic J, Devanand DP, et al. A prospective, randomized, double-blind comparison of bilateral and right unilateral ECT at different stimulus intensities. *Arch Gen Psychiatry.* 2000;57:425–434.

9. A computerized tomographic (CT) scan of the brain prior to ECT

   a. Is indicated as part of the routine work-up
   b. Should not be obtained because magnetic resonance imaging (MRI) scans are more sensitive
   c. Should be obtained every 6 months during maintenance ECT

d. Should be performed if other data suggest the presence of a central nervous system (CNS) abnormality

e. Is never indicated because electroencephalograms (EEGs) are cheaper and equally useful

The answer is d.

Brain CT or MRI scans are not routinely necessary prior to a course of ECT. They should be considered if other data from the history or physical exam suggest a brain abnormality that may be relevant to decision making regarding ECT.

Reference

American Psychiatric Association. *The Practice of Electroconvulsive Therapy: Recommendations for Treatment, Training and Privileging.* 2nd ed. Washington, DC: American Psychiatric Association; 2000.

10. Which nonpsychiatric conditions listed below may benefit from a course of ECT?

a. Pheochromocytoma
b. Hyperthyroidism
c. Parkinson disease
d. Asthma
e. Hypertension

The answer is c.

There is now abundant case report and case series literature supporting the utility of ECT in improving motor symptoms of Parkinson disease, with or without concurrent depression.

References

Kellner CH, Bernstein HJ. ECT as a treatment for neurologic illness. In: Coffey CE, ed. *The Clinical Science of Electroconvulsive Therapy.* Washington, DC: American Psychiatric Press; 1993:183–210.

Krystal AD, Coffey CE. Neuropsychiatric considerations in the use of electroconvulsive therapy. *J Neuropsychiatry Clin Neurosci.* 1997;9:283–292.

Rasmussen K, Abrams R. Treatment of Parkinson's disease with electroconvulsive therapy. *Psychiatr Clin North Am.* 1991;14:925–933.

Wengel SP, Burke WJ, Pfeiffer RF, et al. Maintenance electroconvulsive therapy for intractable Parkinson's disease. *Am J Geriatr Psychiatry.* 1998;6: 263–269.

Chapter 30
Psychopharmacology

1. Which of the following physiological changes associated with aging influences the pharmacodynamic responses to psychiatric medications?

   a. Decreased renal plasma flow
   b. Decreased hepatic blood flow
   c. Decreased plasma albumin
   d. Decreased striatal dopamine neurons
   e. Decreased activity of the P450 2D6 isoenzyme system

   The correct answer is d.

   Both the hepatic blood flow and the activity of the P450 enzyme system can affect the metabolism of psychiatric medications. The levels of plasma proteins (e.g., albumin, α-acid glycoprotein) to which psychotropic drugs are bound influence the distribution of a drug in the plasma (i.e., the ratio of bound vs. unbound form). All the above are examples of pharmacokinetic processes except for answer d. The decreased number of dopamine neurons in the striatum, on the other hand, can affect the tissue response to a given concentration of drug and is an example of a pharmacodynamic process that may influence the response to psychiatric medications. Furthermore, none of the examples of aging-related changes in pharmacokinetic processes, with the possible exception of a decreased binding of benzodiazapines to albumin, are thought to influence in vivo responses to psychiatric medications that occur in association with aging.

   Reference

   Sadavoy J. Introduction. In: *Psychotropic Drugs and the Elderly: Fast Facts.* New York, NY: Norton; 2004:3–21.

2. Which side effect of selective serotonin uptake inhibitors (SSRIs) is thought to occur more frequently in older patients than young adults?

   a. Diarrhea
   b. Syndrome of inappropriate antidiuretic hormone secretion (SIADH)
   c. Insomnia
   d. Diminished memory
   e. Akathisia

   The correct answer is b.

   SSRI treatment has been associated with an increased risk of developing SIADH, especially in the elderly. There is no evidence that any of the other side effects mentioned are any more prevalent in the elderly treated with SSRIs.

References

Fabian TJ, Amico JA, Kroboth PD, et al. Paroxetine-induced hyponatremia in older adults: a 12-week prospective study. *Arch Int Med.* 2004;164:327–332.

Kirby D, Ames D. Hyponatraemia and selective serotonin re-uptake inhibitors in elderly patients. *Int J Geriatr Psychiatry.* 2001;16:484–493.

Pillans PI, Coulter DM. Fluoxetine and hyponatraemia: a potential hazard in the elderly. *N Z Med J.* 1994;107:85–86.

3. Based on randomized, controlled studies, which of the following statements about the treatment of psychiatric symptoms associated with dementia of the Alzheimer type with atypical antipsychotic medications is correct?

   a. Efficacy for psychosis is greater than for behavioral symptoms
   b. The minimum efficacious dose of risperidone is generally 0.5 mg/day
   c. The minimum efficacious dose of olanzapine is 5 mg/day
   d. Efficacious doses are also associated with a significantly greater incidence of worsening of cognition than occurs in association with placebo
   e. Are more efficacious than conventional antipsychotic medications

The correct answer is c.

Both olanzapine at doses of 5 to 10 mg/day and risperidone at doses of 1 to 1.5 mg/day have been associated with significant improvement in psychopathology among nursing home patients with dementia, including both behavioral disturbances and levels of psychosis. These dose ranges were not associated with worsening of cognition or statistically significant increases in other side effects.

References

Katz IR, Jeste DV, Mintzer JE, et al. Comparison of risperidone and placebo for psychosis and behavioral disturbances associated with dementia: a randomized, double-blind trial. Risperidone Study Group. *J Clin Psychiatry.* 1999;60:107–115.

Street JS, Clark WS, Gannon KS, et al. Olanzapine treatment of psychotic and behavioral symptoms in patients with Alzheimer disease in nursing care facilities: a double-blind, randomized, placebo-controlled trial. The HGEU Study Group. *Arch Gen Psychiatry.* 2000;57:968–976.

4. Which of the following medications will most likely cause increased alprazolam levels?

a. Nefazodone
b. Fluoxetine
c. Nortriptyline
d. Buproprion
e. Venlafaxine

The correct answer is a.

Nefazodone is a potent inhibitor of the P450 3A4 system and can increase the levels of triazolobenzodiazepines that are substrates of this system, including alprazolam, midazolam, estazolam, and triazolam. The manufacturer of nefazodone recommends a 50% reduction in dose of alprazolam. Fluoxetine is only a moderate inhibitor of 3A4, and although the theoretical risk exists of interactions with triazolobenzodiazepines, it has not been implicated in clinically significant interactions with alprazolam. Nortriptyline, venlafaxine, and bupropion do not affect the P450 3A4 system.

References

Owen JR, Nemeroff CB. New antidepressants and the cytochrome P450 system: focus on venlafaxine, nefazodone, and mirtazapine. *Depression Anxiety.* 1998;7(suppl 1:24–32.
Bristol-Myers Squibb. Serzone package insert. Princeton, NJ: Bristol-Myers Squibb; 1995.

5. Which of the following factors confounds treatment studies of the depression associated with Alzheimer disease?

a. High placebo response rates
b. High rates of treatment resistance
c. High incidence of somatic side effects
d. Low prevalence of syndrome
e. Worsening of cognition during antidepressant treatment

The correct answer is a.

In most treatment studies of depression in the context of Alzheimer's disease, a large placebo response is noted. This may be caused by the instability of mood symptoms in demented patients and may account for the absence of drug–placebo differences. Clearly, this is a confounding factor that hinders the interpretation of these studies.

There is no evidence that treatment of depression associated with Alzheimer's disease is associated with high rates of treatment resistance or more pronounced somatic side effects. Controlled treatment studies have demonstrated that active treatment is associated with significant improvement rather than worsening of cognition, including trials with tricyclic antidepressants.

References

Lyketsos CG, DelCampo L, Steinberg M, et al. Treating depression in Alzheimer disease: efficacy and safety of sertraline therapy, and the benefits of depression reduction: the DIADS. *Arch Gen Psychiatry.* 2003;60:737–746.

Petracca GM, Chemerinski E, Starkstein SE. A double-blind, placebo-controlled study of fluoxetine in depressed patients with Alzheimer's disease. *Int Psychogeriatr.* 2001;13:233–240.

Reifler BV, Teri L, Raskind M, et al. Double blind trial of imipramine in Alzheimer's disease in patients with and without depression. *Am J Psychiatry.* 1989;146:45–49.

6. The maxim to "start low and go slow" when treating geriatric patients with psychotropic medication is based on

   a. Evidence that older patients require lower doses to respond
   b. Evidence that older patients require a longer time to respond
   c. The increased incidence of idiopathic sensitivity to side effects among older patients
   d. The assumption that older patients will tolerate and adhere to medications better if doses are increased gradually
   e. The assumption that identifying side effects early in treatment will decrease the risk of aging-related serious adverse drug reactions

The correct answer is d.

The available evidence does not support the generalization that older patients require lower doses of psychotropic medications to respond. Similarly, there is no evidence of increased incidence of idiopathic or severe side effects in elderly psychiatric patients or evidence that mild side effects place patients at increased risk for serious drug reactions. There is some evidence that, for some types of geriatric depression and some subsets of other disorders, older patients may respond more slowly than younger patients. This does not logically support the maxim of slow dose increments; if anything, a slower response rate would argue for more aggressive dosing. Theoretically, treatment-emergent side effects would be less severe at lower doses, such that starting low and going slow would enable elderly patients to develop a tolerance to these reactions and increase the likelihood of medication adherence if doses are increased gradually.

Reference

Jacobson SA, Pies RW, Greenblatt DJ. *Handbook of Geriatric Psychopharmacology.* Washington, DC: American Psychiatric Publishing; 2002.

7. Which of the following is the strongest risk factor for the development of torsades de pointes (TdP)?

   a. PR interval greater than 0.2
   b. History of myocardial infarction
   c. QTc interval above 450 ms
   d. History of hypertension
   e. Electrocardiographic evidence of left ventricular hypertrophy

The correct answer is c.

TdP (or "twisting of the points") is a unique, potentially life-threatening form of ventricular tachycardia associated with QT interval prolongation, irregular R-R intervals, and QRS complexes that appear to twist on the electrocardiogram axis. Any condition that lengthens the QT interval can cause TdP, although the specific length that triggers the arrhythmia is not known. The prolonged QT interval can develop during an acute myocardial infarction or result from other conditions associated with a wide QRS complex, such as intraventricular conduction disorders, electrolyte abnormalities, and certain medications. In all cases, however, the proximal risk factor for the development of TdP is prolongation of the QT interval. The greater the duration, the more likely TdP becomes, but 450 ms has frequently been used as a cutoff because longer QTc interval measures are associated with substantially higher risk.

References

El-Sherif N, Turitto G. Torsade de pointes. *Current Opin Cardiol.* 2003;18:6–13.
Glassman AH, Bigger JT Jr. Antipsychotic drugs: prolonged QTc interval, torsade de pointes, and sudden death. *Am J Psychiatry.* 2001;158:1774–1782.

8. Elevation of lithium levels is most likely to occur in association with daily treatment with which of the following medications?

   a. Furosemide
   b. Theophylline
   c. Nifedipine
   d. Potassium hydrochloride
   e. Ibuprofen

The correct answer is e.

Furosemide has limited effect on lithium clearance, whereas theophylline increases it. No effects on lithium levels have been described with either nifedipine or potassium salts. In contrast, some nonsteroidal antiinflammatory agents (including ibuprofen) diminish lithium clearance by 50% and can precipitate lithium toxicity.

References

Crabtree BL, Mack JE, Johnson CD, Amyx BC. Comparison of the effects of hydrochlorothiazide and furosemide on lithium disposition. *Am J Psychiatry.* 1991;148:1060–1063.

Jacobson SA, Pies RW, Greenblatt DJ. *Handbook of Geriatric Psychopharmacology.* Washington, DC: American Psychiatric Publishing; 2002.

Jefferson JW, Greist JH. Lithium: interactions with other drugs. In: David JM, Greenblatt D, eds. *Psychopharmacology Update.* New York, NY: Grune and Stratton; 1979:81–104.

Jefferson JW, Greist JH, Baudhuin M. Lithium: interactions with other drugs. *J Clin Psychopharmacol.* 1981;1:124–131.

Sadavoy J. *Psychotropic Drugs and the Elderly: Fast Facts. Mood Stabilizers. Lithium.* New York, NY: Norton; 2004:516–538.

For questions 9–13, match each of the P450 enzymes listed with the atypical antipsychotic medication for which it is the primary metabolic pathway. An answer may be used once, more than once, or not at all.

9.	1A2	a.	Olanzapine
10.	2D6	b.	Risperidone
11.	3A4	c.	Ziprasidone
12.	2C9	d.	Quetiapine
13.	2C19	e.	Clozapine

The correct answers are 9, a; 10, b; 11, c; 12, c; and 13, a.

Olanzapine is metabolized in multiple ways, but mainly through the P450 1A2 system. Risperidone is metabolized mainly by 2D6 and secondarily by 3A4. Quetiapine is metabolized mainly by 3A4, with minor contribution from other pathways. Drugs that inhibit the 3A4 system can reduce the metabolism of ziprasidone, which is primarily metabolized by this system. The major P450 system involved in clozapine's metabolism is 1A2, although 3A4 and 2D6 are also involved.

Reference

Cozza KL, Armstrong SC: *Concise Guide to the Cytochrome P450 System: Drug Interaction Principles for Medical Practice.* Washington, DC: APPI; 2001.

14. Which statement regarding venlafaxine-associated hypertension is true?

    a. Occurs despite concomitant treatment with antihypertensives
    b. Increased risk occurs at doses of greater than 200 mg/day

c. Risk is greatest among patients with hypertension preceding venlafaxine
d. Primarily involves elevation of diastolic blood pressure
e. Occurs more commonly with increased age

The correct answer is b.

Venlafaxine has been associated with increases in systolic blood pressure. This infrequent side effect occurs primarily at doses over 200 mg/day. Baseline hypertension does not predict subsequent blood pressure elevations, and taking an antihypertensive for preexisting hypertension appears to decrease the risk of developing elevated blood pressure during treatment.

References

Feighner JP. The role of venlafaxine in rational antidepressant therapy. *J Clin Psychiatry.* 1994;55:62–68.
Thase ME. Effects of venlafaxine on blood pressure: a meta-analysis of original date from 3,744 depressed patients. *J Clin Psychiatry.* 1998;59:502–508.

15. Which of the following characterizes secondary amine tricyclic antidepressants (TCAs) as contrasted with tertiary amine TCAs?

a. Greater orthostatic hypotensive effects
b. Less anticholinergic effect
c. Higher plasma concentrations per milligram dose
d. Less efficacy in elderly patients
e. Greater efficacy for comorbid anxiety symptoms

The correct answer is b.

There is no evidence that the secondary TCAs differ in terms of their antidepressant efficacy from the tertiary TCAs. As for their efficacy in anxiety disorders, most of the available studies have been conducted with tertiary agents (e.g., clomipramine treatment for panic and obsessive-compulsive disorder, imipramine for panic disorder, etc.), but there are no systematic comparisons of the anxiolytic efficacy of secondary amine TCAs with that of the tertiary agents. Although there is evidence that the metabolism of tertiary amine TCAs such as imipramine may decrease in association with aging, there is no consistent evidence that aging influences either the plasma level per dose ratios or the general antidepressant efficacy of secondary amine agents. Although both secondary and tertiary amine TCAs antagonize the muscarinic, histaminergic, and the α-adrenergic receptors, the former exhibit a lower level of antagonism. This is the basis of the improved side-effect profile (including less orthostatic hypotension and de-creased anticholinergic phenomena) of the secondary TCAs compared to their tertiary counterparts, particularly among elderly patients.

References

Mulsant BH, Pollock BG, Nebes D, et al. A double-blind randomized compari-son of nortriptyline and paroxetine in the treatment of late-life depression: 6 week outcome. *J Clin Psychiatry.* 1999;60:16–20.
Nelson JC, Jatlow P, Mazure C. Desipramine plasma levels and response in elderly melancholic patients. *J Clin Psychopharmacol.* 1985;5:217–220.
Richelson E. Pharmacology of antidepressants in use in the United States. *J Clin Psychiatry.* 1982;43:4–13.

16. Which of the following side effects of benzodiazepine use is greater in elderly patients than in young adults?

    a. Diminished recent memory
    b. Withdrawal seizures
    c. Psychological dependence
    d. Displacement of other medications from α-acid glycoprotein
    e. Bleeding caused by interactions with warfarin

The correct answer is a.

Elderly patients seem to be particularly vulnerable to the cognitive side effects of benzodiazepines. In particular, "therapeutic" doses of benzo-diazepines can impair learning performance in older persons. There is no evidence that geriatric patients have an increased risk of withdrawal seizures or psychological dependence from benzodiazapines. In con-trast to most antidepressants and antipsychotic medications, benzodia-zapines are bound primarily by albumin and are not known to affect α-acid glycoprotein binding or to affect bleeding time in patients re-ceiving warfarin.

Reference

Pomara N, Tun H, DaSilva D, Hernando R, et al. The acute and chronic performance effects of alprazolam and lorazepam in the elderly: relation-ship to duration of treatment and self-rated sedation. *Psychopharmacol Bull.* 1998;34:139–153.

17. Which of the following anticholinergic side effects is most likely to lead to discontinuation of a psychiatric medication in older patients?

    a. Constipation
    b. Bradycardia
    c. Delirium

d. Decreased working memory
e. Elevated intraocular pressure

The correct answer is a.

Elderly patients do not generally develop clinically apparent memory impairment or frank delirium when treated with modest dosages of drugs with anticholinergic properties. Patients with poorly compensated heart disease may develop tachycardia during tricyclic antidepressant treatment, but bradycardia is not an anticholinergic effect. Care should also be exercised in prescribing any medication with anticholinergic properties to patients with angle-closure glaucoma. However, this form of glaucoma is far less common than open-angle glaucoma. Sensitivity to less-serious anticholinergic side effects such as constipation is more common in older patients, and worsening constipation more commonly results in the discontinuation of a psychiatric medication because of anticholinergic side effects.

References

Muller-Lissner S. General geriatrics and gastroenterology: constipation and faecal incontinence. *Best Pract Res Clin Gastroenterol.* 2002;16:115–133.
Pollack MH, Rosenbaum JF. Management of antidepressant-induced side effects: a practical guide for the clinician. *J Clin Psychiatry.* 1987;48:3–8.

18. Which of the following is the most practical method to enhance adherence to antidepressant treatment of elderly patients?

    a. Dividing the dose to be taken with meals
    b. Involving a visiting nurse service
    c. Simplifying the dosage to once daily
    d. Explaining the need not to miss doses
    e. Ensuring that the patient's primary care physician is aware of the rationale

The correct answer is c.

Dividing the dose is associated with poorer adherence in both elderly and younger patients. Studies of other medical conditions (e.g., hypertension, arthritis) requiring chronic pharmacological treatment found an inverse linear relation between the number of doses a patient is expected to take a day and adherence.

References

Bloom BS. Daily regimen and compliance with treatment. *BMJ.* 2001;323:647.
Goff DC, Jenike MA. Treatment-resistant depression in the elderly. *J Am Geriatr Soc.* 1986;34:63–70.

19. The least frequent consequence of neuroleptic treatment in elderly patients is

a. Dystonia
b. Pseudoparkinsonism
c. Tardive dyskinesia
d. Akathisia
e. Hip fracture

The correct answer is a.

Elderly patients receiving antipsychotic medications seem to be less vulnerable to acute dystonic reactions compared to younger patients. In contrast, they are more prone to the development of tardive dyskinesia as well as parkinsonian side effects. The latter may be one of the mechanisms leading to the increased risk of falls and related morbidity in the elderly. The incidence of akathisia is not greatly affected by aging.

References

Caligiuri M, Jeste DV, Lacro JP. Antipsychotic induced movement disorders in the elderly: epidemiology and treatment recommendations. *Drugs Aging.* 2000;17:363–384.

Jeste DV, Wyatt RJ. Aging and tardive dyskinesia. In: Miller NE, Cohen GD, eds. *Schizophrenia and Aging.* New York, NY: Guilford; 1987.

Magnuson TM, Roccaforte WH, Wengel SP, Burke WJ. Medication-induced dystonias in nine patients with dementia. *J Neuropsychiatry Clin Neurosci.* 2000;12:219–225.

Ray WA, Griffin MR, Schaffner W, et al. Psychotropic drug use and the risk of hip fracture. *N Engl J Med.* 1987;316:363–369.

20. Regarding management of elderly patients with manic states, which of the following statements is true?

a. Sodium valproate increases the hepatic metabolism of concomitant psychotropic agents
b. Plasma lithium levels should be targeted routinely at less than 0.4 mEq/L
c. Divalproex sodium should be dosed to achieve target levels that are 50% lower than those used to treat young adults
d. Dosage should be reduced gradually following remission of symptoms
e. Continuation pharmacotherapy should be provided routinely

The correct answer is e.

Sodium valproate tends to inhibit, not augment, the hepatic metabolism of concomitant psychotropic medications because of its effects on the P450 enzyme system. There are no prospective randomized trials indicating that low plasma concentrations of mood-stabilizing agents are routinely effective in geriatric patients with mania. Similarly, no evidence exists that reduced concentration of mood stabilizers after an acute response will provide adequate continuation efficacy. Finally, in geriatric patients with mania, as in younger patients, episodes tend to be recurrent, and continuation pharmacotherapy should be routine practice.

References

Burke WJ, Wengel SP. Late-life mood disorders. *Clin Geriatr Med.* 2003;19: 777–797.

Young RC, Gyulai L, Mulsant BH, et al. Pharmacotherapy of bipolar disorder in old age: review and recommendations. *Am J Geriatr Psychiatry.* 2004; 12:342–357.

21. What is the most common side effect associated with cholinesterase inhibitors?

    a. Nausea
    b. Insomnia
    c. Dizziness
    d. Muscle cramps
    e. Elevated transaminase levels

The correct answer is a.

Nausea is the side effect that most frequently complicates treatment with cholinesterase inhibitors. Nausea occurs with each of the approved agents in this class, particularly early in treatment. The gradual upward dose titration of these agents is used to facilitate the development of tolerance to nausea. Nausea may result from inhibition of peripheral acetylcholinesterase or by an increased release of dopamine centrally by enhancing cholinergic activity.

References

Farlow M. A clinical overview of cholinesterase inhibitors in Alzheimer's disease. *Int Psychogeriatr.* 2002;14:93–126.

Physician's Desk Reference. 56th ed. Medical Economics; 2002.

22. Which of the following best describes the role of memantine in the treatment of Alzheimer's disease?

    a. Memantine is most effective in slowing the rate of decline of Alzheimer's disease in mildly impaired patients

b. Memantine is contraindicated in patients who are receiving donepezil
c. The action of memantine is related to cholinesterase inhibition
d. Among patients with severe impairment, improvement is greater than that of placebo on global measures of functioning, activities of daily living, and cognition
e. Memantine is thought to act by stimulating nerve growth factor

The correct answer is d.

Memantine, the newest addition to the armamentarium for the treatment of Alzheimer's disease, has a different mechanism of action compared to the cholinesterase inhibitors. Memantine belongs to a class of agents that antagonizes glutamate at the N-methyl-D-aspartate (NMDA) receptor. Glutamate is an excitatory neurotransmitter that has been implicated in neuronal loss in degenerative diseases. Memantine has been shown to slow the rate of cognitive and functional decline in patients with Alzheimer's disease with moderate-to-severe dementia. Combining memantine with the cholinesterase inhibitor donepezil increased the cognitive benefits and did not affect the metabolism of either medication.

References

Reisberg B, Doody R, Stoffler A, Schmitt F, Gerris S, Mobius HJ for the Memantine Study Group. Memantine in moderate to severe Alzheimer's disease. *N Engl J Med.* 2003;348:1333–1341.

Tariot PN, Farlow MR, Grossberg GT, Graham SM, McDonald S, Gergel I for the Memantine Study Group. Memantine treatment in patients with moderate to severe Alzheimer disease already receiving donepezil: a randomized controlled trial. *JAMA.* 2004;291:317–324.

23. Based on placebo-controlled studies, which of the following statements about the efficacy of maintenance treatment for late-life depression is correct?

a. Patients between ages 60 and 70 years have a greater recurrence rate than those older than 70 years of age
b. Long-term SSRI treatment is more efficacious than maintenance nortriptyline
c. Monthly maintenance psychotherapy does not affect recurrence rates
d. Impaired memory is associated with a higher likelihood of recurrence
e. Impaired executive functioning is associated with an increased risk of recurrence

The correct answer is e.

Among geriatric patients, those over age 70 years have been found to have a more brittle response and higher recurrence rates during active antidepressant treatment and while receiving placebo. Monthly inter-personal psychotherapy alone or in combination with antidepressants has been shown to decrease recurrence rates, particularly in the older-old. Impaired performance on tests of executive functioning but not on those of memory has been found to increase the rate of recurrence. There is no evidence of differences in prophylactic efficacy between SSRIs and tricylic antidepressants. Empirical data are consistent with the maxim that patients who require long-term treatment should con-tinue receiving the dose and medication that was associated with re-covery.

References

Alexopoulos GS, Meyers BS, Young RC, et al. Executive dysfunction worsens the long-term outcome of geriatric depression. *Arch Gen Psychiatry.* 2000; 57:285–290.

Bump GM, Mulsant BH, Pollock BG, et al. Paroxetine versus nortriptyline in the continuation and maintenance treatment of depression in the elderly. *Depression Anxiety.* 2001;13:1338–1344.

Reynolds CF, Frank E, Perel JM, et al. Nortriptyline and interpersonal psycho-therapy as maintenance therapies for recurrent major depression: a ran-domized controlled trial in patients older than 59 years. *JAMA.* 1999;281: 39–45.

Chapter 31
Individual Psychotherapy

1. An 83-year-old woman of Chinese descent who emigrated to New York in 1963 presents to her general practitioner with symptoms of grief following the death of her husband of 52 years. It is most likely that this patient

   a. Prefers to see a mental health professional
   b. Will be referred by her general practitioner for psychotherapeutic treatment
   c. Is too old to benefit from insight-oriented therapy
   d. Will preferentially respond to cognitive-behavioral therapy (CBT)
   e. Will at first complain of physical problems

   The correct answer is e.

Patients from Chinese and other minority cultures often present emotional problems early on in a somatized fashion. Because of suspicion of the mainstream system and unfamiliarity with psychiatric care and the stigma attached to mental disorders, they frequently reject mental health professionals. Family doctors have a low rate of recognition of depressive disorders and often fail to refer appropriate patients for psychotherapeutic treatment. This is especially true for patients of minority cultures. Age is not a barrier to insight-oriented therapy provided the patient has sufficient cognitive capacity, a willingness to engage in the process, and the physical ability to deal with the problems of therapy such as transportation. CBT is an effective form of therapy in grief treatments, but there is no evidence that it is superior to other forms of brief or longer-term therapy. CBT may be initially unfamiliar and mystifying to patients of other cultures and requires the preliminary development of a common ground of understanding and therapeutic relationship before its introduction.

Reference

Lee E. Chinese American families. In: Lee E, ed. *Working With Asian Americans.* New York, NY: Guilford Press; 1997:46–77.

2. An 81-year-old woman presents with a 6-month history of depressed mood, sleeplessness, new-onset anxiety, and suicidal ideation. She also reports diurnal variation of mood, apparently unrealistic ruminations about being abandoned by her children, and a history of unstable and chaotic interpersonal relationships through her adult life. Her family doctor diagnosed depressive disorder and referred her to a psychiatrist. Based on the best evidence available on therapeutic efficacy for this condition, the most effective recommendation would be

a. CBT alone
b. Selective serotonin reuptake inhibitor (SSRI) medication with intermittent monitoring follow-up
c. SSRI medication with psychotherapy
d. Interpersonal therapy (IPT) alone

The correct answer is c.

The work of Reynolds et al. (1999) strongly suggested that psychotherapy in combination with an antidepressant is the most effective treatment. Although that study was conducted with nortriptyline, SSRIs are currently the antidepressants of choice. CBT and IPT, although effective in depression, are probably not as effective as combination therapy. Antidepressant therapy with intermittent follow-up does not seem to be as effective as combined medication and psychotherapy.

References

Miller MD, Wolfson L, Frank E, et al. Using interpersonal psychotherapy in a combined psychotherapy/medication research protocol with depressed elders. *J Psychother Pract Res.* 1988;7:47–55.

Reynolds CF 3rd, Frank E, Perel JM, et al. Nortriptyline and interpersonal psychotherapy as maintenance therapies for recurrent major depression: a randomized controlled trial in patients older than 59 years. *JAMA.* 1999; 281:39–45.

3. A 68-year-old woman is referred to a therapy clinic by her family doctor; at the clinic, she sees a psychiatric resident. She comes to therapy about 6 months after the sudden, unexpected death of her husband. Her family doctor had treated her for many years, during which time she spoke to him frequently about the angry conflicts she had with her husband and her mixed feelings for him. The physician correctly judged that she was at higher risk for complicated grief because of her agitation, anxiety, and failure to return to her usual activities 6 months following the death of her husband, together with her history of trauma and loss in her childhood. She had always relied on her husband to look after the problems of their home and rarely had taken the lead in solving problems. This pattern of deferring to others was present in all her relationships. During long-term therapy, her psychiatrist notes that their relationship is characterized by behaviors that he found annoying and difficult, such as calling between sessions and expressions of clinging and obvious distress when each session ended. The most accurate way for him to understand his patient's behavior is that

   a. It is most likely an enactment of a realistic reaction to the therapist's failure to provide the patient with appropriate support
   b. It is most likely an enactment of feelings deriving from childhood abandonment by her parents and now her husband
   c. It is most likely an enactment of a fear that she will be institutionalized because she cannot look after herself
   d. It is most likely an enactment of a disguised form of anger caused by her belief that the therapist is too young to understand her problems.

The correct answer is b.

Clinging behavior and anxious phone calling between sessions are most likely an expression of abandonment anxiety. In this patient, it probably stems from childhood experiences exacerbated by a reenactment of these experiences through the loss of her husband. Maintenance of a therapeutic schedule with appropriate limits does not constitute failure of appropriate support unless the therapist is inappropriately remote. Unless reality testing is significantly impaired, a patient of this age under these circumstances is unlikely to fear institutionalization. Rather, anxiety is related to feelings of abandonment and the desperate search for a replacement for the lost other, acted out with the therapist. Although patients of this type may believe that younger therapists cannot understand them and may be ineffective, this is usually a preliminary form of resistance to confronting the underlying abandonment conflicts.

Reference

Sadavoy J. Character disorders in the elderly: an overview. In: Sadavoy J, Leszcz M, eds. *Treating the Elderly With Psychotherapy: The Scope for Change in Later Life*. Madison, CT: International Universities Press; 1987: 175–229.

4. Psychotherapy with patients from a culture different from that of the therapist can be a challenging process calling on the therapist to use a variety of skills and techniques. Recommended therapeutic approaches in these cases include

a. Actively encouraging the patient to integrate with the dominant culture
b. Using background information from seminars on cross-cultural therapy to provide the main basis for understanding the patient's struggles
c. Beginning a brief, structured form of psychotherapy early on, after educating the patient about the biological and social basis of their problem
d. Exploring the patient's relationship to the dominant culture, including racism

The correct answer is d.

Patients from minority cultures often struggle with uncertainty and mistrust of the dominant culture and have often had this feeling reinforced by significant experiences of racism directed either at them or others in their immediate environment. This poses a significant barrier to trust in the therapeutic relationship and needs to be addressed early on. It is inappropriate to actively encourage such patients to integrate with the dominant culture as this may reinforce some of the patient's mistrust and cause them to feel that their cultural beliefs are being rejected or devalued. Background information from academic sources such as seminars or readings can be helpful, but the core of understanding in the psychotherapeutic context is based on the patient's personal experience. It is crucial that the therapist allow the patient to educate the therapist to his or her belief structure and life view rather than relying on generalities. Beginning a formal process of psychotherapy too early may conflict with the patient's belief system. Many patients from other cultures do not share the biological and social etiological understanding that is common in Western thought and science. Failure to inquire about and develop a common base of understanding in this regard will alienate the patient and interfere with or prevent the utilization of psychotherapeutic techniques.

Reference

Tang NM. Psychoanalytic Psychotherapy with Chinese Americans. In: Lee E, ed. *Working With Asian Americans*. New York, NY: Guilford Press; 1997: 323–341.

5. Cognitively impaired elders in institutions are often depressed, anxious, lonely, unconnected, and abandoned. In these situations,

   a. Reminiscence therapy generally provokes increased feelings of loss
   b. Psychodynamic understanding adds little to the management of problems
   c. Touch and attending to nonverbal cues are important to treatment
   d. The patient is calmed and reassured by the structure of cognitive mental status questions at the beginning of each meeting with the therapist

The correct answer is c.

There is a high incidence of cognitive impairment combined with physical frailty in institutional settings, especially long-term care. Verbal expression may be limited, and it is necessary for the therapist to hone personal observational skills to extract meaning from the nonverbal behaviors of the patient. Similarly, for many patients who are regressed and cut off by cognitive or other impairments, appropriate direct physical touch can be comforting and an effective means of communication. For those patients who are able to communicate verbally, reminiscence is generally a comforting self-enhancing process that puts them in touch with past experiences of competence or loving relationships. Psychodynamic understanding is a crucial adjunct to understanding the behavioral presentation of patients and putting it in the context of their psychological past. Introducing formal structured cognitive mental status testing too early in the relationship with a cognitively impaired patient often mobilizes feelings of incompetence and agitation rather than calming and reassuring the patient.

Reference

Duffy M. Individual therapy in long term care institutions. In: Molinari V, ed. *Professional Psychology in Long Term Care*. New York, NY: Hatherleigh; 1997.

Chapter 32
Group Therapy

1. In considering the recommendation of group psychotherapy for an 82-year-old man under treatment for a major depressive episode, the most important factor to consider regarding group composition is

   a. Age of other members
   b. Level of physical functioning
   c. Marital status
   d. Level of cognitive functioning
   e. Gender

   The correct answer is d.

   The geriatric population is very heterogeneous. Age alone does not determine or define the individual. Hence, particular attributes and capacities must be considered in constructing a psychotherapy group because the groups that are the most effective are those that become cohesive quickly. An important factor that fosters the development of group cohesion is the positive identification patients make with one another. Mixing patients with variable levels of cognitive functioning is likely to create a group in which cohesion is impaired because some patients will be overwhelmed by the group task and others will feel slowed down, impeded by the compromised cognitive functioning of more impaired patients. Furthermore, a counteridentification may ensue, with a wish to flee the group for fear of recognizing one's worst fears for the future in the evident cognitive decline.

   Reference

   Leszcz M. Geriatric group therapy. In: Kaplan HI, Sadock BJ, eds. *Comprehensive Textbook of Psychiatry*. Vol. 8. New York, NY: Williams and Wilkins; 2004.

2. Cognitive-behavioral group approaches with elderly patients generally do not emphasize

   a. Role playing
   b. Relaxation exercises
   c. Log book and homework assignments
   d. Psychoeducation
   e. Interpretation of conflict

   The correct answer is e.

Unlike psychodynamic approaches that emphasize the internal psychological experience of the individual and the group members, cognitive-behavioral group therapy emphasizes problems with impaired information processing, shaped by and having an impact on one's fundamental beliefs about oneself in relationship to the world. The group setting is utilized to foster self-efficacy by helping patients monitor their mood, alter behavior such that they increase pleasurable activities, and log the relationship between thoughts, behaviors, and attitudes to correct distortions in thinking. Behavioral practice is directly encouraged, making use of group support to foster patient participation in the therapeutic task. Little attention is placed on the process within the group or on here-and-now interpersonal dynamics, conflicts, or resistances.

References

Thompson LW, Gantz F, Florsheim M, et al. Cognitive-behavioural therapy in affective disorders in the elderly. In: Myers WA, ed. *New Techniques in the Psychotherapy of Older Patients*. Washington, DC: American Psychiatric Press; 1991:3–19.

Thompson LW, Powers DP, Coon DW, Takagi K, McKibbin C, Gallagher-Thompson D. Older adults. In: White JR, Freeman AS, eds. *Cognitive-Behavioural Group Therapy for Specific Problems and Populations*. Washington, DC: American Psychological Association; 2000:235–262.

3. In developing a group psychotherapeutic approach that is aimed at improving cognitive and behavioral functioning in patients who suffer from cognitive impairment, it is essential to

   a. Provide frequent opportunities for unstructured social interaction
   b. Discourage reminiscing in the group
   c. Examine group process and the group dynamics within the group
   d. Coordinate a compatible, ongoing reality orientation approach on the ward

The correct answer is d.

Groups that aim at improving cognitive and behavioral functioning in cognitively impaired patients must be a component of an integrated approach to treatment that involves staff outside the group itself and family members regarding ongoing reinforcement. Gains that are otherwise made are likely to be transient and lost in the absence of this ongoing reinforcement. Structured reminiscing and an approach in which the experience of the individual patient is respected and made sense of are important ingredients of effective treatment. While empirical data are not available, clinical experience suggests that approaches that raise anxiety, such as an emphasis on interpretation and exploration of group process, are likely to be useless at best and potentially harmful at worst.

References

Gerber GJ, Prince PN, Snider MC, et al. Group activity and cognitive improvement among patients with Alzheimer's disease. *Hosp Community Psychiatry.* 1991;42:843–845.

Lantz MS, Buchalter E, McRea L. The wellness group: a novel intervention for coping with disruptive behaviour in elderly nursing home residents. *Gerontologist.* 1997;37:551–556.

Spector A, Davies S, Woods B, Orrell M. Reality orientation for dementia: a systematic review of the evidence for effectiveness from randomized controlled trials. *Gerontologist.* 2000;40:206–212.

4. Therapist interventions that make use of the concept of "prizing" are frequently associated with

a. Increasing undue dependence in patients
b. Enhancing patient self-concept
c. Therapist countertransference
d. Impeding group cohesion
e. Increased idealization of the therapist

The correct answer is b.

Common resistances to participation in group psychotherapy among the elderly relate to problems with self-esteem, self-worth, and the reverberating projection of self- and other devaluation. Often, this reflects both the depression and the response to societal attitudes that are at times prejudiced against the worth of the elderly. A number of reviews of the recommended therapist posture emphasize the importance of respect and the maximum use of nonspecific therapeutic factors, such as genuine warmth, empathy, and "prizing," that is, unconditional positive regard, at a technical level, in ensuring that the group experience is a nonfailure one for each participant. An experience of devaluation within the group is likely to lead to premature termination of treatment. Group cohesiveness is likely to be fostered rather than hampered, and as the group becomes more cohesive, patients' sense of competence and effectiveness is similarly favorably improved.

References

Leszcz M. Integrated group psychotherapy for the treatment of depression in the elderly. *Group.* 1997;21:89–107.

Tross S, Blum JE. A review of group therapy with the older adult: practice and research. In: MacLennan BW, Saul S, Bakur Weiner M, eds. *Group Psy-*

chotherapies for the Elderly. Madison, CT: International Universities Press; 1988:3–29. American Group Psychotherapy Association Monograph 5.

Williams-Barnard CL, Lindell AR. Therapeutic use of "prizing" and its effect on self-concept of elderly clients in nursing homes and group homes. *Issues Ment Health Nurs.* 1992;13:1–17.

5. Psychosocial interventions for burdened caregivers, including the provision of structured group experiences have demonstrated

   a. No improvement in measures of caregiver burden despite high subjective valuation of the group experience
   b. Some improvement in measures of caregiver burden and a 1-year reduction in rates of institutionalization of the identified patient of up to 50%
   c. Little impact on rates of institutionalization
   d. Improved psychosocial functioning in the identified care receiver

The correct answer is b.

The area of investigating interventions for caregiver burden is complicated by the complexities of measuring objective and subjective burden in the context of a situation in which there is likely to be a progressive functional deterioration of the care receiver. The meta-analysis performed by Knight et al. (1993), however, has shown that distressed caregivers receiving structured group interventions in general show a small, positive effect on caregiver burden and dysphoria and are highly valued by participants. There is also evidence that comprehensive treatment, including family counseling and peer support groups, coupled with individual counseling, can reduce and significantly delay rates of institutionalization.

References

Knight BG, Lutzky SM, Macofsky-Urban F. A meta-analytic review of interventions for caregiver distress: recommendations for future research. *Gerontologist.* 1993;33:240–243.

Mittelman MS, Ferris SH, Steinberg G, et al. An intervention that delays institutionalization of Alzheimer's disease patients: treatment of spouse caregivers. *Gerontologist.* 1993;33:730–740.

6. Two men, both in their late 70s and bereaved, participating in a partial hospitalization program for depression are noted to be spending a great deal of time together outside the treatment groups. Concern is raised by a staff member that a subgrouping phenomenon is taking place that could have a deleterious impact on the rest of the patients in group therapy. A first consideration to employ in response to this concern is

a. Restrict extragroup contact
b. It is benign and should not be addressed
c. Interpret other group members' envy of the closeness achieved by these two men
d. It reflects a self-object transference and should be interpreted
e. Explore in the group the meaning and experience of this special relatedness

The correct answer is e.

Extragroup contact is an inevitable component of partial hospitalization and day hospital programming. Therefore, rather than trying to prevent subgrouping, it is often most useful to examine within the group its meaning, impact, and value. It may well reflect a form of self-object transference that serves an important function regarding restoration of self-esteem and self-worth. There is therapeutic benefit in examining it from the vantage point of potentially supporting it and viewing it as a reflection of the importance of social connection and the possibility of making deeply meaningful social connections again.

References

Leszcz M. Geriatric group therapy. In: Kaplan HI, Sadock BJ, eds. *Comprehensive Textbook of Psychiatry.* Vol. 7. New York, NY: Williams and Wilkins; 1999:1327–1331.

Lothstein LM, Zimet G. Twinship and alter ego self-object transferences in group therapy with the elderly: a reanalysis of the pairing phenomenon. *Int J Group Psychother.* 1988;38:303–317.

7. In establishing a group therapy program within an institutional setting, an often-neglected but important consideration within the system in which treatment is provided relates to

a. The therapist-to-patient relationship
b. The patient-to-patient relationship
c. The relationship between the patient and group
d. The relationship between the cotherapists
e. The relationship between the group and the institution

The correct answer is e.

In establishing a group therapy program, it is important to look at the system as a whole. Group therapy will not flourish without administrative support and understanding of the importance of establishing set times and protocols for group therapy. Interdisciplinary rivalries and subtle overvaluing and devaluing of the roles that staff have within the institution are often expressed around the establishment of new therapeutic interventions. The more obvious therapeutic relationships are generally addressed regarding patient-to-patient and patient-to-therapist interaction, but systemic issues are often neglected at the peril of the group.

References

Klausner EJ, Alexopoulous GS. The future of psychosocial treatments for elderly patients. *Psychiatr Serv.* 1999;50:1198–1204.

Toseland RW. *Group Work With the Elderly and Family Caregivers.* New York, NY: Springer; 1995.

8. Effects of pregroup preparation for patients entering group therapy include

   a. Reducing patient anxiety
   b. Increasing patient hopefulness
   c. Facilitating the therapeutic alliance
   d. Improving patient adherence to the group task
   e. All of the above

The correct answer is e.

Entering into a psychotherapy group is an anxiety-provoking experience for virtually all patients. This is even more so for seniors, who may have had little exposure to the principles of psychotherapy earlier in their lives. Demystifying the process of treatment through the provision of information serves the function of orienting patients to the treatment. This allows them to engage more fully and tolerate some of the initial uncertainty and puzzlement that frequently can occur in group therapy. Greater clarity about how to work in the group increases hope and patient confidence.

References

Leszcz M. Geriatric group therapy. In: Kaplan HI, Sadock BJ, eds. *Comprehensive Textbook of Psychiatry.* Vol. 7. New York, NY: Williams and Wilkins; 1999:1327–1331.

Yalom ID. *The Theory and Practice of Group Psychotherapy.* 4th ed. New York, NY: Basic Books; 1995.

Chapter 33
Family Issues in Mental Disorders of Late Life

1. Which of the following *less consistently* influences whether an elderly person is likely to live with his or her family?

a. Race and ethnicity
b. Sex
c. Age
d. Chronic health conditions

The correct answer is d.

In the United States, the chance that an older person lives with family members is influenced by age, sex, race, and ethnicity. The evidence that chronic conditions influence living arrangements is less consistent. Some studies suggest that chronic conditions facilitate intergenerational coresidence, but other studies found little evidence for this. The proportion of older people living alone rises with age, especially in elders 85 years or older. The proportion of elders 85 years and older living alone is about double the proportion of those aged 65 to 74 years. At all ages, women are about twice as likely to be living alone as men. Race and ethnicity also enter into this picture. At any age, African American and Hispanic women are more likely to live with other relatives than non-Hispanic white women. On the other hand, older African American men are considerably more likely to live alone than other men.

References

Al-Hamad A, Flowerdew R, Hayes, L. Migration of elderly people to join existing households: some evidence from the 1991 Household Sample of Anonymised Records. *Environ Plan.* 1997;29:1243–1255.

Choi NG. Living arrangements and household compositions of elderly couples and singles: a comparison of Hispanics and blacks. *J Gerontol Soc Work.* 1999;31:41–61.

Commonwealth Fund. *The Unfinished Agenda: Improving the Well-Being of Elderly People Living Alone.* New York, NY: Commonwealth Fund; 1993.

Ebly EM, Hogan DB, Rockwood K. Living alone with dementia. *Dement Geriatr Cogn Dis.* 1999;10:541–548.

Lefley HP. Aging parents as caregivers of mentally ill adult children: an emerging social problem. *Hosp Community Psychiatry.* 1987;38:1063–1070.

2. Which groups of relatives are most likely to be involved in caring for a demented, elderly person?

a. Siblings
b. Aunts and uncles
c. Sons and daughters-in-law
d. Spouse and daughters

The correct answer is d.

Families of demented elderly patients, as a rule, take responsibility for a wide range of caregiving tasks, such as transportation, nutrition, personal care, and finances (Marin et al, 2000). Spouses and daughters usually assume a leading role in providing this care (Sparks et al., 1998).

References

Marin DB, Dugue M, Schmeidler J, et al. The Caregiver Activity Survey (CAS): longitudinal validation of an instrument that measures time spent caregiving for individuals with Alzheimer's disease. *Int J Geriatr Psychiatry.* 2000;15:680–686.
Sparks MB, Farran CJ, Donner E, Keane-Hagerty E. Wives, husbands, and daughters of dementia patients: predictors of caregivers' mental and physical health. *Sch Inq Nurs Pract.* 1998;12:221–234.

3. Family caregiving for an elderly chronically mentally ill patient can produce serious subjective burden on caregivers, such as medical (e.g., immune function disturbance) and psychosocial morbidity (e.g., depression) and deterioration in family relations and work-related performance. All of these factors have been shown to predict subjective burden except

   a. Presence of behavioral disturbances
   b. Lack of availability of informal social support
   c. Cognitive or functional status of the patient
   d. Cultural and ethnic background

The correct answer is c.

The relationship between subjective and objective burden (i.e., patient's needs and deficits) has been a productive area of research. For example, Coen et al. (1997) studied predictors of caregiver burden among patients diagnosed with Alzheimer's disease (AD) and found that daughters who were primary caregivers were particularly prone to suffer from high levels of subjective burden. In this study, neither cognitive nor functional status of the patient predicted caregiver burden, but behavioral disturbances and lack of social support were independent predictors. Harwood et al. (1998) found a higher prevalence of depressive symptoms in white Hispanics (45%) compared to white non-Hispanics (36%).

References

Coen RF, Swanwick GR, O'Boyle CA, Coakley D. Behavior disturbance and other predictors of caregiver burden in Alzheimer's disease. *Int J Geriatr Psychiatry.* 1997;12:331–336.
Harwood D, Barker W, Cantillon M, et al. Depressive symptomatology in

first-degree family caregivers of Alzheimer disease patients: a cross-ethnic comparison. *Alzheimer Dis Assoc Disord.* 1998;12:340–346.

Stuckey JC, Neundorfer MM, Smyth KA. Burden and well-being: the same coin or related currency. *Gerontologist.* 1996;36:686–693.

Zarit SH, Todd PA, Zarit JM. Subjective burden of husbands and wives as caregivers: a longitudinal study. *Gerontologist.* 1986;26:260–266.

4. When confronted with family units that hold opposing points of view, the clinician should

   a. Ally him- or herself with the main caregiver to ensure the patient gets appropriate care
   b. Remain neutral and facilitate the family in resolving their issues
   c. Take a clear position on the issues and encourage the family to unite and debate the conflict with the clinician
   d. Develop a strong alliance with the most influential member of the family to ensure a therapeutic decision

The correct answer is b.

Clinicians who work with families should be attuned to the possible presence of opposing family units of power. At times of elevated anxiety, these opposing units are active and visible in the family. There is increased pressure on the clinician to take sides in a family disagreement even though doing so can decrease his or her value as a family resource. By communicating appreciation of the various alignments and allegiances within the family, the clinician should attempt to maintain neutrality. This is not to say the clinician has no opinion; rather, the emphasis should be to allow the family to resolve the differences. Families may resolve differences if they have a "concerned outsider" to whom they can communicate their thoughts and feelings without judgment or criticism. According to some theories, the effort by the clinician aimed at keeping the conflict within the family, rather than between the family and the therapist, can be crucial.

Reference
Bowen M. *Family Therapy in Clinical Practice.* Washington, DC: Aronson; 1978.

5. In-home respite care has been shown in one study to have

   a. Little effect on "upset" in caregiver spouses
   b. Little effect on self-efficacy of caregivers managing difficult behaviors
   c. Little effect on self-efficacy in managing functional dependency
   d. All of the above
   e. None of the above

Correct answer is e.

Gitlin et al. (2001) provided home respite care in the form of occupational therapy support in a controlled randomized study. The intervention of five 90-minute home visits reduced feelings of "upset" in caregiver spouses and enhanced efficacy of caregivers managing difficult behaviors and functional dependency.

Reference

Gitlin L, Corcoran M, Winter L, et al. A randomized, controlled trial of a home environmental intervention: effect on efficacy and upset in caregivers and on daily function of persons with dementia. *J Consult Clin Psychol.* 2001;41:4–14.

Chapter 34
Psychiatric Aspects of Long-Term Care

1. Epidemiological studies reveal that the prevalence of psychiatric disorders in nursing homes is

   a. Less than 50%
   b. Between 50% and 60%
   c. Between 65% and 75%
   d. Greater than 80%

The correct answer is d.

Studies conducted since 1986 have consistently found diagnosable psychiatric disorders in 80%–94% of nursing home residents. These prevalence rates include patients with a diagnosis of dementia, which accounts for approximately two thirds of all psychiatric disorders in the nursing home setting.

References

Chandler JD, Chandler JE. The prevalence of neuropsychiatric disorders in a nursing home population. *J Geriatr Psychiatry Neurol.* 1988;1:71–76.

Rovner BW, Kafonek S, Filipp L, et al. Prevalence of mental illness in a community nursing home. *Am J Psychiatry.* 1986;143:1446–1449.

Tariot PN, Podgorske CA, Blazina L, et al. Mental disorders in the nursing home: another perspective. *Am J Psychiatry.* 1993;150:1063–1069.

2. Most psychiatric consultations requested in the nursing home are for evaluation and treatment of

   a. Depression
   b. Psychosis
   c. Behavioral disturbances

d. Anxiety

e. Insomnia

The correct answer is c.

Although symptoms of depression, anxiety, and insomnia are common, the problems that most often trigger a request for a psychiatric consultation in the nursing home setting are behavioral disturbances, most of which occur in patients with dementia. Behavioral disturbances are among the most common reasons that patients with dementia are admitted to nursing homes, and they frequently complicate care after admission.

References

Cohen-Mansfield J, Marx MS, Rosenthal AS. A description of agitation in a nursing home. *J Gerontol.* 1989;44:M77–M84.

Fenton J, Raskin A, Gruber-Baldini AL, et al. Some predictors of psychiatric consultation in nursing home residents *Am J Geriatr Psychiatry.* 2004;12: 297–304.

Loebel JP, Borson S, Hyde T, et al. Relationships between requests for psychiatric consultations and psychiatric diagnoses in long term care facilities. *Am J Psychiatry.* 1991;148:898–903.

Steele C, Rovner BW, Chase GA, Folstein MF. Psychiatric symptoms and nursing home placement in Alzheimer's disease. *Am J Psychiatry.* 1990;147: 1049–1051.

3. Evidence from research conducted in nursing home residents indicates that depression in this setting is associated with

   a. Poor nutrition

   b. Increased pain complaints

   c. Disability

   d. Increased mortality

   e. All of the above

The correct answer is e.

Studies of residents of nursing homes have shown an association between depression and biochemical markers of undernutrition (such as low serum albumin levels), increased pain complaints, diminished performance of activities of daily living (disability), and mortality rates that are 1.5 to 3 times higher than the rates in nondepressed nursing home elders.

References

Katz IR, Beaston-Wimmer P, Parmelee PA, et al. Failure to thrive in the elderly: exploration of the concept and delineation of psychiatric components. *J Geriatr Psychiatry Neurol.* 1993;6:161–169.

Parmelee PA, Katz IR, Lawton MP. Depression and mortality among institutionalized aged. *J Gerontol Psychol Sci.* 1992;47:P3–P10.

Parmelee PA, Katz IR, Lawton MP. The relation of pain to depression among institutionalized aged. *J Gerontol Psychol Sci.* 1991;46:15–21.

Rovner BW, German PS, Brant LJ, et al. Depression and mortality in nursing homes. *JAMA.* 1991;265:993–996.

4. Among the many factors that prompted Congress to pass the Nursing Home Reform Act as part of the Omnibus Budget Reconciliation Act in 1987 was pressure from various consumer groups. The greatest concern of patient advocacy groups was

   a. Inadequate recognition and undertreatment of depression
   b. Inappropriate admission of acutely psychotic patients to nursing homes
   c. Attempts to shift the cost of nursing home care from the states to the federal government
   d. Inappropriate use of physical and chemical restraints

The correct answer is d.

Congress was responding to several concerns when it passed the Nursing Home Reform Act in 1987. The Institute of Medicine had issued a report in 1986 citing the undertreatment of depression. The General Accounting Office had raised concerns about the transfer of geriatric patients from state hospitals (many of which were closing) to nursing homes, thereby shifting a large portion of the cost of their care from the states to the federal government. However, the greatest concern of consumers and patient advocacy groups, such as the Alzheimer's Association and the National Citizens' Coalition for Nursing Home Reform, stemmed from reports of the widespread misuse of physical and chemical restraints.

References

Elon R, Pawlson LG. The impact of OBRA on medical practice within nursing facilities. *J Am Geriatr Soc.* 1992;40:958–963.

Institute of Medicine, Committee on Nursing Home Regulation. *Improving the Quality of Care in Nursing Homes.* Washington, DC: National Academy Press; 1986.

National Center for Health Statistics. *The National Nursing Home Survey.* Washington, DC: US Government Printing Office; 1979. DHEW Publication PHS 79–1794.

5. Federal guidelines permit the use of physical restraints in nursing homes if

   a. The patient has severe motor restlessness from any cause
   b. There is documentation that the use of restraints is necessary to enhance body positioning

c. The patient has a history of falls when trying to get out of bed

d. The nursing home is not staffed to provide 1:1 supervision for an agitated patient

The correct answer is b.

The federal guidelines for nursing home care specifically prohibit the use of physical restraints for purposes of discipline or convenience and when they are not required to treat the resident's medical symptoms. It must be documented in the nursing home clinical record that the use of restraints is essential to prevent harm to self or others or that it enables the resident to achieve or maintain a higher level of function. If restraints are deemed necessary to enhance body positioning or improve mobility, a consultation note from a physical or occupational therapist should document this need.

References

Health Care Financing Administration. Medicare and Medicaid; requirements for long term care facilities, final regulations. *56(187) Federal Register* 48865–48921 (September 26, 1991).

Health Care Financing Administration. *State Operations Manual: Provider Certification, Transmittal No. 250.* Washington DC: US Government Printing Office; April 1992.

6. After implementation of federal regulations in the early 1990s,

a. The use of antipsychotic medications declined, then plateaued

b. The use of antidepressant drugs increased

c. Anxiolytic prescriptions increased to replace antipsychotic agents

d. There was no change in psychotropic prescribing until 1995, when the use of atypical antipsychotics increased dramatically

The correct answer is b.

After implementation of federal regulations regarding psychotropic drugs, antipsychotic drug use declined significantly in the early 1990s, but with the availability of atypical agents, there is recent evidence that the rate of antipsychotic prescriptions has been increasing since the mid-1990s. There is no evidence for an increase in anxiolytic prescriptions, which might have been expected as a substitute for antipsychotic drugs. The most consistent trend has been the increase in prescription of antidepressants.

References

Lasser RA, Sunderland T. Newer psychotropic medication use in nursing home residents. *J Am Geriatr Soc.* 1998;46:202–207.

Rovner BW, Edelman BA, Cox MP, Shmuely Y. The impact of antipsychotic drug regulations (OBRA 1987) on psychotropic prescribing practices in nursing homes. *Am J Psychiatry.* 1992;149:1390–1392.

Shorr RI, Fought RL, Ray WA. Changes in antipsychotic drug use in nursing homes during implementation of the OBRA-87 regulations. *JAMA.* 1994; 271:358–362.

7. Randomized, placebo-controlled trials of which of the following drugs have demonstrated efficacy for treatment of psychosis specifically in nursing home patients with dementia?

   a. Clozapine and olanzapine
   b. Risperidone and olanzapine
   c. Risperidone and quetiapine
   d. Carbamazepine and divalproex

   The correct answer is b.

   Randomized, controlled studies showing efficacy of drug treatment for psychosis in demented nursing home patients include multicenter trials of risperidone and olanzapine. There are no published controlled studies of clozapine, quetiapine, or ziprasidone in nursing home populations. There is some evidence that carbamazepine and divalproex reduce agitated behavior in demented nursing home patients, but not mania or psychosis.

   References

   Katz IR, Jeste DV, Mintzer JE, et al. Comparison of risperidone and placebo for psychosis and behavioral disturbances associated with dementia: a randomized, double-blind trial. *J Clin Psychiatry.* 1999;60:107–115.

   Street JS, Clark WS, Gannon KS, et al. Olanzapine treatment of psychotic and behavioral symptoms in patients with Alzheimer disease in nursing care facilities: a double-blind, randomized, placebo-controlled trial. The HGEU Study Group. *Arch Gen Psychiatry.* 2000;57:968–976.

   Tariot PN, Erb R, Podgorski CA, et al. Efficacy and tolerability of carbamazepine for agitation and aggression in dementia. *Am J Psychiatry.* 1998;155: 54–61.

8. Which of the following statements is true regarding serotonin reuptake inhibitors (SRIs) in nursing home patients?

   a. A large-scale, randomized, controlled nursing home trial demonstrated efficacy for treatment of depression
   b. They are equally effective in depressed patients with dementia and those who are cognitively intact
   c. They are consistently tolerated without significant adverse effects, even in the oldest, most frail residents

    d. They are associated with a nearly two-fold increase in risk of falls in nursing home residents

The correct answer is d.

To date, there have been no randomized controlled studies that demonstrate the efficacy of SRIs in nursing home populations. Open-label studies in nursing home residents with depression have shown mixed results, with some suggesting they may be less effective for depression in patients with dementia compared to those who are cognitively intact. Although many elderly patients appear to tolerate these drugs, it has been shown that their use in nursing home residents is associated with a two-fold increase in the risk of falls.

References

Oslin DW, Streim JE, Katz IR, et al. Heuristic comparison of sertraline with nortriptyline for the treatment of depression in frail elderly patients. *Am J Geriatr Psychiatry*. 2000;8:141–149.

Rosen J, Mulsant BH, Pollock BG. Sertraline in the treatment of minor depression in nursing home residents: a pilot study. *Int J Geriatr Psychiatry*. 2000;15:177–180.

Thapa PB, Gideon P, Cost CW, Milam AD, Ray WA. Antidepressants and the risk of falls among nursing home residents. *N Engl J Med*. 1998;339:875.

9. Low agitation levels on special care units (SCUs) in nursing homes are correlated with

    a. Low rate of physical restraint use
    b. Greater functional dependency among residents
    c. A high proportion of residents who are out of bed during the day
    d. High comorbid illness burden among residents
    e. Large unit size

The correct answer is a.

Knowledge about the essential elements of SCUs is limited, and evidence for their effectiveness has not been adequately demonstrated. However, a study of the independent correlates of low agitation levels included favorable scores on measures of physical environment and unit activities, low rates of physical restraint use, a high proportion of residents in bed during the day, small unit size, fewer comorbid conditions, and low levels of functional dependency. This suggests that low levels of agitated behavior on some SCUs are not necessarily attributable to a case mix with a high proportion of medically ill, debilitated, bed-bound, or restrained patients.

References

Leon J, Ory M. Effectiveness of special care unit (SCU) placements in reducing physically aggressive behaviors in recently admitted dementia nursing home residents. *Am J Alzheimer's Dis.* 1999;14:270–277.

Sloane PD, Mathew LS, Scarborough M, Desai JR, Koch GG, Tangen C. Physical and pharmacologic restraint of nursing home patients with dementia: impact of specialized units. *JAMA.* 1991;265:1278–1282.

Sloane PD, Mitchell CM, Preisser JS, Phillips C, Commander C, Burker E. Environmental correlates of resident agitation in Alzheimer's disease special care units. *J Am Geriatr Soc.* 1998;46:862–869.

Chapter 35
Psychogeriatric Programs: Inpatient Hospital Units and Partial Hospital Programs

1. The characteristics of patients admitted to geriatric psychiatry inpatient units have changed over the past 10 years. Which of the following characteristics of hospitalized patients have become more common?

   a. They are older
   b. They are more likely to be demented
   c. They are more likely to have psychotic symptoms
   d. They are more likely to have severe medical problems
   e. All of the above

The correct answer is e.

Aging of the population over the past decade accounts for changes in the demographic and clinical characteristics of inpatients. Because the population is older, characteristics associated with age become more prevalent. Patients are more likely to be demented (the prevalence of dementia doubles with every 5-year increment in age), to be admitted for treatment of psychotic symptoms (which are the main reason for admission), and to have medical problems that increase in complexity and severity with age. Thus, the answer to this question is all of the above.

References

Weintraub D, Mazour I. Clinical and demographic changes over ten years on a psychogeriatric inpatient unit. *Ann Clin Psychiatry.* 2000;12:227–231.

Zubenko GS, Marino LJ, Sweet RA, et al. Medical co-morbidity in elderly psychiatric inpatients. *Biol Psychiatry.* 1997;41:724–736.

2. An 85-year-old woman with a progressive dementia syndrome is admitted to a geriatric psychiatry inpatient unit because of combativeness. Which of the following factors will determine how long she is hospitalized?

   a. Her comorbid medical problems
   b. Her personal financial resources
   c. Her caregiver's level of stress
   d. Her compliance with medications
   e. All of the above.

The correct answer is e.

Although the length of stay on geriatric psychiatry inpatient units has decreased with changes in reimbursement mechanisms, a number of risk factors for increased length of stay have been identified. For example, Draper and Luscombe (1998) identified high levels of caregiver stress as an important factor accounting for variance in length of stay. Behavioral issues during hospitalization will also influence length of stay: Patients failing to comply with treatments delay time to remission, which prolongs hospital stay. Comorbid medical problems are a known determinant of length of stay because they complicate psychiatric treatment, require consultant visits, and at times necessitate medical transfers and eventual returns to the psychiatric unit. Limited financial resources also can delay discharge because of restrictions in care options (assisted living facilities are often private pay based). The limited availability of Medicaid beds in general nursing homes (especially for demented patients with behavioral disorders) further implicates financial resources as a determinant of hospital length of stay.

Reference

Draper B, Luscombe G. Quantification of factors contributing to length of stay in an acute psychogeriatric ward. *Int J Geriatr Psychiatry.* 1998;13: 1–7.

3. Patients admitted to a geriatric psychiatry unit for the treatment of major depression vary in their long-term affective outcomes. Which admission characteristic best predicts continued depressive symptoms after discharge?

   a. Being introverted
   b. Being unable to walk
   c. Having a urinary catheter
   d. Having pain complaints
   e. Being widowed

The correct answer is d.

The correct response derives from empirical data on older patients admitted to a geriatric inpatient unit with follow-up data over 1 year. The data indicated that elevated depression scores, worse instrumental activities of daily living functioning, poor self-rated health, and high levels of pain intensity predicted poor long-term affective outcomes. Personality traits, marital status, and physical functioning were not predictive.

References

Casten RJ, Rovner BW, Pasternak RE, Pelchat R. A comparison of self-reported function assessed before and after depression treatment among depressed geriatric inpatients. *Int J Geriatr Psychiatry.* 2000;15:813–818.

Casten RJ, Rovner BW, Shmuely-Dulitzki Y, Pasternak RE, Pelchat R, Ranen N. Predictors of recovery from major depression among geriatric psychiatry inpatients: the importance of caregivers' beliefs. *Int Psychogeriatr.* 1999; 11:149–157.

4. A substantial proportion of older patients admitted to geriatric psychiatry inpatient units have a personality disorder (PD). The most frequently diagnosed PD among older psychiatrically hospitalized patients is

   a. Dependent
   b. Narcissistic
   c. Hysterical
   d. Borderline
   e. Schizoid

The correct answer is a.

A number of studies have identified rates of different PD diagnoses among older patients admitted to geriatric psychiatry units. Consistently, they have found that the majority are from the anxious cluster and identify dependent PD as the most common.

References

Kunik ME, Mulsant BH, Rifai AH, Sweet RA, Pasternak R, Zubenko GS. Diagnostic rate of comorbid personality disorder in elderly psychiatric inpatients. *Am J Psychiatry.* 1994;151:603–605.

Molinari V, Kunik ME, Mulsant B, Rifai AH. The relationship between patient, informant, social worker, and consensus diagnoses of personality disorder in elderly depressed inpatients. *Am J Geriatr Psychiatry.* 1998;6:136–144.

5. Among older patients with major depression admitted to a geriatric psychiatry inpatient unit, patients with comorbid PDs are more likely to have which of the following characteristics compared with patients without PDs?

a. Later age of onset of depression
b. Comorbid psychotic symptoms
c. History of mania
d. Previous suicide attempts
e. Longer length of stay

The correct answer is d.

Kunik et al. (1993) evaluated older patients admitted with major depression who met *Diagnostic and Statistical Manual of Mental Disorders, Third Edition, Revised (DSM-III-R*; American Psychiatric Association; 1990) criteria for a PD. Compared to patients without PDs, those with PD had higher rates of previous suicide attempts. Other characteristics were that they had never married or were separated or divorced. The investigators did not find that age of onset of depression, comorbid psychotic symptoms, history of mania, or longer length of stay were associated characteristics.

Reference

American Psychiatric Association. *Diagnostic and Statistical Manual of Mental Disorders*. 3rd ed., rev. Washington, DC: American Psychiatric Association; 1987.

Kunik ME, Mulsant BH, Rifai AH, et al. Personality disorders in elderly inpatients with major depression. *Am J Geriatr Psychiatry*. 1993;1:38–45.

Chapter 36
Geriatric Consultation-Liaison Psychiatry

1. The evaluation of competency in a medical setting must

a. Be completed at the time of admission
b. Determine if a patient is legally competent to make all decisions
c. Include evaluation of the patient's financial status
d. Assess a patient's ability to understand the choices and the consequences of a decision.

The correct answer is d.

The evaluation of competency can occur at any time during the admission. A patient may be competent to make some decisions regarding care but incompetent for others. Assessment of financial competence is not necessarily a part of the competency evaluation during a medical hospitalization. Competency evaluations must assess the patient's ability to understand the choices and their consequences.

Reference

Appelbaum BC, Appelbaum PS, Grisso T. Competence to consent to voluntary psychiatric hospitalization: a test of a standard proposed by APA. American Psychiatric Association. *Psychiatr Serv.* 1998;49:1193–1196.

2. Psychiatric consultation for geriatric inpatients requires special geriatric skills because

   a. About 40% of elderly inpatients have some psychiatric disorder
   b. Elderly patients are more likely to have drug interactions than younger patients
   c. Elderly patients with medical illness are at high risk for suicide
   d. All of the above

The correct answer is d.

Elderly patients are more likely to have dementia and delirium than younger patients. Depression is more common in the medically burdened elders. Drug interactions and suicide are both more common in the elderly.

References

Conwell Y, Olsen K, Caine ED, Flannery C. Suicide in later life: psychological autopsy findings. *Int Psychogeriatr.* 1991;3:59–66.
De Leo D, Spathonis K. Suicide and euthanasia in late life. *Aging Clin Exp Res.* 2003;15:99–110.
Popkin MK, Mackenzie TB, Callies AL. Psychiatric consultation to geriatric medically ill inpatients in a university hospital. *Arch Gen Psychiatry.* 1984; 41:703–707.
Wetterling T, Junghanns K. Affective disorders in older inpatients. *Int J Geriatr Psychiatry.* 2004;1:487–492.

3. Consultation always includes

   a. Examining the patient
   b. Discussing findings with family
   c. Teaching the nursing staff
   d. Comprehensive evaluation of the patient

The correct answer is a.

Consultation may involve family and, when combined with a liaison model, education for the nursing staff. A consultation can be brief and focused or comprehensive, depending on the request and clinical need. In all cases, the patient must be examined.

Reference

Lipowski ZJ. Consultation-liaison psychiatry 1990. *Psychother Psychosom.* 1991;55:62–68.

4. When an elderly patient suddenly becomes delirious in a medical setting, the first thing that should be done is

   a. A complete medical and pharmacological assessment
   b. Give haloperidol to reduce the agitation
   c. Leave the lights on to prevent "sundowning"
   d. Have the family bring in familiar objects from home

The correct answer is a.

A new onset of delirium reflects a change in the patient's physical condition. This may be caused by a change in their medical or pharmacological status or environmental factors such as sensory deprivation or the stress of being in an intensive care unit. Ruling out a new medical problem or serious drug interaction is the first step.

References

Lipowski ZJ. Delirium, clouding of consciousness and confusion. *J Nerv Ment Dis.* 1967;145:227–255.
Lipowski ZJ. Review of consultation psychiatry and psychosomatic medicine. I. General principles. *Psychosom Med.* 1967;29:153–171.
Weber JB, Coverdale JH, Kunik ME. Delirium: current trends in prevention and treatment. *Intern Med J.* 2004;34:115–121.

5. Which of the following are risk factors for persistent depression following hospital discharge?

   a. History of dysthymia or depression
   b. Stressful life events in the year prior to the index admission
   c. Greater number of active medical diagnoses
   d. Patient's perception of severity of depression
   e. All of the above
   f. None of the above

Correct answer is e.

All of these factors are probable risk factors for persistent postdischarge depression. Unfortunately, despite the treatability of depression and evidence for effectiveness of psychiatric consultation in curbing depressive symptoms and their negative impact on medical outcomes, both risk factors for depression and the disorder itself remain markedly underdiagnosed in medical settings.

References

Koenig H, George L. Depression and physical disability outcomes in depressed medically ill hospitalized older adults. *Am J Geriatr Psychiatry*. 1998;6: 247.

Lesprance F, Frasure-Smith N. Depression in patients with cardiac disease: a practical review. *J Psychosom Res*. 2000;48:379–391.

Chapter 37
Integrated Community Services

1. Which of the following would be an appropriate service for an older person with a moderate level of functional impairment?

   a. Foster grandparent program
   b. Skilled nursing facility
   c. Assisted living
   d. Retired Seniors Volunteer Program

The correct answer is c.

Assisted living is typically designed for persons who cannot live independently but require some assistance with daily living. Programs such as Foster Grandparents or Retired Senior Volunteers are for active, independent older persons. Finally, nursing homes are typically for severely impaired older persons who require 24-hour nursing care and medical coverage as well as assistance in basic activities of daily living, such as bathing, eating, grooming, or dressing.

References

Administration on Aging page. Department of Health and Human Services Web site. Available at: http://www.aoa.dhhs.gov/eldfam/Housing/Housing. asp. Accessed December 24, 2004.

Cantor M, Little V. Aging and social care. In: Binstock RH, Shanas E, eds. *Handbook of Aging and the Social Sciences*. 2nd ed. New York, NY: Van Nostrand Reinhold; 1985.

Hawes C, Rose M, Phillips CD, et al. *A National Study of Assisted Living for the Frail Elderly. Results of a National Survey Facilities*. Washington, DC: US Dept of Health and Human Services/Assistant Secretary for Planning and Evaluation; December 1999.

2. Congregate meal programs are provided under which governmental program?

   a. Title XVIII of the Social Security Act
   b. Title V of the Older American Act
   c. Title III of the Older American Act
   d. Title XIX of the Social Security Act

The correct answer is c.

Title III of the Older Americans Act (OAA) was originally passed in 1965. Although services vary by state, this provision encourages the provision of congregate meals, home-delivered meals, chore services, senior centers, and home health care. Title XVIII of the Social Security Act created Medicare in 1965; Title XIX of the Social Security Act (1965) created Medicaid. Title V of the OAA created community employment and volunteer programs for older persons.

References

Administration on Aging page. Department of Health and Human Services Web site. Available at: http://www.aoa.dhhs.gov. Accessed December 24, 2004.

Gelfand DE. *The Aging Network Programs and Services*. 5th ed. New York, NY: Springer; 1999.

3. Area agencies on aging

   a. Primarily provide information and referral
   b. Generally provide direct services
   c. Were created under Title V of the OAA
   d. All of the above

The correct answer is a.

As part of Title III of the OAA, each state is required to designate an agency for aging services. In most states, the state aging agency designates smaller geographic centers called area agencies on aging. Their principal purpose is to provide information and referral, and they are forbidden to provide direct services unless absolutely necessary.

References

Administration on Aging page. Department of Health and Human Services Web site. Available at: www.aoa.dhhs.gov. Accessed December 24, 2004.

Gelfand DE. *The Aging Network Programs and Services*. 5th ed. New York, NY: Springer; 1999.

4. The three case management approaches that are commonly used to secure and coordinate services are

   a. Social, benefits, and educational models
   b. Brokering, service management, and managed-care models
   c. Quality-of-life, utilization, and screening models
   d. Mobility, seedling, and developmental models

The correct answer is b.

The three most common case management approaches are the brokering model (the case manager identifies an appropriate service package from community resources), the service management model (the case manager authorizes services and the client's service budget), and the managed-care model (services are provided by a managed-care health organization).

Reference

Westhoff LJ. Care management: quelling the confusion. *Health Prog.* 1992; 73:43–46.

5. In most states, adult protective services (APS) serve persons who may have all the following problems *except*

   a. Incapable of performing functions necessary to meet basic physical requirements
   b. Incapable of managing finances
   c. Exhibiting behavior that brings them into conflict with society
   d. Neglect and abuse occurring in nursing homes

The correct answer is d.

APS are used for persons who may be incapable of performing functions to meet basic physical and health requirements, incapable of managing finances, are dangerous to self or others, or exhibit behavior that brings them into conflict with the community. In most states, APS is responsible for community-dwelling older persons, but the state ombudsman on aging is responsible for abuse or exploitation in nursing homes.

References

Lachs MS, Williams C, O'Brien S, et al. Older adults: an 11-year longitudinal study of adult protective service use. *Arch Intern Med.* 1996;156:449–453.
Wolf RS. Adult protective services. In: Maddox GL, ed. *The Encyclopedia of Aging.* 3rd ed. New York, NY: Springer; 2001: 26–28.

6. All of the following governmental programs provide specifically for in-home services *except*

   a. Medicaid
   b. Title III of the OAA
   c. Social Services Block Grant
   d. Supplemental Security Income

The correct answer is d.

Medicaid, Title III of the OAA, and the Social Services Block Grant of 1981 can all potentially provide for in-home services, although the level of services varies by state. Supplemental Security Income, which was implemented in 1970, is a supplemental income program for the disabled, aged, and blind.

References

Administration on Aging page. Department of Health and Human Services Web site. Available at: www.aoa.dhhs.gov. Accessed December 24, 2004.
Gelfand DE. *The Aging Network Programs and Services*. 5th ed. New York, NY: Springer; 1999.

7. Of the various respite programs, which of the following has been found to most consistently achieve its goals for relieving the distress and improving the mood of caregivers?

   a. In-home services
   b. Adult day programs
   c. Overnight respite
   d. Adult homes

The correct answer is a.

An extensive review by Zarit and colleagues (1999) found that in-home service was the only respite program that consistently benefited caregivers' mood, level of distress, and time spent in caregiving activities. Reports of caregivers' satisfaction are high for day programs and day hospitals, but there seems to be little positive long-term effect on caregivers' mood and distress.

Reference

Zarit SH, Gaugler JE, Jarrot SE. Useful services for families: research findings and directions. *Int J Geriatr Psychiatry*. 1999;14:165–177.

8. Which of the following is true about mental health services for older adults?

   a. The 1981 federal block grant mandated that treatment of elderly persons be a required psychiatric service for mental health centers
   b. Outreach services have not been very effective in addressing mental health needs of older persons
   c. The existence of a specialized outpatient unit for older adults does not seem to enhance utilization of services
   d. The two basic types of vocational rehabilitation programs are sheltered employment and transitional employment

The correct answer is d.

Although vocational programs underserve older persons, two basic types are available: sheltered employment, which provides work opportunities for individuals who are not ready for competitive employment, and transitional employment, which provides real work jobs under supervision of a rehabilitation professional. The 1981 federal block grant actually eliminated an earlier mandate that mental health centers serve elderly persons. The review by Lebowitz (1988) demonstrated that a specialized outpatient unit for older adults will enhance utilization of services. A series of studies of underserved populations (e.g., rural elderly persons, homeless elderly individuals, older persons in public housing, mentally ill older adults in suburban communities) has demonstrated the effectiveness of outreach interventions, increasing services, and improving well-being.

References

Cuijpers P. Psychological outreach programmes for the depressed elderly: a meta-analysis of effects and dropout. *Int J Geriatr Psychiatry.* 1998;13: 41–48.

Jacobs HE. Vocational rehabilitation. In: Lieberman RP, ed. *Psychiatric Rehabilitation of Chronic Mental Patients.* Washington, DC: American Psychiatric Press; 1988:245–284.

Lebowitz B. Correlates of success in community mental health programs for the elderly. *Hosp Community Psychiatry.* 1988;39:721–722.

Morrissey JP, Goldman HH. Cycles of reform in the care of the chronically mentally ill. *Hosp Community Psychiatry.* 1984;35:785–793.

9. All of the following are true about senior centers *except*

   a. About one third of seniors attend senior centers
   b. Race is not associated with participation
   c. Centers are used by "less-advantaged" seniors
   d. Title III of the OAA provides support for centers

The correct answer is a.

Approximately 15% of all seniors use centers nationwide. Title III of the OAA, as amended in 1973, provided for the acquisition, renovation, or construction and operation of senior centers. Krout's survey (1995) found that centers are used by older persons with lower family income, those living alone, women, and persons who have no college education. Contrary to earlier studies, race is not associated with participation. Krout concluded that senior centers are used by the less advantaged but not the "least advantaged."

References

Krout JA. Senior centers and services for the frail elderly. *J Aging Soc Policy.* 1995;7:59–76.

Krout JA, Cutler S, Coward R. Correlates of senior center participation: a national analysis. *Gerontologist.* 1990;30:72–79.

10. Which of the following is true about housing for older adults?

    a. About one fifth of older adults live in planned housing (i.e., housing specifically for the aging)
    b. Funding levels for senior housing under Section 202 has remained stable over the past 20 years
    c. Assisted living is designed to accommodate frail elderly
    d. Congregate housing typically does not provide any health services or other support services

The correct answer is c.

The Administration on Aging states that assisted living is designed for the *frail elderly*, who are defined as persons 62 years of age or older who are unable to perform at least three activities of daily living. Lawton (2001) estimated that about 10% of older persons live in "planned housing" (i.e., housing specifically targeted to older people). Federal funding levels for Section 202 senior housing has declined substantially since 1980. Congregate housing consists of apartment houses or group accommodations that provide limited health services and support services to functionally impaired older persons who do not require nursing home care.

References

Administration on Aging page. Department of Health and Human Services Web site. Available at: http://www.aoa.dhhs.gov. Accessed December 24, 2004.

Lawton MP. Housing. In: Maddox GL, ed. *The Encyclopedia of Aging.* 3rd ed. New York, NY: Springer; 2001.

11. Which is true about Natural Occurring Retirement Communities (NORCs)?

   a. They include any building or neighborhood where more than one third of residents are over age 60 years
   b. About two fifths of elderly persons live in NORCs
   c. NORCs typically include social and health supports
   d. They are the most common form of retirement community in the United States

The correct answer is d.

NORCs are generally defined as any building or neighborhood where more than 50% of the residents are age 60 years or older. These are now the most common form of retirement community in the United States; that is, 27% of elderly persons live in NORCs. Most NORCs do not provide any health or social services, although there is increased recognition that services may be needed.

Reference

Bassuk K. NORC supportive service programs: effective and innovative programs that support seniors living in the community. *Case Manage J.* 1999; 1:132–137.

V Medical-Legal, Ethical, and Financial Issues

Chapter 38
Legal and Ethical Issues

1. Which of the following statements about incompetency is not correct?

   a. It can be used interchangeably with "impaired decisional capacity"
   b. It requires evaluation of functional abilities
   c. It may be partial and apply only to specific areas of functioning
   d. It can indicate that the patient is at risk for harm

The correct answer is a.

Competency is a legal term, and decisional capacity (or incapacity) is a clinical determination. Every adult is presumed to be competent until something triggers a question of mental incapacity. Incompetence is determined only by a judge's express ruling, usually in probate court.

Reference
Kapp MB. *Geriatrics and the Law*. 3rd ed. New York, NY: Springer; 1999: 31.

2. Which of the following is not true regarding decisional capacity?

   a. It can fluctuate
   b. It can be evaluated using the MacArthur Competence Assessment Tool (MacCAT)
   c. It has clearly defined standards depending on the jurisdiction
   d. It can be enhanced by therapeutic interventions

The correct answer is c.

There is no single test or scale of "competency" or capacity. This owes partly to the inherent characteristics of decisional capacity assessments, their specificity, complexity, and the flexibility needed for application across a limitless range of treatment scenarios. Of the numerous capacities relevant to competency described in the literature, four major elements of competency have reached general consensus. These are (a) the ability to express a choice, (b) the ability to reason about the risks and benefits of options, (c) the ability to understand relevant information, (d) the ability to appreciate the nature of one's situation, including the consequences of one's choices, this being the most stringent standard. Most of the literature supports using a sliding scale model that selects capacity standards according to the risk of the decision at hand, with greater risks or fewer benefits requiring higher standards.

References

Grisso T, Appelbaum PS. Comparison of standards for assessing patients' capacities to make treatment decisions. *Am J Psychiatry*. 1995;152:1033–1037.
Drane JF. The many faces of competency. *Hastings Center Rep*. 1985;15:17–21.

3. Proxy decision making for decisionally incapacitated persons

   a. Only can be performed after a court finding of incompetence
   b. Has been found to correlate inadequately with decisions the impaired person would make for himself
   c. Should follow the "best interests" standard
   d. Serves as an adequate safeguard for research participation

The correct answer is b.

Proxy decision making using substituted judgment is difficult, often inaccurate, and fraught with ethical dilemmas. Studies showed that often proxies never discussed the wishes of patients and frequently guessed inaccurately. Accurate substituted judgment requires that the proxy know the patient's preferences, extrapolate them to the situations at hand, and have the courage to carry them out even when the decision might not appear to be in the patient's best interest. It is especially difficult for a proxy when decisions for the patient are in conflict with their own interests.

References

Caralis PV. Ethical and legal issues in the care of Alzheimer's patients. *Med Clin North Am*. 1994;78:877–893.
Fellows LK. Competency and consent in dementia. *J Am Geriatr Soc*. 1998; 46:922–926.

4. The Patient Self Determination Act (PSDA) requires that

   a. A standard advance directive format be used nationally
   b. The facility to which a person is being admitted is responsible to inform the person about its policy concerning which directives it will and will not honor
   c. The primary care doctors familiarize patients with advance directives in office and nursing home settings
   d. Incompetent patients have guardians assigned

The correct answer is b.

According to the provisions of the PSDA of 1991 (42 USC Sections 1395 cc and 1396 a Supp. 1991), all persons entering a health care facility must be asked if they have an advance directive, and the directive (or documentation that none exists) must be entered into the record. The facility is also responsible to inform the person about its policy concerning which directives it will and will not honor. A shortcoming of the PSDA is that it does not apply to outpatient settings, which would be more suitable for discussion and encouragement of advance directives.

Reference

Grossberg GT. Advance directives, competency evaluation, and surrogate management in elderly patients. *Am J Geriatr Psychiatry.* 1998;6:S79–S84.

5. Disclosure of the diagnosis of probable Alzheimer's disease (AD)

   a. Enables advance directives regarding future research participation to be formulated
   b. Is recommended by the Alzheimer's Disease and Related Disorders Association (ADRDA)
   c. Can both enhance and disrupt family dynamics
   d. All of the above

The correct answer is d.

Diagnostic truth telling about a diagnosis of "probable AD" should be the current standard of care and is strongly recommended by the Alzheimer's Association (formerly ADRDA). Informing the person of the AD diagnosis enables the person to (a) plan to optimize experiences and relationships in his or her time of relative intactness; (b) prepare advance directives including durable power of attorney; (c) consider possible participation in AD research; (d) participate in AD support groups; (e) make an informed decision about antidementia agents; and (f) attend to estate and will issues.

References

Alzheimer's Disease and Related Disorders Association. *Ethical Consideration: Issues in Diagnostic Disclosure.* Chicago, IL: ADRDA; 1997.

Post SG. The fear of forgetfulness: a grassroots approach to an ethics of Alzheimer's disease. *J Clin Ethics.* 1998;9:71–80.

6. The following is true regarding the guardianship process:

   a. It is often expensive and time consuming
   b. It is required before any significant surgical procedure is performed on an incapacitated person
   c. It ensures that the ward will not be subject to abuse
   d. It can be arranged by psychiatrists working in conjunction with attorneys

The correct answer is a.

Guardianship involves the judicial appointment of a guardian empowered to make personal or financial decisions for an incompetent individual (referred to as the *ward*). The judge determines that a person is fully or partially incompetent, with limited forms of guardianship taking over only the compromised areas of decision making. The guardianship process is expensive and time consuming, usually requiring an attorney, court time, and monitoring. It is a court procedure, and a psychiatrist cannot legally arrange guardianship with an attorney. An individual incompetent to decide on a surgical procedure will require a substitute decision maker, not a guardian. Guardianship needs to be monitored as it is no guarantee in itself that the guardian or other person will not abuse the subject in some way.

Reference

Grossberg GT. Advance directives, competency evaluation, and surrogate management in elderly patients. *Am J Geriatr Psychiatry.* 1998;6:S79–S84.

7. Which of the following statements is not true regarding research with older subjects?

   a. It usually does not differ from research with younger subjects
   b. It requires special safeguards for cognitively impaired subjects
   c. When it involves nursing home residents, it is best conducted by nursing home staff familiar to them
   d. Incapacitated patients who refuse should not be included even if their proxy decision makers have given permission

The correct answer is c.

Nursing home residents considered for research participation are particularly vulnerable to exploitation. In addition to the difficulties obtaining informed consent because of cognitive impairments, valid informed consent is jeopardized by encroachments on autonomy inherent in the setting. Life within a "total institution" challenges the ability of even the cognitively intact to make free, voluntary decisions, such as the refusal of participation in research. This is also problematic if the nursing home staff or doctors conduct the research.

Reference

Sachs GA, Cohen HJ. Ethical challenges to research. In: Cassel CK, Cohen HJ, Larson EB, et al., eds. *Geriatric Medicine*. 3rd ed. New York, NY: Springer; 1996:1029.

8. Which of the following is *not true* of older drivers?

   a. They often compensate for changes by reducing mileage and refraining from night driving
   b. Compared with other seniors, drivers with mild AD generally do not yet show declines in their driving skills
   c. They experience significantly more crashes, more severe injuries, and more fatalities after age 65 years
   d. They often react with profound feelings of loss if driving privileges are revoked

The correct answer is b.

Studies of the risk of accidents among drivers with AD have yielded conflicting results. Unlike nondemented elders, cognitively impaired persons tend not to take corrective steps to compensate for their aging changes, such as reducing mileage or refraining from driving at night. Unfortunately, patients with dementia are typically not aware of their relevant deficits and tend to characterize themselves as safe drivers even when they are deemed "unsafe" on structured driving evaluations. Evidence suggests that drivers with mild AD Clinical Dementia Rating (CDR) of 0.5 ("possible AD, slight forgetfulness and slight impairment of activities") pose a danger, and those with a CDR of 1.0 or more have a substantially increased rate of accidents and driving errors and should be advised not to drive. More research is needed to determine whether there are subsets of people with mild AD who can drive safely with certain restrictions.

References

Bonn D. Patients with mild Alzheimer's disease should not drive. *Lancet*. 2000;356:49.

Dubinsky RM, Stein AC, Kelly L. Practice parameter: risk of driving and Alzheimer's disease (an evidence-based review): report of the quality standards subcommittee of the American Academy of Neurology. *Neurology*. 2000; 54:2205–2211.

Hunt L, Morris JC, Edwards D, et al. Driving performance in persons with mild senile dementia of the Alzheimer type. *J Am Geriatr Soc*. 1993;41: 747–753.

Chapter 39
Financial Issues

1. A 78-year-old man with hypertension, hypercholesterolemia, and diabetes developed severe depression after having right knee surgery 4
   weeks earlier. A trial of an antidepressant was initiated, but the patient
   continued to deteriorate. The patient was hospitalized on a geropsychiatric unit and improved but continued to have significant anxiety, depression, and anhedonia. The patient also needed encouragement to
   dress and groom himself, go to the dining room for meals, and engage
   in activities during the day rather than retreating to his bed. Nursing
   expressed concerns that he was so apathetic that he would not take all
   of his medications correctly. The dietician had developed an American
   Diabetes Association diet for the patient to which he could adhere in
   the hospital because his meals were prepared for him, but the dietician
   expressed grave reservations about whether the patient would be able
   to maintain a proper diet at home. The physical therapist believed that
   the patient would benefit from additional physical therapy for his right
   knee, but that he needed extra encouragement to participate. The patient insisted that he wanted to get well but lacked the confidence to
   "make it" at home.

   Following his knee surgery, the patient had spent 20 days on a rehabilitation unit. The patient has Medicare Parts A and B and Medicare
   supplemental insurance that would cover skilled nursing facility copay-
   ments. Which of the discharge aftercare plan options would best serve
   the patient and be covered by his insurance plans?

   a. Subacute rehabilitation
   b. Transitional care unit
   c. Discharge home with referral to the local visiting nurse association
   d. Acute rehabilitation hospitalization

   The correct answer is a.

   This patient would benefit from rehabilitative and psychiatric care services provided through a subacute rehabilitative facility. A subacute
   rehabilitative facility is considered by Medicare to be a skilled nursing
   facility and is often located in a nursing home setting. A transitional
   care unit, also a skilled nursing facility, is a possible disposition for
   this patient, but typically transitional care units have a postacute, restorative, and rehabilitative focus. Each subacute rehabilitative facility
   is unique and may offer a different range of specific services and admission requirements, so it would be important for the patient and
   family members to consider a variety of facilities carefully.

   Because the patient spent 20 days in a rehabilitative unit following his knee surgery and 60 days had not yet passed since the patient was discharged from the rehabilitative unit, the patient would be required to pay a copayment ($109.50 per day in 2004); this copayment may be covered by the patient's Medicare supplemental insurance, depending on the policy. After day 100 of skilled nursing care, the patient would have to cover all costs. Medicare will not pay for care classified as custodial care if it is the only type of care needed. *Custodial care* means help with the activities of daily living, such as bathing, getting in and out of bed, dressing, eating, and using the bathroom.

The patient, if discharged home with visiting nurse support, would be likely to fail. He may be able to receive time-limited nursing care with limited medication monitoring, occupational therapy, physical therapy, home health care, and meals assistance referral through the visiting nurse association. However, he continues to experience significant anhedonia and apathy, and under this arrangement, he would not be able to receive the level of cueing and support that he needs to care for himself safely and adequately and to take medications and adhere to a diabetic diet reliably throughout the day.

References

Medicare Fee-for-Service page. Department of Health and Human Services, Center for Medicare and Medicaid Services Web page. Available at: http://www.cms.hhs.gov/providers/default.asp. Accessed November 16, 2003.

Medicare Information Resource page. Department of Health and Human Services, Center for Medicare and Medicaid Services Web page. Available at: http://www.cms.hhs.gov/medicare. Accessed December 24, 2004.

2. An 81-year-old female nursing home long-term care resident with dementia, recurrent delirium, and associated behavioral difficulties has required three geropsychiatric hospitalizations totaling 110 days in the past year. During this time, there has been no continuous out-of-hospital period longer than 60 days. The patient has Medicare and Medicaid insurance. The patient is again admitted to a geropsychiatric unit because she developed behavior problems that the nursing home staff could not manage safely. Which of the following are true?

   a. Medicare will cover the patient's hospital costs indefinitely
   b. Medicare and Medicaid will cover the full cost of the patient's hospitalization
   c. The patient would have all her Medicare lifetime reserve days available for use in the future
   d. Medicare will not cover hospital services costs beyond hospitalization day 150

The correct answer is d.

Medicare Part A insurance is intentionally limited to coverage of relatively brief inpatient stays for stabilization of acute conditions. Regulations provide coverage for spells of illness. A *spell* is defined as an inpatient episode that begins with inpatient admission and ends with the close of the first period of 60 consecutive days after discharge. It is possible for a patient to be discharged and readmitted on several occasions during a given episode of illness and still be considered to be in the same spell as long as 60 days have not elapsed between discharge and admission. For admission to general hospitals, there is no limit on the number of spells or total lifetime days covered. However, the maximum number of covered days during a single spell is 150.

There are different levels of coverage for various lengths of hospitalization. For hospitalization days 1–60, Medicare pays in full after a deductible equal to the average cost of 1 day of hospitalization has been paid by the patient. For days 61–90, the patient covers 25% per hospital day copayment. For days 91–150, the patient covers 50% per hospital day copayment. For hospitalization days over 150, the patient is responsible for all costs.

Days 91–150 are considered lifetime reserve days; coverage for these days may be used electively during any episode but may be used only once during a patient's lifetime. Patients may elect to save these days for future prolonged hospitalizations and to use other financial resources for payment of any part of the costs of days 91–150.

Medicaid is a state-administered program and would provide Medicare copayment coverage according to state regulations. Each state sets its own guidelines subject to federal rules and guidelines. Title XIX of the Social Security Act requires that certain basic services must be offered to the categorically needy population in any state program for the state to receive federal matching funds. These basic services include inpatient hospital services, physician services, and laboratory and radiographic services. States may also receive federal funding if they elect to provide other optional services, such as prescription drug coverage or prosthetic devices.

Within broad federal guidelines, the states determine the amount, duration, and scope of services offered under Medicaid programs. Although the services must be sufficient to reasonably achieve their purpose, the states may limit a Medicaid service based on medical necessity or utilization control. Providers participating in Medicaid must accept the Medicaid reimbursement level as payment in full. Therefore, Medicare and Medicaid may not fully cover the costs of the patient's hospitalization.

References

Medicare Fee-for-Service page. Department of Health and Human Services, Center for Medicare and Medicaid Services Web page. Available at: http://www.cms.hhs.gov/providers/default.asp. Accessed December 24, 2004.

Medicare Information Resource page. Department of Health and Human Services, Center for Medicare and Medicaid Services Web page. Available at: http://www.cms.hhs.gov/medicare/. Accessed December 24, 2004.

Medicaid Services page. Department of Health and Human Services, Center for Medicare and Medicaid Services Web page. Available at: http://www.cms.hhs.gov/medicaid/mservice.asp. Accessed December 24, 2004.

3. Which of the following statements about entitlement to Medicare health benefits is correct?

   a. Recent legislation ensures that the payment of full Social Security benefits and Medicare coverage will continue to begin at age 65 years for future retirees
   b. Individuals who are younger than age 65 years are not be eligible for Social Security or Medicare benefits
   c. Part B benefits are reimbursed only for treatments delivered in a licensed facility
   d. Benefits for mental health treatment are limited to covered services
   e. Medicare coverage is limited to patients who are entitled to Social Security benefits

   The correct answer is d.

   Recent legislative changes have mandated a phased-in delay of eligibility for full Social Security benefits to begin after the age of 65 years. Eligibility for Medicare, which is a social insurance program that was initiated under the 1966 Social Security Act to provide health cost insurance coverage, is not affected by the delay in Social Security retirement benefits. Medicare will continue to begin at the customary age of 65 years. Medicare was expanded subsequently to insure younger individuals who are disabled. Americans who are not entitled to Social Security benefits may receive Medicare as well, but they must pay a monthly premium to be eligible. Part B Medicare benefits provide insurance coverage for health provider services. Psychiatric benefits cover designated services regardless of the setting in which a patient is seen. Medicare procedures and their corresponding billing codes are described in the Current Procedural Terminology (CPT). Social Security legislation also relates to non-health-related payments made to older Americans. Although these cash benefits have customarily begun at age 65 years, the age at which Medicare health insurance takes effect, recent legislation has phased in delays in the initiation of benefits to take trends toward later retirements into account.

4. Which of the following statements about reimbursement paid to providers under Medicare is correct?

   a. Billing by providers who have not signed Medicare contracts is also subject to Medicare regulations

b. Participating Medicare providers are prohibited from billing Medicare recipients for copayment of covered services

c. Limiting charges for participating providers are lower than those for providers who do not participate

d. Nonparticipating providers may accept assignment for Medicare covered services

e. Nonparticipating providers are not required to accept assignment for patients who have both Medicare and Medicaid coverage

The correct answer is d.

Medicare regulations regarding billing apply only to physicians who have signed contracts with Medicare. Although physicians who have not signed Medicare contracts are allowed to bill all of their patients who have Medicare privately at whatever fee has been agreed on, Medicare does not allow physicians who do not have Medicare contracts to seek Medicare reimbursement for themselves or their patients on a case-by-case basis. The use of Medicare is precluded for all of the services delivered to Medicare patients by physicians who do not have Medicare contracts. In the case of physicians who do have Medicare contracts, Medicare billing rules must be followed for all of the physician's Medicare patients. For example, physicians with Medicare contracts are prohibited from having arrangements with some patients that would bill for services at rates higher than Medicare allows.

Participating providers are those with Medicare contracts who agree to accept assignment (or direct payment from Medicare) for their covered services. Participating providers are expected to bill their patients or their patients' secondary carriers for the copayment portion of the costs for these services. In return for this arrangement, participating providers are paid 100% of the Medicare allowable amount; nonparticipating providers are only paid 95% of the Medicare allowable for services when they accept assignment. Nonparticipating providers have the option of accepting or not accepting assignment (or direct payment from Medicare) for their services. Nevertheless, assignment must be accepted in the case of all impoverished patients who have both Medicare and Medicaid coverage. In these cases, patients may not be billed directly for any portion of physician provider services.

Reference

www.cms.hhs.gov (click on Professional tab, click on Providers, click on Physicians, click on Billing/Payment) Accessed December 24, 2004.

5. Which of the following statements about reimbursement to institutions for Part A Medicare services is correct?

a. Prospective payment systems (PPSs) are customarily used to specify the Medicare limits of hospital coverage for the treatment of patients in psychiatric hospitals

b. Reimbursement for inpatient stays at psychiatric hospitals are determined by the patient's diagnosis related group (DRG)

c. Capitation rates determined under the Tax Equity and Fiscal Responsibility Act (TEFRA) limit reimbursement for the hospital stay of individual patients to costs anticipated for the treatment of the patient's diagnosis

d. Capitation of institutional payments has been shown to improve the quality of care rendered to psychiatric patients

e. Medicare reimbursement rates for psychiatric treatments rendered to patients in freestanding psychiatric hospitals, psychiatric units in general hospitals, and general hospital scatter beds are all subject to federally mandated limitations

The correct answer is e.

As with medical diagnoses, the determination of institutional reimbursement rates for patients treated in general hospital scatter beds is made using a prospective payment system that is based on a patient's diagnosis. However, these methodologies are not applied currently to determine reimbursement rates for inpatient treatment rendered on either designated psychiatric DRG-exempt units in general hospitals or for treatments rendered in freestanding psychiatric hospitals. TEFRA is a method used by Medicare to contain the costs of inpatient treatment of psychiatric disorders in psychiatric hospitals by taking into account the costs incurred for inpatient treatment previously. The uses of DRGs and capitation rates are methods used by the federal government to limit the Medicare rates for inpatient psychiatric treatment across types of hospital bed settings.

6. Which of the following statements about possible local variations in Part B reimbursement under Medicare is correct?

a. Federal legislation determines the details of the allowed frequency at which specific provider services may be reimbursed

b. States are required to follow federally mandated Medicare fee schedules

c. Medicare reimbursement rates to providers are always higher than those provided through coverage available to Medicaid recipients

d. Local carriers interpret federal guidelines in determining which services are allowable for reimbursement under the "medical necessity" provision of Medicare regulations

The correct answer is d.

Local insurance companies or carriers have the authority to interpret the details of Medicare Part B reimbursement in collaboration with state government agencies and in consultation with local provider groups. Therefore, fee schedules for provider services may vary across and within states, taking into account the costs incurred by providers in delivering service and reimbursement rates for nonpsychiatrist providers in specific geographic areas. Federal legislation regulates the proportion of specific mental health services that may be reimbursed through Medicare but does not determine the dollar amount of allowable charges. The dollar amount is determined locally. Local carriers may also limit the number of services that it deems medically necessary and therefore eligible for reimbursement. States participate in determining both Medicare and Medicaid reimbursement rates. In some states, reimbursement rates under Medicaid may exceed those under Medicare.

Reference

www.cms.hhs.gov (the Medicare and choice payment methodology) Accessed March 3, 2005.

7. Which of the following statements about Medicare Part B coverage for provider services is correct?

   a. The Omnibus Budget Reconciliation Acts (OBRA) refers to legislation passed to regulate provider reimbursement under Medicare
   b. OBRA legislation limits the annual dollar amount of reimbursement of outpatient mental health treatment
   c. Psychiatrists are prohibited from billing under the evaluation and management (E and M) codes utilized by most primary care physicians
   d. Psychiatrists, psychologists, and social workers are eligible to become participating Medicare providers
   e. Psychotherapy provided by psychologists and social workers in inpatient and nursing home settings is covered by Medicare

The correct answer is d.

OBRA refers to the Omnibus Budget Reconciliation Acts passed to reconcile differences between the annual budgets passed by the Senate and House of Representatives. Since 1987, important provisions about Medicare reimbursement have been included in OBRA legislation. Psychiatrists are allowed to bill under the E and M codes used by other physicians if the criteria for the specified levels of service are appropriately documented. OBRA laws have expanded services that are covered by Medicare such that the outpatient annual limit has been removed, and psychologists and social workers are accepted as Medicare providers. Nevertheless, psychotherapy provided by social workers in nursing homes cannot be billed under Part B of Medicare.

Reference
OBRA-89. HR 3299 pub L No. 101–239.

Chapter 40
Private Practice Issues

1. The average net annual income for psychiatrists

   a. Has risen faster than the average increase for all physicians in the decade 1989–1999
   b. Was about $126,000 in 1999
   c. Is approximately in the middle for the top 20 medical specialties
   d. Has risen faster than the inflation rate for the decade 1989–1999

   The correct answer is b.

   For psychiatrists in general, 1999 median annual gross income was $167,090 (a 2.6% decrease from 1998), but annual net income was $125,790 (a 6.0% increase from 1998, which in turn was a 4.33% increase over their 1997 net income). This income is the second lowest among office-based specialties.

   Reference
   Goldberg J. Yikes! Primary care earnings plummet. *Med Econ.* 2000;18:140.

2. All of the following statements about psychiatrists in the United States are true *except*

   a. Over 2,500 have subspecialty certification in geriatric psychiatry
   b. Of American psychiatrists, 18% have geriatric caseloads exceeding 20% of their practices
   c. Psychiatrists with larger geriatric caseloads spend proportionately more time in their offices seeing patients than those seeing fewer geriatric patients
   d. Psychiatrists with larger geriatric caseloads average more patient visits per week and a longer average work week than those seeing fewer geriatric patients

   The correct answer is d.

When psychiatrists who provide a higher proportion of geriatric services (more than 20% of their case load) were compared to those who were low geriatric providers), it was found that the high geriatric providers spent proportionately less time in their offices (although still spending most of their time in their offices), more time in hospitals, and significantly more time in nursing homes than low geriatric providers. The mean percentage of patients over 65 years seen by high geriatric providers was 43.9% ± 20.9% during 44.3 ± 28.4 patient visits/week in a total work week of 50.3 ± 17.5 hours compared to the percentage over 65 years seen by the low geriatric providers of 7.4% ± 6.8% during 35.6 ± 25.1 patient visits/week in a work week of 46.3 ± 16.0 hours.

Reference

Colenda CC, Pincus H, Tanielian TL, et al. Update of geriatric psychiatry practices among American psychiatrists; analysis of the 1996 national survey of psychiatric practice. *Am J Geriatr Psychiatry.* 1999;7:279–288.

3. Medicare billing for psychiatric services requires the exclusive use of

a. The 908xx psychiatric services coding system
b. The *Diagnostic and Statistical Manual of Mental Disorders, Fourth Edition* (DSM-IV; American Psychiatric Association, 1994) diagnostic coding system
c. The *International Classification of Diseases, Ninth Revision–Clinical Modification* (ICD-9-CM; 2000) coding system
d. The American Medical Association's evaluation and management (E and M) coding system

The correct answer is c.

The *ICD-9-CM* (2000) is a classification of all medical conditions, including listings of mental and emotional disorders that are similar to, but not identical with, the listings in *DSM-IV*. It is the standard coding nomenclature for diseases. (The next version, *ICD-10*, is in preparation and will supplant *ICD-9*.) All Medicare intermediaries and most other insurers utilize the coding terminology in the *ICD-9* books exclusively for reimbursement for services.

Reference

World Health Organization. *ICD-9-CM 2001, International Classification of Diseases, 9th Revision—Clinical Modification, 2001 Edition.* Dover, DE: American Medical Association; 2000.

4. Billing for services under "incident to" provisions

   a. Is paid at 85% of the physician's fee schedule
   b. Requires a physician to be available by telephone
   c. Can be performed by nurse practitioners and physician assistants (PAs) but not psychologists or social workers
   d. Can only be provided by the physician's employees

The correct answer is d.

"Incident to" services must be performed by a bona fide employee of the physician.

Reference
Grant DW. *Part B Answer Book*. Rockville, MD: Part B News Group; 2000.

5. Medicare

   a. Pays 62.5% of fees for psychotherapy performed during nursing home visits
   b. Was created in 1959
   c. Requires acceptance of Medicare assignment from patients who are also Medicaid recipients and those below the federal poverty level
   d. Pays only 50% of the fee for office-based consultation services even if you send a report back to the referring physician

The correct answer is c.

Both participating and nonparticipating providers must accept assignment from Medicare beneficiaries who are also Medicaid recipients or who are at or below the federal poverty level. Medicare was created in 1965.

Reference
OBRA 89. *Omnibus Budget Reconciliation Act of 1989 Reform: Annual Report to Congress*. Washington, DC: US Government Printing Office; 1989.

6. Which of the following is true?

   a. Participating providers have their claims sent automatically to the patient's Medigap provider
   b. Participating providers may bill up to 115% of the Medicare fee schedule
   c. Nonparticipating providers are not required to submit Medicare insurance claims for their services

d. Nonparticipating providers may not accept Medicare assignment because of the "limiting charge"

The correct answer is a.

There are several advantages to participating in Medicare. These include higher fee schedule payments; many claims will be automatically sent to the patient's Medigap insurer (crossover), which can be a tremendous saving of paperwork; and your name is published in any Medicare participating physician/supplier directory.

Reference
Grant DW. *Part B Answer Book*. Rockville, MD: Part B News Group; 2000.

7. E and M service codes

   a. May be used to code initial psychiatric office visits
   b. May not be coded in combination with psychiatric diagnosis codes
   c. Are dependent on the time spent providing them
   d. Are documented according to rules that are updated annually

The correct answer is a.

E and M codes can be used for initial visits with a patient or follow-up visits for ongoing evaluation and management. They can be used for patients of your own or patients of another physician whom you are seeing in consultation.

Reference
Grant DW. *Part B Answer Book*. Rockville, MD: Part B News Group; 2000.

8. All of the following are important steps to take in setting up a geriatric practice *except*

   a. Creating a practice brochure and other written materials using large fonts
   b. Have comfortable, deep, soft chairs in your office to make your older patients feel at ease because many will be unfamiliar with psychiatric treatment and may be anxious
   c. Deciding whether to register as a participating physician with Medicare
   d. Evaluating transportation issues; stairs, ramps, and elevators; proximity to senior housing, activity centers, and to other doctors

The correct answer is b.

The office seating should be appropriate for the elderly, including sturdy chairs with arms to assist in sitting or standing and firm seats that are at an appropriate height (not low "comfortable" chairs that an older person will have difficulty getting in and out of). Also, consider fabrics and carpets that are waterproof and stain proof.

Reference

Stein, EM. Geriatric psychiatry in office and clinic. *J Appl Gerontol.* 1983;2: 102–111.

Chapter 41
Psychiatry at the End of Life

1. Mrs. B is an 83-year-old woman with advanced gastrointestinal cancer and extensive liver metastases who was admitted to home hospice 3 weeks ago. She is bed bound because of her illness, and the hospice medical director estimates that her survival is less than 2 weeks. She has been steadily less interested in activities such as reading and watching TV, which she found pleasurable even 2 weeks ago. She is more listless and tired, and her sleep is very poor. This morning she is tearful, agitated, and distraught and complains of vivid dreams of her late husband in which he seemed to be touching her. What should you do first?

   a. Start 5 mg methylphenidate bid
   b. Test her attention, concentration, and memory
   c. Explain to the family that these are normal symptoms that are part of the letting go process at the end of life
   d. Send her to the emergency room for further evaluation, including neuroimaging
   e. Start 1 mg lorazepam tid

   The correct answer is b.

   The most appropriate first step is to determine if she has delirium, which is the most common mental disorder in the final weeks of life and often presents in elderly patients with substantial depressive symptoms. Delirium is common, but often treatable, and needs to be addressed in patients who have new agitation. Methylphenidate and lorazepam may worsen the symptoms of delirium. For this hospice patient, the need to evaluate and treat her symptoms must be weighed against the obligation to avoid excessively burdensome, aggressive medical treatment. As such, emergency room evaluation is usually reserved for severe symptoms that impair quality of life and cannot be managed in another setting.

References

Breitbart W, Marotta R, Platt MM, et al. A double-blind trial of haloperidol, chlorpromazine, and lorazepam in the treatment of delirium in hospitalized AIDS patients. *Am J Psychiatry*. 1996;153:231–237.

Farrell K, Ganzini L. Misdiagnosing delirium as depression in medically ill elderly patients. *Arch Intern Med*. 1995;155:2459–2464.

Lipowski ZJ. *Delirium: Acute Confusional States*. New York, NY: Oxford University Press; 1990:175–188.

2. Mr. R is a 65-year-old man with advanced lung cancer who has been in home hospice for 4 weeks. Within the last 2 days, he has been increasingly fearful, confused, agitated, and paranoid. He denies pain and is receiving only very low doses of morphine. He is still drinking fluids well and is able to take oral medications. His family caregivers are distressed by these changes but are coping well, able to get breaks from his care, and able to sleep at night. His favorite brother is expected to arrive by plane tomorrow to say his goodbyes. Which approach would you advise?

  a. Counsel the family that death is imminent and the risks and burdens of any treatment outweigh the benefits
  b. Start 25–50 mg diphenhydramine po bid/tid
  c. Start 0.5–1.0 mg clonazepam po bid/tid
  d. Start 1.0–3.0 mg haloperidol po bid/tid
  e. Start 2.5–5.0 mg olanzapine qhs

The correct answer is d.

Mr. R has an agitated delirium that should be treated with haloperidol. There are no clear benefits to more expensive medications such as olanzapine. Diphenhydramine and clonazepam may worsen delirium and diminish the patients' opportunity for meaningful interactions with his brother.

References

Breitbart W, Marotta R, Platt MM, et al. A double-blind trial of haloperidol, chlorpromazine, and lorazepam in the treatment of delirium in hospitalized AIDS patients. *Am J Psychiatry*. 1996;153:231–237.

Fainsinger RL, Tapper M, Bruera E. A perspective on the management of delirium in terminally ill patients on a palliative care unit. *J Palliat Care*. 1993;9:4–8.

3. Mr. R is a 76-year-old widowed man with advanced colon cancer and difficulties with pain control in hospice. He is bed bound, and his internist estimates less than a month of survival. His mood has been increasingly low for several weeks, he has lost interest in other activities, his appetite is poor, and he is hopeless and apathetic. On examination, he scores 28/30 on the Mini-Mental State Examination. He refuses some of his oral morphine because he does not like the sedation. Medications you might consider to treat him include

a. 20 mg citalopram qd
b. 1 mg lorazepam tid
c. 7.5 mg mirtazapine qhs
d. 20 mg fluoxetine qd
e. 5 mg methylphenidate at 8:00 AM and noon

The correct answer is e.

Mr. R appears depressed, with no evidence of delirium. In the context of life expectancy of less than 1 month, a trial of methylphenidate is warranted. With methylphenidate treatment, he may tolerate higher dosages of morphine, thus improving his pain control.

References

Breitbart W, Strout D. Delirium in the terminally ill. *Clin Geriatr Med.* 2000; 16:357–372.
Olin J, Masand P. Psychostimulants for depression in hospitalized cancer patients. *Psychosomatics.* 1996;37:57–62.

4. In the United States, what percentage of people who die receive hospice service before death?

a. 7%
b. 17%
c. 29%
d. 42%

The correct answer is c.

About 29% of all deaths in the United States occur in hospice.

Reference

National Hospice and Palliative Care Organization. *Facts and Figures on Hospice Care in America.* Alexandria, VA: National Hospice and Palliative Care Organization; September, 2000.

5. Which of the following is *not* associated with interest in assisted suicide or hastened death in cancer patients?

   a. Hopelessness
   b. Low religiousness
   c. Sense of burden to others
   d. Female gender

The correct answer is d.

Hopelessness and sense of burden to others have been shown to be risk factors for interest in assisted suicide. Religious affiliation and religiousness protect against interest in assisted suicide.

References

Breitbart W, Rosenfeld BD, Passik SD. Interest in physician-assisted suicide among ambulatory HIV infected patients. *Am J Psychiatry*. 1996;153:238–242.

Emanuel EJ, Fairclough DL, Emanuel LL. Attitudes and desires related to euthanasia and physician-assisted suicide among terminally ill patients and their caregivers. *JAMA*. 2000;284:2460–2468.

Ganzini L, Nelson HD, Schmidt TA, Kraemer DF, Delorit MA, Lee MA. Physicians' experiences with the Oregon Death With Dignity Act. *N Engl J Med*. 2000;342:557–563.

6. Based on qualitative studies of dying patients, which one of the following is among the most important goals for patients at the end of life?

   a. To die quickly without warning
   b. To achieve transcendence
   c. To separate from loved ones
   d. To obtain good pain and symptom control

The correct answer is d.

Qualitative studies by Steinhauser et al. (2000) and Singer et al. (1999) demonstrated that pain and symptom control is a priority for most dying patients. Patients are more interested in strengthening relationships to loved ones than separating and having an opportunity to achieve closure rather than die quickly without warning.

References

Singer PA, Martin DK, Kelner M. Quality end-of-life care: patients' perspectives. *JAMA*. 1999;281:163–168.

Steinhauser KE, Clipp EC, McNeilly M, Christakis NA, McIntyre LM, Tulsky JA. In search of a good death: observations of patients, families, and providers. *Ann Intern Med*. 2000;132:825–832.

7. Which one of the following is *not* covered under the Medicare hospice benefit?

   a. Bereavement services for the family after the patient's death
   b. Home health aide services
   c. Medications for pain
   d. Respite care
   e. Emergency services for life-threatening medical events

The correct answer is e.

Reference

Medicare Rights Center. *A Technical Guide to the Medicare Home Health Benefits: Care for People With Advanced Illnesses.* New York, NY: Medicare Rights Center; 1998.

8. Mr. X is a 65-year-old patient you have treated for depression with psychotherapy and 100 mg sertraline qd. He is now in hospice care, terminally ill with multiple myeloma. You have not seen him for 4 months because of his worsening medical status. His hospice nurse calls you with the following information. His pain is well controlled, his cognition is unimpaired, he continues to take the sertraline, but he is very weak from anemia and illness. He has been tearful several times when talking about missing his grandson's growing up. His appetite is poor, and his sleep impaired. He was formerly an active gardener and feels bad about not being able to help his wife in the garden. He worries that his care is a burden to her. He denies feeling depressed but has mentioned your name several times. He still takes pleasure in seeing family and has been actively working toward closure in many of his relationships. His nurse asks you what should be done. What is the best recommendation?

   a. Increase sertraline to 150 mg
   b. Start 5 mg methylphenidate bid
   c. Tell your secretary to arrange for him to come to your office within the next 2 weeks
   d. Arrange to visit the patient at home

The correct answer is d.

Mr. X has symptoms of a severe medical illness, anticipatory grieving, and concerns common in many persons who are dying. He does not appear to have core symptoms of depression. He is actively working for closure in his relationships, and your relationship with him is important. He is too ill to tolerate an office visit. Visit him at home to evaluate further for treatable psychiatric symptoms and attend to the patient's desire to say goodbye.

Reference

Chochinov HM. Psychiatry and terminal illness. *Can J Psychiatry.* 2000;45: 143–150.

9. Which of the following is *not* true about hospice care in the United States?

   a. The median stay in community hospice in the United States is less than 6 weeks
   b. Experts believe patients and families benefit from hospice stays of greater than 3 months
   c. Physicians are more likely to underestimate than overestimate survival of hospice patients
   d. In the United States, most hospice care is delivered in patients' residences

The correct answer is c.

Physicians are more likely to overestimate than underestimate survival in hospice patients.

References

Christakis NA, Lamont EB. Extent and determinants of error in doctors' prognoses in terminally ill patients: prospective cohort study. *BMJ.* 2000;320: 469–473.

National Hospice and Palliative Care Organization. *Facts and Figures on Hospice Care in America.* Alexandria, VA: National Hospice and Palliative Care Organization; September, 2000.

10. All but one of the following support the use of psychostimulants such as methylphenidate for the treatment of depressive syndromes in terminally ill cancer patients:

    a. Augmentation of opioid analgesia
    b. Diminished opioid sedation
    c. Response within 1 to 3 days
    d. Support of efficacy demonstrated in several randomized clinical trials among terminally ill patients

The correct answer is d.

Although methylphenidate is recommended for depressed patients with less than 1 month to live, its efficacy has not been demonstrated in randomized clinical trials.

Reference

Breitbart W, Strout D. Delirium in the terminally ill. Clin Geriatr Med. 2000; 16:357–372.

11. Among patients with Alzheimer's disease who have lost function in an ordinal fashion on the Functional Assessment Strategy Scale (FAST), median life expectancy of 3 months is associated with the presence of which characteristic?

   a. Patient has one word or less of speech
   b. Psychosis
   c. Hypoalbuminemia
   d. Aggressive behavior

The correct answer is a.

Median life expectancy is 3 months in patients with Alzheimer's disease when such patients are mute and dependent in all activities of daily living, including ambulation.

Reference

Luchins DJ, Hanrahan P, Murphy K. Criteria for enrolling dementia patients in hospice. *J Am Geriatr Soc.* 1997;45:1054–1059.

12. Which one of the following statements regarding patients with Alzheimer's disease in hospice is true?

   a. Approximately 15% of all patients in hospice have Alzheimer's disease as the terminal diagnosis
   b. Most geriatricians do not support the concept of hospice in end-stage Alzheimer's disease
   c. Difficulties in predicting survival in Alzheimer's disease have constituted a major impediment to enrollment if Alzheimer's patients are in hospice

The correct answer is c.

References

Christakis NA, Escarce JJ. Survival of Medicare patients after enrollment in hospice programs. *N Engl J Med.* 1996;335:172–178.
Luchins DJ, Hanrahan P. What is the appropriate level of health care for end-stage dementia patients? *J Am Geriatr Soc.* 1993;41:25–30.
Volicer L. Hospice care for dementia patients. *J Am Geriatr Soc.* 1997;45: 1147–1149.

13. Which one of the following is true about delirium in terminally ill patients?

    a. Delirium is the third most common psychiatric disorder in dying patients
    b. With expert management, sedation is rarely required to treat delirium in terminally ill patients
    c. Delirium improves pain control
    d. Delirium improves about half the time in the final weeks of life, sometimes even without intervention

The correct answer is d.

Delirium is the most common psychiatric disorder in patients near the end of life. Even with expert management, sedation is sometimes required. Delirium worsens pain control. Delirium that occurs in the final weeks of life will resolve in many patients before death.

References

Fainsinger RL, Landman W, Hoskings M, Bruera E. Sedation for uncontrolled symptoms in a South African hospice. *J Pain Symptom Manage.* 1998;16: 145–152.

Gagnon P, Allard P, Masse B, DeSerres M. Delirium in terminal cancer: a prospective study using daily screening, early diagnosis and continuous monitoring. *J Pain Symptom Manage.* 2000;19:412–426.

Lawlor PG, Gagnon B, Mancini IL, et al. Occurrence, causes, and outcomes of delirium in patients with advanced cancer. *Arch Intern Med.* 2000;160: 786–794.

14. Which of the following is a good treatment recommendation for major depressive disorder in terminally ill cancer patients in hospice?

    a. Consider using a psychostimulant if the patient has less than 2 months to live
    b. Because of the risks of medications, give a trial of psychotherapy before a trial of antidepressants
    c. Psychotherapeutic approaches that focus on psychological understanding and developmental issues are recommended
    d. Because of the high risk of brain metastasis, neuroimaging should be a routine part of the evaluation of depression in hospice patients

The correct answer is a.

Psychostimulants are recommended for depressed terminally ill cancer patients in the final weeks of life. Because of diminished life expectancy, medical trials should start concurrently with psychotherapy.

Psychotherapy should focus on active coping strategies that focus mostly on working through issues about the disease. Neuroimaging is not routinely indicated in hospice patients.

Reference

Chochinov HM. Psychiatry and terminal illness. *Can J Psychiatry.* 2000;45: 143–150.